ACETYLSALICYLIC ACID

Acetylsalicylic Acid

New Uses for an Old Drug

Editors

H. J. M. Barnett, M.D., F.R.C.P.(C), F.A.C.P., F.R.C.P.
Department of Clinical Neurological Sciences
University of Western Ontario
London, Ontario, Canada

J. Hirsh, M.D., F.R.A.C.P., F.R.C.P.(C)
Vice-Chairman and Professor
Department of Pathology
McMaster University
Coordinator, Hamilton District Coordinating Committee for Hematology
McMaster University Medical Centre
Hamilton, Ontario, Canada

J. Fraser Mustard, M.D., Ph.D.
Faculty of Health Sciences
McMaster University
Hamilton, Ontario, Canada

Raven Press ■ New York

Raven Press, 1140 Avenue of the Americas, New York, New York 10036

© 1982 by Raven Press Books, Ltd. All rights reserved. This book is protected by copyright. No part of it may be reproduced, stored in a retrieval system, or transmitted, in any form or by any means, electronic, mechanical, photocopying, recording, or otherwise, without the prior written permission of the publisher.

Made in the United States of America

International Standard Book Number 0-89004-647-6
Library of Congress Catalog Number 81–48333

Great care has been taken to maintain the accuracy of the information contained in the volume. However, Raven Press cannot be held responsible for errors or for any consequences arising from the use of the information contained herein.

Preface

This book represents the proceedings of a conference exploring the role of prostaglandins in disease, the mechanism of action of acetylsalicylic acid as a therapeutic agent, and its clinical uses, principally in the management of thromboembolic disease. Each topic is discussed in depth by recognized experts in the field.

The book is divided into two main sections. The first reviews the roles of prostaglandins in inflammation and in hemostasis and thrombosis, the pharmacokinetics and mode of action of acetylsalicylic acid, and its pharmacological effects on the gastrointestinal tract, on platelet–vessel wall interactions, on smooth muscle and the patent ductus and the uterus during parturition, on pain, and on temperature regulation.

The second section reviews the clinical applications of acetylsalicylic acid as an antithrombotic agent and provides an in-depth discussion of the reported side effects of the drug. This section includes a comprehensive account of the results of clinical trials of acetylsalicylic acid in patients with cerebrovascular disease and with coronary artery disease, in the prevention of venous thrombosis, and in patients with other thrombovascular disorders. Unresolved issues arising from these trials are considered, including the important questions of optimal dosage and frequency of administration of acetylsalicylic acid and the interesting sex difference reported between males and females regarding the effectiveness of acetylsalicylic acid as an antithrombotic agent.

It is hoped that this volume will prove useful to all scholars of medicine, particularly in the fields of internal medicine, cardiology, neurology, rheumatology, and hematology.

Acknowledgments

This volume represents the proceedings of the First Canadian Conference on Acetylsalicylic Acid: New Uses for an Old Drug, held in Banff, Alberta, Canada, in April 1980. The conference was co-sponsored by The Canadian Heart Foundation, The Canadian Cardiovascular Society, and The Canadian Stroke Society.

Manuscripts for this volume were prepared with the editorial assistance of MEDI-EDIT Limited, Toronto, Canada.

Contents

Contributors

H. J. M. Barnett
Department of Clinical Neurological
Sciences
University of Western Ontario
London, Ontario, Canada N6A 5A5

M. R. Buchanan
Department of Pathology
McMaster University
Hamilton, Ontario, Canada L8S 3Z5

Cedric J. Carter
Faculty of Health Sciences
McMaster University
Hamilton, Ontario, Canada L8S 3Z5

John R. G. Challis
Departments of Obstetrics, Gynecology, and
Physiology
University of Western Ontario
London, Ontario, Canada N6A 4V2

Flavio Coceani
Research Institute and Division of
Cardiology
The Hospital for Sick Children
Toronto, Ontario, Canada M5B 1X8

Keith E. Cooper
Division of Medical Physiology
The University of Calgary
Calgary, Alberta, Canada T2N 1N4

Michael Gent
Faculty of Health Sciences
McMaster University
Hamilton, Ontario, Canada L8S 3Z5

Edward Genton
Faculty of Health Sciences
McMaster University
Hamilton, Ontario, Canada L8S 3Z5

William H. Harris
Departments of Surgery and Orthopedics
Harvard Medical School
Beth Israel Hospital and
Massachusetts General Hospital
Boston, Massachusetts 02215

J. Hirsh
Department of Pathology
McMaster University
Hamilton, Ontario, Canada L8S 3Z5

Hershel Jick
Boston Collaborative Drug Surveillance
Program
Boston University Medical Center
Boston, Massachusetts 02154

N. W. Kasting
Division of Medical Physiology
The University of Calgary
Calgary, Alberta, Canada T2N 1N4

John G. Kelton
Department of Pathology and Medicine
McMaster University Medical Centre
Hamilton, Ontario, Canada L8S 3Z5

John W. D. McDonald
Department of Medicine
University of Western Ontario
London, Ontario, Canada N6A 5A5

J. Fraser Mustard
Faculty of Health Sciences
McMaster University
Hamilton, Ontario, Canada L8S 3Z5

Philip Needleman
Departments of Pharmacology and Medi-
cine
Jewish Hospital and Washington Univer-
sity Medical School
St. Louis, Missouri 63110

Peter M. Olley
Research Institute and Division of
Cardiology
The Hospital for Sick Children
Toronto, Ontario, Canada M5B 1X8

Marian A. Packham
Department of Biochemistry
Faculty of Medicine
University of Toronto
Ontario, Canada M5S 1A8 and
Department of Pathology
McMaster University
Hamilton, Ontario, Canada L8S 3Z5

John E. Patrick
Departments of Obstetrics, Gynecology, and
Physiology
University of Western Ontario
London, Ontario, Canada N6A 4V2

Edwin W. Salzman
Departments of Surgery and Orthopedics
Harvard Medical School
Beth Israel Hospital and
Massachusetts General Hospital
Boston, Massachusetts 02215

Jake James Thiessen
Faculty of Pharmacy
University of Toronto
Toronto, Ontario, Canada

John Turk
Departments of Pharmacology and Medi-
cine
Jewish Hospital and Washington Univer-
sity Medical School
St. Louis, Missouri 63110

W. L. Veale
Division of Medical Physiology
The University of Calgary
Calgary, Alberta, Canada T2N 1N4

Gerald Weissmann
Division of Rheumatology
Department of Medicine
New York University
School of Medicine and
University Hospital and
Bellevue Hospital
New York, New York 10016

Tony L. Yaksh
Departments of Neurologic Surgery and
Pharmacology
Mayo Clinic
Rochester, Minnesota 55901

Acetylsalicylic Acid: New Uses for an Old Drug,
edited by H. J. M. Barnett, J. Hirsh, and
J. F. Mustard. Raven Press, New York © 1982.

Prostaglandins in Disease: Modification by Acetylsalicylic Acid

J. Fraser Mustard

Faculty of Health Sciences, McMaster University, Hamilton, Ontario, Canada

The medicinal history of salicylic acid dates back centuries to the use of powdered willow bark for treatment of inflammation. Salicylates were introduced into clinical medicine in 1899. The synthetic derivative, acetylsalicylic acid, which is the least toxic and irritating of the compounds, has remarkable analgesic, anti-inflammatory, antipyretic, and antirheumatic properties. Its use is widespread and it is estimated that 25 to 50 million pounds of acetylsalicylic acid are consumed annually in North America.

During the early 1930s, Goldblatt and von Euler isolated vasodepressor substances from human and sheep seminal vesicles; later, these were purified by Bergström and called prostaglandins E and F. Prostaglandins are synthesized from polyunsaturated fatty acids such as dihomogammalinolenic acid, arachidonic acid, and eicosapentaenoic acid. Arachidonic acid, the most ubiquitous precursor of prostaglandins, can be freed from most tissues when they are stimulated. Cyclo-oxygenase, a key enzyme in the synthesis of prostaglandins, is inhibited by nonsteroidal anti-inflammatory drugs; in particular, acetylsalicylic acid acetylates the enzyme irreversibly. The discovery that both stable and unstable prostaglandins participate in smooth muscle contraction and relaxation, platelet aggregation, and secretion from a number of cell types led to widespread interest in prostaglandins as local mediators of biological reactions and in the role of acetylsalicylic acid in modifying these responses. Nonsteroidal anti-inflammatory drugs such as acetylsalicylic acid have been used to close patent ductus arteriosus, to alter renal function, and in attempts to prevent the thromboembolic complications of venous and arterial vessel disease.

The antipyretic properties of powdered willow bark have been recognized for centuries, and it was used by the Reverend Edward Stone in 1763 to treat fever and inflammation. Salicylates were isolated from willow bark and several other sources during the 1800s and eventually synthesized (122). Acetylsalicylic acid was synthesized by Gerhardt (33) in 1853. However, the potential therapeutic uses of this compound were not recognized until the turn of the century, when Felix Hoffman, an employee of the Bayer Company, administered it to his father, who did not tolerate sodium salicylate well. The observation that acetylsalicylic acid provided considerable relief to this individual suffering from rheumatoid arthritis led Dreser (24), at the time the Bayer Company's director of pharmacological research, to develop acetylsalicylic acid as a pharmaceutical product. The work led to the further

1

observation that in treating some aspects of inflammation, acetylsalicylic acid was more effective than sodium salicylate. The reason for this difference became known only during the last 10 years.

In the latter part of the 1960s, advances in the understanding of arachidonic acid metabolism, and of the formation of prostaglandins from arachidonic acid, led to the demonstration that nonsteroidal anti-inflammatory drugs such as acetylsalicylic acid inhibited prostaglandin formation. Smith and Willis (119) and Vane (128) demonstrated that acetylsalicylic acid prevented the formation of prostaglandins, and it was later shown that it inhibits cyclo-oxygenase, which is involved in the conversion of arachidonic acid to the prostaglandin endoperoxide, PGG_2 (106). As a result, a wide interest developed in the role of prostaglandins in inflammation and in the role of nonsteroidal anti-inflammatory drugs in inhibiting prostaglandin formation and relieving some of the symptoms of inflammation (79).

ARACHIDONIC ACID AND PROSTAGLANDINS

Prostaglandins are formed from long-chain unsaturated fatty acids; in mammalian tissues the principal one appears to be arachidonic acid. Arachidonic acid is freed from membrane phospholipids by the action of phospholipases (6,32,102). It may then be incorporated into triglycerides or phospholipids. The lipoxygenase pathway leads to formation of 12-L-hydroperoxy-5,8,10,14-eicosatetraenoic acid (HPETE) and 12-L-hydroxy-5,8,10,14-eicosatetraenoic acid (HETE) (62); the prostaglandin pathway results in the formation of prostaglandins and related products (71,79). In leukocytes, arachidonic acid undergoes oxidation to form a variety of compounds that appear to be involved in inflammation (50,81). Theoretically, disorders of function could occur because of abnormalities in any or all of these pathways. The main effect of acetylsalicylic acid and other nonsteroidal anti-inflammatory drugs is the inhibition of conversion of arachidonic acid to prostaglandins and related products.

The first step leading to prostaglandin synthesis is the hydrolysis of arachidonic acid from the second position of the glycerol moiety of membrane phospholipids. Figure 1 illustrates two possible routes by which arachidonic acid is freed from phospholipids. First, when the phospholipase A_2 present in many cells is activated, it catalyzes the release of arachidonic acid, producing a lysophospholipid as well (32). In another reaction, phospholipase C can split the phosphoryl bond at the third carbon of glycerol, giving rise to 1,2-diacylglycerol (102). It is then possible for diglyceride lipase to free arachidonic acid from the 1,2-diacylglycerol, giving rise to monoacylglycerol and arachidonic acid (6). In some cells, specific phospholipids seem to be hydrolyzed during the early stages of the response to stimuli. In platelets, the inositol phospholipids (as well as phosphatidylcholine and phosphatidylserine) appear to be involved in these changes (7,71,107). The significance of this is not understood at the present time.

Obviously, activation of the phospholipases is the first step of the arachidonate-prostaglandin pathway. A number of stimuli have been identified as having the capacity to cause various cells to form prostaglandins. These stimuli include epi-

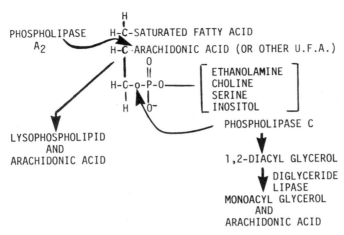

FIG. 1. Arachidonic acid is liberated from membrane phospholipids by the action of phospholipase A_2 or by phospholipase C followed by diglyceride lipase.

nephrine (94), angiotensins II (8) and III (9), bradykinin (84, 129), histamine (3), thrombin (21,22,136), collagen (117), slow-reacting substance (73), and thyrotropin (46). What is not known in all cases is the specificity of these stimuli for certain cells and whether specific receptors are involved in the process of activation. One can speculate that there may be deficiencies in some of these pathways in certain individuals. In addition to specific stimuli, both ischemia and mechanical injury can stimulate prostaglandin release from cells (52,85). Ischemia and injury appear to have this effect on all cells that have been examined.

Lipoxygenase Pathway

A pathway not directly affected by acetylsalicylic acid is the conversion of arachidonic acid, through the action of lipoxygenase and a peroxidase, to the hydroxy acid HETE (43,71) (Fig. 2). Acetylsalicylic acid and salicylic acid do not inhibit the conversion of arachidonic acid to HPETE. However, Siegel and his co-workers (111,112) have recently reported that high concentrations of acetylsalicylic acid and sodium salicylate will inhibit the conversion of HPETE to HETE. Another speculation relating to this pathway, and to some of the problems that will be discussed, is that if HPETE escapes from cells it can inhibit the prostaglandin synthetase involved in conversion of prostaglandin endoperoxides to PGI_2 (41). However, it has recently been shown that HPETE does not escape from cells such as platelets unless they lyse (P. Needleman, *personal communication*); therefore the amount of PGI_2 inhibition that can be caused by HPETE is probably limited by the amount of cell lysis that occurs in an area of thrombosis.

In white blood cells, arachidonate is converted to 5-HPETE, which gives rise to a group of compounds called leukotrienes. At least three have been identified, i.e., leukotrienes A, B, and C; leukotriene C is a cysteinyl derivative of arachidonic

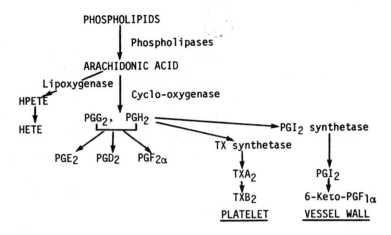

FIG. 2. Arachidonic acid can be converted to prostaglandin G_2 (PGG$_2$) by cyclo-oxygenase. PGG$_2$ gives rise to PGH$_2$. In platelets, PGH$_2$ is converted to thromboxane A$_2$ (TXA$_2$), PGD$_2$, PGE$_2$, and PGF$_{2\alpha}$. TXA$_2$ is rapidly converted to TXB$_2$. In the vessel wall, PGH$_2$ is converted to prostacyclin (PGI$_2$), an unstable compound that gives rise to 6-keto-PGF$_{1\alpha}$. In platelets, arachidonic acid can also be acted upon by lipoxygenase, giving rise to HPETE, which is converted to HETE.

acid (83). This compound has been identified as the slow-reacting substance believed to be an important mediator of release reactions and airway reactivity during an-aphylaxis in experimental animals and asthma attacks in man (1,28,83). It has been suggested that when the prostaglandin pathway is inhibited, more arachidonic acid enters the lipoxygenase pathway (28,71). In asthma, the formation of increased amounts of slow-reacting substance is considered to be potentially damaging (1), and acetylsalicylic acid therapy has been shown to increase respiratory problems in asthmatics (125,132), possibly because of increased leukotriene formation.

PROSTAGLANDIN FORMATION

Figure 2 summarizes the prostaglandin pathways as we understand them at present (71,79). Arachidonic acid is converted by cyclo-oxygenase to PGG$_2$, which is converted to PGH$_2$. Thromboxane A$_2$ is a short-lived product formed from the prostaglandin endoperoxides and is rapidly converted to its stable, relatively inactive endproduct, thromboxane B$_2$. Four prostaglandins can be formed: PGI$_2$, PGD$_2$, PGE$_2$, and PGF$_{2\alpha}$. PGD$_2$, PGE$_2$, and PGF$_{2\alpha}$ are reasonably stable end-products, whereas PGI$_2$ is unstable and is rapidly converted to its stable and relatively inert end-product 6-keto-PGF$_{1\alpha}$. There is some evidence that under some circumstances PGE$_2$ may be converted to PGF$_{2\alpha}$ in man (62). In addition, a hydroxy fatty acid, 12-L-hydroxy-5,8,10-heptadecatrienoic acid (HHT), and malondialdehyde are formed. The relative importance of all these products is not understood, but some are involved in controlling biological reactions.

EFFECTS OF PROSTAGLANDINS

Prostaglandins and related compounds have many effects on biological processes. Thromboxane A_2 has been shown to cause bronchial constriction (42), vasoconstriction (86,124), cell aggregation, and cell secretion (44). It appears to activate contractile processes. In contrast, PGI_2 increases cyclic AMP levels in cells that have receptors for PGI_2 (36,127), which tends to inhibit cell aggregation (75), secretion (78), and contraction (25); to cause vasodilatation (97); and to inhibit chemotaxis (51,135). PGD_2 also increases cyclic AMP levels in cells with the appropriate receptors (108) and can inhibit cell aggregation and secretion (118). It also tends to cause bronchoconstriction (131) and vasodilatation in the systemic circulation (54). PGE_2 causes bronchial dilatation (105), vasodilatation in some vascular beds (26), and contraction of uterine tissue (92). $PGF_{2\alpha}$ is interesting in that it appears to cause bronchial constriction and pulmonary vasoconstriction, in contrast with the effects of PGE_2 (53,54). Theoretically, inhibition of the formation of these products should affect the biological reactions in which they participate, and defects in the enzymes involved in their formation should lead to an abnormal response.

Inhibition of cyclo-oxygenase with nonsteroidal anti-inflammatory drugs such as acetylsalicylic acid prevents the formation of thromboxane A_2 and all of the prostaglandins. Inhibition of thromboxane synthetase by substances such as imidazole or its derivatives (74,87,126) prevents the formation of thromboxane A_2 but does not inhibit the formation of prostaglandins. One of the advantages of inhibiting thromboxane synthetase, of course, is that this does not interfere with the formation of PGI_2 from prostaglandin endoperoxides. Prostacyclin synthetase can be inhibited by tranylcypromine (38) or by lipid peroxides (38,41,76). There is some speculation that in diseased atherosclerotic vessels, lipid peroxides present in the lesions may inhibit PGI_2 synthesis by the diseased vessel wall (23,78).

PROSTAGLANDINS IN DISEASE

Little is known concerning deficiencies in the prostaglandin pathway and disease states. A few cases of cyclo-oxygenase deficiency in platelets, associated with platelet dysfunction and mild bleeding, have been reported (61,70,133). The fact that in such subjects no symptoms other than a mild bleeding defect were found is of interest, particularly if other tissues were also deficient in cyclo-oxygenase activity. Unfortunately, no evidence was presented in regard to this point. At this time, it is not possible to determine from these reports whether the condition is acquired or congenital. Weiss and Lages (133) have also reported the case of a patient in whom a deficiency of thromboxane synthetase activity appeared to be the cause of a hemorrhagic disorder. These observations illustrate that defects in the prostaglandin pathway seem to be associated only with a mild impairment of the hemostatic mechanism. Recently, it was found that a patient with a mild bleeding tendency who lacked the ability to form thromboxane A_2 or PGI_2 did not have a thrombotic tendency (95).

A condition in which there is evidence of increased prostaglandin production is Bartter's syndrome (34). In 1962, Bartter and his colleagues (4) described two patients with growth retardation and hypertrophy and hyperplasia of the juxtaglomerular apparatus of the kidney. These patients had increased amounts of circulating angiotensin II, aldosteronism, hypokalemic alkalosis, and normal blood pressure. They showed a decreased pressure response to the intravenous infusion of angiotensin II (65). This condition is relatively rare, but in the affected individuals who have been studied, increased urinary prostaglandin excretion has been observed (31,35). It is not clear whether the increased urinary excretion of prostaglandins is a consequence of increased production by tissues such as the kidney or increased renal clearance. The observation that nonsteroidal anti-inflammatory drugs such as indomethacin, ibuprofen, and acetylsalicylic acid can correct the hyperreninemia and aldosteronism and decrease urinary excretion of prostaglandins provides some evidence that increased prostaglandin production, possibly in the kidney, plays a part in this condition (90,123). It is, however, of interest that inhibition of prostaglandin synthesis does not correct the hypokalemia in these patients (10), which may indicate that the increased prostaglandin excretion by the kidney is a consequence of a more primary mechanism. It has recently been reported that platelets from patients with Bartter's syndrome show a defect in platelet aggregation in response to such agents as ADP and that this is associated with a plasma factor, probably a prostaglandin, that could be the cause of the increased cyclic AMP concentrations found in platelets from such patients (93,123). This plasma factor does not appear to be PGI_2 but rather a stable prostaglandin (123).

Severe uremia is another condition in which increased prostaglandin levels, in this case possibly PGI_2, have been associated with abnormal platelet function and a bleeding tendency (99).

INHIBITION OF CYCLO-OXYGENASE IN DISEASE

Evidence of the relationship between prostaglandins and abnormal physiology in disease is derived, to a large extent, from an examination of the effects of inhibition of cyclo-oxygenase. Most of this information has been obtained from studies using nonsteroidal anti-inflammatory drugs such as acetylsalicylic acid.

It is well documented that side effects of inhibition of the prostaglandin pathway include ulceration of the gastric mucosa and bleeding (16,115,138). In the case of acetylsalicylic acid, it is not clear whether there are multiple effects on the gastric mucosa or whether these effects simply result from inhibition of PGI_2 production (40,80). Some studies have indicated that acetylsalicylic acid may have a direct effect on the gastric mucosa (16,37). Cells of the gastric mucosa produce PGI_2, which inhibits the increased acid secretion induced by pentagastrin (137). PGI_2 also causes vasodilatation of the stomach mucosa (60,137), and inhibition of PGI_2 formation by the gastric mucosa appears to make the lining more vulnerable to ulceration by gastric secretions.

As discussed in relation to Bartter's syndrome, prostaglandins are involved in the control of renal blood vessels and renal tubules (67). Inhibition of prostaglandin production is thought to be a factor in the development of the nephrotoxicity caused by nonsteroidal anti-inflammatory drugs (11). However, there is very little evidence that acetylsalicylic acid, which strongly inhibits cyclo-oxygenase in most tissues, causes nephrotoxicity (138). High blood pressure may also be related to the effects of prostaglandins on the kidney and arteries. Although relatively little is known at present, there is good reason to suspect that prostaglandins may play a role in the control of blood pressure (69,130). Since the vessel wall can produce PGI_2 and because the normal direction of diffusion of PGI_2 is into the wall or through it, any PGI_2 formed by the endothelium will likely be transported into the wall. Furthermore, PGI_2 can be produced by smooth muscle cells in the vessel wall (2,52,77,114) and thereby exert a strong local effect. Chronic treatment of rabbits with indomethacin causes a progressive rise in arterial pressure (17). A number of investigators have speculated that production of prostaglandins and their effects on vessels may be abnormal in essential hypertension (64,66,130).

Prostaglandins are known to be important in the physiology of the reproductive system. They are involved in the control of uterine blood flow and modulate uterine contractions (55,79). Inhibition of cyclo-oxygenase prevents the production of uterine prostaglandins and can cause delayed parturition (19). Prostaglandins play a role in maintaining the patency of the ductus arteriosus (15). When the blood oxygen tension increases at birth, prostaglandin production falls, and this is one of the factors in closure of the ductus arteriosus (89). Administration of nonsteroidal anti-inflammatory drugs in doses that inhibit prostaglandin production can cause closure of a patent ductus (110). Some investigators have speculated that the administration of nonsteroidal anti-inflammatory drugs late in pregnancy might cause premature closure (45,109).

Dysmenorrhea is a common cause of temporary disability in females. Increased prostaglandin production by the uterus is thought to be a major factor, because of the increased levels of prostaglandins found in the menstrual fluid in association with dysmenorrhea (14,96). Inhibition of prostaglandin synthesis with ibuprofen, indomethacin, mefenamic acid, and naproxen sodium rapidly relieves the symptoms (13,48). In contrast, acetylsalicylic acid has not been reported to be effective (72); the reason for its failure to relieve the symptoms has not been established. It may be related to the rapid hydrolysis of acetylsalicylic acid, so that insufficient drug reaches the cells of the uterus to acetylate the cyclo-oxygenase. This raises the important question of the pharmacology of acetylsalicylic acid and its distribution in the body, particularly in relation to its capacity to acetylate cyclo-oxygenases in the various tissues. It has also been suggested that agents such as mefenamic acid may block prostaglandin receptors (J. E. Patrick, *personal communication*).

PROSTAGLANDINS AND THROMBOSIS

A subject of considerable interest at present is the effect of inhibition of the prostaglandin pathway on thromboembolic events in man. Thromboxane A_2 and PGI_2 have central roles in this process.

There is reasonably good evidence that PGI_2 is important in maintaining the integrity of the microvascular circulation (68,104). Some patients with deficient PGI_2 production by the vessel wall show enhanced platelet thromboembolism in the microcirculation (100). The two conditions in which this may be important are thrombotic thrombocytopenic purpura and hemolytic-uremic syndrome (47,68,101). In hemolytic-uremic syndrome, a plasma factor appears to be involved in prostaglandin production. One view holds that the plasma normally contains a factor that stimulates the vessel wall to produce PGI_2 and when this is deficient, the failure of PGI_2 production together with a stimulus to platelet aggregation causes microthrombi to form, leading to disseminated thrombosis in the microcirculation (101). If this hypothesis is correct, then it is interesting to speculate that in circumstances where there are stimuli causing microcirculatory thromboemboli, the use of drugs that further inhibit PGI_2 synthesis could make the condition worse. However, no experimental or clinical evidence exists to support this idea.

It should be emphasized that several pathways are involved in thrombosis in large vessels. Initiation of thrombosis may not be mediated solely by exposed collagen in the vessel wall (5). In some circumstances, the capacity of the wall to promote the generation of thrombin may be critical to the initiation and growth of thrombi (58). At least three pathways (59) can induce platelet aggregation. These include an ADP pathway, thromboxane A_2, and a thrombin pathway that is independent of either thromboxane A_2 or released ADP. Thus, blocking thromboxane formation does not inhibit all the pathways for platelet aggregation. Increasing platelet cyclic AMP levels tends to inhibit all the pathways, but the thrombin pathway is the most difficult to inhibit, even when cyclic AMP levels are increased (59). The importance of PGI_2 formation by the vessel wall, particularly when it is injured, in preventing or limiting thrombus formation is also under active investigation (56,71,75,78–80). There is no doubt that PGI_2 is a powerful inhibitor of platelet aggregation, although it is only a weak inhibitor of platelet adherence to damaged vessel walls under conditions of low shear (12,49,134). As discussed in greater detail elsewhere, when vessels are injured and blood flow is arrested, PGI_2 production may have sufficient influence that its inhibition leads to increased thrombosis (57).

DIETARY FATTY ACIDS AND PROSTAGLANDIN SYNTHESIS

An area of potential importance is the modification of fatty acids in membrane phospholipids by changes in diet. Such an approach has the obvious advantage that it can be achieved by food supplementation and is simpler than attempting to affect prostaglandin synthesis by the regular administration of drugs. The ω-3 polyunsaturated fatty acids have been shown to bind to cyclo-oxygenase and to be competitive inhibitors of the enzyme (20,63). Recent studies have confirmed that these fatty acids inhibit the conversion of arachidonic acid to thromboxane A_2 and PGI_2 (88,98). Although Lands and his associates (20,63) had shown that eicosapentaenoic acid (EPA) and other ω-3 fatty acids were competitive inhibitors of cyclo-oxygenase, it was proposed that EPA is converted to thromboxane A_3 (a weak platelet-aggregating agent) and PGI_3 (a strong inhibitor of platelet aggregation) (27,39). The most recent evidence indicates that diets rich in EPA exert an antithrombotic effect by inhibiting the conversion of arachidonic acid to thromboxane A_2 (20,88,113). It has been postulated that the apparently low incidence of atherosclerosis and its complications in Greenland Eskimos results from the high content of EPA in their diet (27).

PROSTAGLANDINS AND INFLAMMATION

As discussed in greater detail in other chapters, many observations have shown that prostaglandins are involved in inflammatory reactions (79). The administration of inhibitors of cyclo-oxygenase such as acetylsalicylic acid has demonstrable effects on fever, pain, and erythema (16,80,115,138). Prostaglandins do not appear to be directly responsible for the swelling associated with inflammation (80) and their role cannot be central, since chronic inhibition of the prostaglandin pathway does not lead to a significant change in the response of individuals to inflammation (103). Inhibition of the cyclo-oxygenase pathway does not appear to change the susceptibility of individuals to infection (30,103). It is generally believed that the role of prostaglandins in inflammation may be facilitation of the action of other mediators that cause fever, pain, and erythema (30,80). In considering the effects of these drugs, one must bear in mind that inhibition of prostaglandin synthesis may not be identical in all tissues because of the presence of isoenzymes (29) and the likely variation in pharmacological distribution of the drugs.

ADDITIONAL EFFECTS OF ACETYLSALICYLIC ACID

An important question that must also be considered is whether drugs such as acetylsalicylic acid have other effects in addition to those related solely to inhibition of cyclo-oxygenase of the prostaglandin pathway (120). There is certainly substantial evidence that in some circumstances sodium salicylate is an effective anti-inflammatory agent and that its action cannot be satisfactorily explained in terms of inhibition of prostaglandin synthesis (18,121). Also, drugs such as acetylsalicylic acid and sodium salicylate produce other effects, such as an increase in fibrinolytic activity when given in moderately high doses (82). It is therefore important, in considering the role of these drugs in the context of prostaglandins and disease, to keep in mind that other unrecognized effects may be important.

Finally, it should be emphasized that the action of a prostaglandin-inhibiting drug in preventing the clinical complications of atherosclerosis may not be related to its effect on platelet function, but may be the result of some other action, e.g., on the prostaglandin pathways in other tissues such as the myocardium (91,116).

REFERENCES

1. Austen, K. F. (1978): Homeostasis of effector systems which can also be recruited for immunologic reactions. *J. Immunol.*, 121:793–805.

2. Baenziger, N. L., Dillender, M. J., and Majerus, P. W. (1977): Cultured human skin fibroblasts and arterial cells produce a labile platelet-inhibitory prostaglandin. *Biochem. Biophys. Res. Commun.*, 78:294–301.

3. Baenziger, N. L., Force, L. E., and Becherer, P. R. (1980): Histamine stimulates prostacyclin synthesis in cultured human umbilical vein endothelial cells. *Biochem. Biophys. Res. Commun.*, 92:1435–1440.

4. Bartter, F. C., Pronove, P., Gill, J. R., Jr., and MacCardle, R. C. (1962): Hyperplasia of the juxtaglomerular complex with hyperaldosteronism and hypokalemic alkalosis. A new syndrome. *Am. J. Med.*, 33:811–828.

5. Baumgartner, H. R. (1977): Platelet interaction with collagen fibrils in flowing blood. I. Reaction of human platelets with a chymotrypsin-digested subendothelium. *Thromb. Haemostas.*, 37:1–16.

6. Bell, R. L., Kennerly, D. A., Stanford, N., and Majerus, P. W. (1979): Diglyceride lipase: A pathway for arachidonate release from human platelets. *Proc. Natl. Acad. Sci. USA*, 76:3238–3241.

7. Bills, T. K., Smith, J. B., and Silver, M. J. (1977): Selective release of arachidonic acid from the phospholipids of human platelets in response to thrombin. *J. Clin. Invest.*, 60:1–6.

8. Blumberg, A. L., Denny, S. E., Marshall, G. R., and Needleman, P. (1977): Blood vessel-hormone interactions: Angiotensin, bradykinin and prostaglandins. *Am. J. Physiol.*, 232:H305–H310.

9. Blumberg, A., Denny, S., Nishikawa, K., Pure, E., Marshall, G. R., and Needleman, P. (1976): Angiotensin III-induced prostaglandin (PG) release. *Prostaglandins*, 11:195–197.

10. Bowden, R. E., Gill, J. R., Jr., Radfar, N., Taylor, A. A., and Keiser, H. R. (1978): Prostaglandin synthetase inhibitors in Bartter's syndrome. *JAMA*, 239:117–121.

11. Brezin, J. H., Katz, S. M., Schwartz, A. B., and Chinitz, J. L. (1979): Reversible renal failure and nephrotic syndrome associated with nonsteroidal anti-inflammatory drugs. *N. Engl. J. Med.*, 301:1271–1273.

12. Cazenave, J-P., Dejana, E., Kinlough-Rathbone, R. L., Richardson, M., Packham, M. A., and Mustard, J. F. (1979): Prostaglandins I$_2$ and E$_1$ reduce rabbit and human platelet adherence without inhibiting serotonin release from adherent platelets. *Thromb. Res.*, 15:273–279.

13. Chan, W. Y., Dawood, M. Y., and Fuchs, F. (1979): Relief of dysmenorrhea with the prostaglandin synthetase inhibitor ibuprofen: Effect on prostaglandin levels in menstrual fluid. *Am. J. Obstet. Gynecol.*, 135:102–108.

14. Chan, W. Y., and Hill, J. C. (1978): Determination of menstrual prostaglandin levels in non-dysmenorrheic and dysmenorrheic subjects. *Prostaglandins*, 15:365–375.

15. Coceani, F., and Olley, P. M. (1973): The response of the ductus arteriosus to prostaglandins. *Can. J. Physiol. Pharmacol.*, 51:220–225.

16. Cohen, L. S. (1976): Clinical pharmacology of acetylsalicylic acid. *Semin. Thromb. Haemostas.*, 2:146–175.

17. Colina-Chourio, J., McGiff, J. C., and Nasjletti, A. (1975): Development of high blood pressure following inhibition of prostaglandin synthesis. *Fed. Proc.*, 34:368.

18. Collier, H. O. J. (1969): A pharmacological analysis of aspirin.[1] *Adv. Pharmacol. Chemother.*, 7:333–405.

19. Collins, E., and Turner, G. (1975): Maternal effects of regular salicylate ingestion in pregnancy. *Lancet*, ii:335–338.

20. Culp, B. R., Titus, B. G., and Lands, W. E. M. (1979): Inhibition of prostaglandin biosynthesis by eicosapentaenoic acid. *Prostaglandins Med.*, 3:269–278.

21. Czervionke, R. L., Hoak, J. C., and Fry, G. L. (1978): Effect of aspirin on thrombin-induced adherence of platelets to cultured cells from the blood vessel wall. *J. Clin. Invest.*, 62:847–856.

22. Czervionke, R. L., Smith, J. B., Hoak, J. C., Fry, G. L., and Haycraft, D. L. (1979): Use of a radioimmunoassay to study thrombin-induced release of PGI$_2$ from cultured endothelium. *Thromb. Res.*, 14:781–786.

23. D'Angelo, V., Villa, S., Mysliwiec, M., Donati, M. B., and de Gaetano, G. (1978): Defective fibrinolytic and prostacyclin-like activity in human atheromatous plaques. *Thromb. Haemostas.*, 39:535–536.

24. Dreser, H. (1899): Pharmakologisches über Aspirin (Acetylsalicylsaure). *Pfluegers Arch. Physiol.*, 76:306–318.

---

[1]In Canada, Aspirin is the registered trade mark of Sterling Drug Ltd., Aurora, Ontario.

25. Dusting, G. J., Moncada, S., and Vane, J. R. (1977): Prostacyclin (PGX) is the endogenous metabolite responsible for relaxation of coronary arteries induced by arachidonic acid. *Prostaglandins*, 13:3–15.

26. Dusting, G. J., Moncada, S., and Vane, J. R. (1979): Prostaglandins, their intermediates and precursors: Cardiovascular actions and regulatory roles in normal and abnormal circulatory systems. *Prog. Cardiovasc. Dis.*, 21:405–430.

27. Dyerberg, J., Bang, H. O., Stoffersen, E., Moncada, S., and Vane, J. R. (1978): Eicosapentaenoic acid and prevention of thrombosis and atherosclerosis? *Lancet*, ii:117–119.

28. Engineer, D. M., Niederhauser, U., Piper, P. J., and Sirois, P. (1978): Release of mediators of anaphylaxis: Inhibition of prostaglandin synthesis of and the modification of release of slow reacting substance of anaphylaxis and histamine. *Br. J. Pharmacol.*, 62:61–66.

29. Ferreira, S. H., and Vane, J. R. (1974): New aspects of the mode of action of nonsteroidal anti-inflammatory drugs. *Annu. Rev. Pharmacol.*, 14:57–73.

30. Ferreira, S. H., and Vane, J. R. (1979): Mode of action of anti-inflammatory agents which are prostaglandin synthetase inhibitors. In: *Anti-inflammatory Drugs*, edited by J. R. Vane and S. H. Ferreira, pp. 348–398. Springer-Verlag, New York.

31. Fichman, M. P., Telfer, N., Zia, P., Speckart, P., Golub, M., and Rude, R. (1976): Role of prostaglandins in the pathogenesis of Bartter's syndrome. *Am. J. Med.*, 60:785–797.

32. Flower, R. J., and Blackwell, G. J. (1976): The importance of phospholipase A_2 in prostaglandin biosynthesis. *Biochem. Pharmacol.*, 25:285–291.

33. Gerhardt, C. F. (1853): Untersuchung über die wasserfreien organischen Sauren. In: *Annalen der Chemie und Pharmacie*, edited by F. Wohler, J. Liebig, and H. Kopp, pp. 149–179. Akademische Verlagsbuchhandlung, Heidelberg.

34. Gill, J. R., Jr. (1980): Bartter's syndrome. *Annu. Rev. Med.*, 31:405–419.

35. Gill, J. R., Jr., Fröhlich, J. C., Bowden, R. E., Taylor, A. A., Keiser, H. R., Seyberth, H. W., Oates, J. A., and Bartter, F. C. (1976): Bartter's syndrome: A disorder characterized by high urinary prostaglandins and a dependence of hyperreninemia on prostaglandin synthesis. *Am. J. Med.*, 61:43–51.

36. Gorman, R. R., Bunting, S., and Miller, O. V. (1977): Modulation of human platelet adenylate cyclase by prostacyclin (PGX). *Prostaglandins*, 13:377–388.

37. Grossman, M. I., Matsumoto, K. K., and Lichter, R. J. (1961): Fecal blood loss produced by oral and intravenous administration of various salicylates. *Gastroenterology*, 40:383–388.

38. Gryglewski, R. J., Bunting, S., Moncada, S., Flower, R. J., and Vane, J. R. (1976): Arterial walls are protected against deposition of platelet thrombi by a substance (prostaglandin X) which they make from prostaglandin endoperoxides. *Prostaglandins*, 12:685–713.

39. Gryglewski, R. J., Salmon, J. A., Ubatuba, F. B. Weatherly, B. C., Moncada, S., and Vane, J. R. (1979): Effects of all Cis-5,8,11,14,17 eicosapentaenoic acid and PGH_3 on platelet aggregation. *Prostaglandins*, 18:453–478.

40. Guth, P. H., Aures, D., and Paulsen, G. (1979): Topic aspirin plus HCl gastric lesions in the rat: Cytoprotective effect of prostaglandin, cimetidine, and probanthine. *Gastroenterology*, 76:88–93.

41. Ham, E. A., Egan, R. W., Soderman, D. D., Gale, P. H., and Kuehl, F. A., Jr. (1979): Peroxidase dependent deactivation of prostacyclin synthetase. *J. Biol. Chem.*, 254:2191–2194.

42. Hamberg, M., Hedqvist, P., Strandberg, K., Svensson, J., and Samuelsson, B. (1975): Prostaglandin endoperoxides. IV. Effects on smooth muscle. *Life Sci.*, 16: 451–462.

43. Hamberg, M., and Samuelsson, B. Prostaglandin endoperoxides. Novel transformations of arachidonic acid in human platelets. *Proc. Natl. Acad. Sci USA*, 71:3400–3404.

44. Hamberg, M., Svensson, J., and Samuelsson, B. (1975): Thromboxanes: a new group of biologically active compounds derived from prostaglandin endoperoxides. *Proc. Natl. Acad. Sci. USA*, 72:2994–2998.

45. Harris, W. H. (1980): The effects of repeated doses of indomethacin on fetal rabbit mortality and on the patency of the ductus arteriosus. *Can. J. Physiolo. Pharmacol.*, 58:212–216.

46. Haye, B., and Jacquemin, C. (1977): Incorporation of [^{14}C] arachidonate in pig thyroid lipids and prostaglandins. *Biochim. Biophys. Acta*, 487:231–242.

47. Hensby, C N., Lewis, P J., Hilgard, P., Mufti, G. J., and Hows, J., and Webster, J. (1979): Prostacyclin deficiency in thrombotic thrombocytopenic purpura letter). *Lancet*, ii:748.

48. Henzl, M. R., and Izu, A. (1979): Naproxen and naproyen sodium in dysmenorrhea: Development from in vitro inhibition of prostaglandin synthesis to suppression of uterine contractions in women and demonstration of clinical efficiency. *Acta Obstet. Gynecol. Scand.*, 87:105–117.

49. Higgs, G. A., Moncada, Vane, J. R., Caen, J. P., Michel, H., and Tobelem, G. (1978): Effect of prostacyclin (PGI₂) on platelet adhesion to rabbit arterial subendothelium. *Prostaglandins*, 16:17–22.

50. Higgs, G. A., McCall, E., and Youlton, L. J. F. (1975): A chemotactic role for prostaglandins released from polymorphonuclear leucocytes during phagocytosis. *Br. J. Pharmacol.*, 53:539–546.

51. Higgs, G. A., Moncada, S., and Vane, J. R. (1978): Prostacyclin (PGI₂) reduces the number of "slow-moving" leukocytes in hamster cheek pouch venules. *J. Physiol.*, 280:55P–56P.

52. Hornstra, G., Haddeman, E., and Don, J. A. (1978): Some investigations into the role of prostacyclin in thromboregulation. *Thromb. Res.*, 12:367–374.

53. Horton, E. W. (1969): Hypotheses on physiological roles of prostaglandins. *Physiol. Rev.*, 49:122–161.

54. Hyman, A. L., Spannhake, E. W., and Kadowitz, R. J. (1978): Prostaglandins and the lung. *Annu. Rev. Resp. Dis.*, 117:111–136.

55. Karim, S. M. M., and Adaikan, P. G. (1979): Some pharmacological studies with prostacyclin in baboon and man. In: *Prostacyclin*, edited by J. R. Vane and S. Bergström, pp. 419–433. Raven Press, New York.

56. Kelton, J. G. (1980): Prostaglandin I (Prostacyclin). *Can. Med. Assoc. J.*, 122:175–179.

57. Kelton, J. G., Hirsh, J., Carter, C. J., and Buchanan, M. R. (1978): Thrombogenic effect of high-dose aspirin in rabbits. Relationship to inhibition of vessel wall synthesis of prostaglandin I₂-like activity. *J. Clin. Invest.*, 62:892–895.

58. Kinlough-Rathbone, R. L., Groves, H. M., Jorgensen, L., Richardson, M., Moore, S., Packham, M. A., and Mustard, J. F. (1980): The role of thrombin in the response of platelets to injury of the rabbit aorta. *Clin. Res.*, 28:548A.

59. Kinlough-Rathbone, R. L., Packham, M. A., Reimers, H J., Cazenave, J P., and Mustard, J. F. (1979): Mechanisms of platelet shape change, aggregation, and release induced by collagen, thrombin, or A23,187. *J. Lab. Clin. Med.*, 90:707–719.

60. Konturek, S. J., Pawlik, W., and Walus, K. (1979): Comparison of the action of prostaglandin E₂ and I₂ on gastric acid secretion and mucosal blood flow in the dog. In: *Prostacyclin*, edited by J. R. Vane and S. Bergström, pp. 173–177. Raven Press, New York.

61. Lagarde, M., Byron, P. A., Vargaftig, B. B., and Dechavanne, M. (1978): Impairment of platelet thromboxane A₂ generation and of the platelet release reaction in two patients with congenital deficiency of platelet cyclo-oxygenase. *Br. J. Haematol.*, 38:251–266.

62. Lands, W. E. M. (1979): The biosynthesis and metabolism of prostaglandins. *Annu. Rev. Physiol.*, 41:633–652.

63. Lands, W. E. M., LeTellier, P. R., Rome, L. H., and Vanderhoek, J. Y. (1973): Inhibition of prostaglandin biosynthesis. *Adv. Biosci.*, 9:15–28.

64. Lee, J. B. (1969): Hypertension, natriuresis and the renal prostaglandins. *Ann. Intern. Med.*, 70:1033–1038.

65. McGiff, J. C. (1977): Bartter's syndrome results from an imbalance of vasoactive hormones. *Ann. Intern. Med.*, 87:369–372.

66. McGiff, J. C., and Itskovitz, H. D. (1973): Prostaglandins and the kidney. *Circ. Res.*, 33:479–488.

67. McGiff, J. C., and Wong, P-Y. K. (1979): Compartmentalization of prostaglandins and prostacyclin within the kidney: Implications for renal function. *Fed. Proc.*, 38:89–93.

68. Machin, S. J., Defreyn, G., Chamone, D. A. F., and Vermylen, J. (1980): Plasma 6-keto-PGF₁α levels after plasma exchange in thrombotic thrombocytopenic purpura (letter). *Lancet*, i:661.

69. Malik, K. U., and McGiff, J. C. (1976): Cardiovascular actions of prostaglandins. In: *Prostaglandins: Physiological, Pharmacological and Pathological Aspects*, edited by S. M. M. Karim, pp. 103–200. MTP Press Ltd., Lancaster, England.

70. Malmsten, C., Hamberg, M., Svensson, J., and Samuelsson, B. (1975): Physiological role of an endoperoxide in human platelets: Hemostatic defect due to platelet cyclo-oxygenase deficiency. *Proc. Natl. Acad. Sci. USA*, 72:1446–1450.

71. Marcus, A. J. (1978): The role of lipids in platelet function: With particular reference to the arachidonic acid pathway. *J. Lipid Res.*, 19:793–826.

72. Marx, J. L. (1979): Dysmenorrhea: Basic research leads to a rational therapy. *Science*, 205:175–176.

73. Mathe, A. A., Strandberg, K., and Yen, S-S. (1977): Prostaglandin release by slow reacting substance from guinea pig and human lung tissue. *Prostaglandins*, 14:1105–1115.

74. Moncada, S., Bunting, S., Mullane, K., Thorogood, P., Vane, J. R., Raz, A., and Needleman, P. (1977): Imidazole—selective inhibitor of thromboxane synthetase. *Prostaglandins*, 13:611–618.

75. Moncada, S., Gryglewski, R., Bunting, S., and Vane, J. R. (1976): An enzyme isolated from arteries transforms prostaglandin endoperoxides to an unstable substance that inhibits platelet aggregation. *Nature*, 263:663–665.

76. Moncada, S., Gryglewski, R. J., Bunting, S., and Vane, J. R. (1976): A lipid peroxide inhibits the enzyme in blood vessel microsomes that generates from prostaglandin endoperoxides the substance (prostaglandin X) which prevents platelet aggregation. *Prostaglandins*, 12:715–737.

77. Moncada, S., Herman, A. G., Higgs, E. A., and Vane, J. R. (1977): Differential formation of prostacyclin (PGX or PGI$_2$) by layers of the arterial wall. An explanation for the antithrombotic properties of vascular endothelium. *Thromb. Res.*, 11:323–344.

78. Moncada, S., Higgs, E. A., and Vane, J. R. (1977): Human arterial and venous tissues generate prostacyclin (prostaglandin X), a potent inhibitor of platelet aggregation. *Lancet*, i:18–20.

79. Moncada, S., and Vane, J. R. (1978): Pharmacology and endogenous roles of prostaglandin endoperoxides, thromboxane A$_2$, and prostacyclin. *Pharmacol. Rev.*, 30:293–331.

80. Moncada, S., and Vane, J. R. (1979): Mode of action of aspirin-like drugs. *Adv. Intern. Med.*, 24:1–22.

81. Morley, J., Bray, M. A., Jones, R. W., Nugteren, D. H., and van Dorp, D. A. (1979): Prostaglandin and thromboxane production by human and guinea-pig macrophages and leucocytes. *Prostaglandins*, 17:730–736.

82. Moroz, L. A. (1977): Increased blood fibrinolytic activity after aspirin ingestion. *N. Engl. J. Med.*, 296:525–529.

83. Murphy, R. S., Hammarström, S., and Samuelsson, B. (1979): Leukotriene C: a slow-reacting substance from murine mastocytoma cells. *Proc. Natl. Acad. Sci. USA*, 76:4275–4279.

84. Nasjletti, A., and Kalik, K. U. (1979): Minireview. Relationships between the kallikrein-kinin and prostaglandin systems. *Life Sci.*, 25:99–110.

85. Needleman, P., Bronson, S. D., Wyche, A., Sivakoff, M., and Nicolaou, K. C. (1978):Cardiac and renal prostaglandin I$_2$. Biosynthesis and biological effects in isolated perfused rabbit tissues. *J. Clin. Invest.*, 61:839–849.

86. Needleman, P., Kulkarni, P. S., and Raz, A. (1977): Coronary tone modulation: formation and actions of prostaglandins, endoperoxides, and thromboxanes. *Science*, 195:409–412.

87. Needleman, P., Raz, A., Ferrendelli, J. A., and Minkes, M. (1977): Application of imidazole as a selective inhibitor of thromboxane synthetase in human platelets. *Proc. Natl. Acad. Sci. USA*, 74:1716–1720.

88. Needleman, P., Raz, A., Minkes, M. S., Ferrendelli, J. A., and Sprecher, H. (1980): Triene prostaglandins: prostacyclin and thromboxane biosynthesis and unique biological properties. *Proc. Natl. Acad. Sci. USA*, 76:944–948.

89. Noel, S., and Cassin, S. (1976): Maturation of contractile response of ductus arteriosus to oxyten and drugs. *Am. J. Physiol.*, 231:240–243.

90. Norby, L., Flamenbaum, W., Lentz, R., and Ramwell, P. (1976): Prostaglandins and aspirin therapy in Bartter's syndrome. *Lancet*, ii:604–606.

91. Ogletree, M. L., Flynn, J. T., Feola, M., and Lefer, A. M. (1977): Early prostaglandin release from the ischemic myocardium in the dog. *Surg. Gynecol. Obstet.*, 144:734–740.

92. Omini, C., Moncada, S., and Vane, J. R. (1977): The effects of prostacyclin (PGI$_2$) on tissues which detect prostaglandins (PG's). *Prostaglandins*, 14:625–632.

93. O'Regan, S., Rivard, G. E., Mongeau, J -G., and Robitaille, P. O. (1979): A circulating inhibitor of platelet aggregation in Bartter's syndrome. *Pediatrics*, 64:939–941.

94. Pace-Asciak, C. R. (1973): Catecholamine-induced increase in prostaglandin E biosynthesis in homogenates of the rat stomach fundus. In: *Advances in the Biosciences*, Vol. 9, edited by S. Bergström and S. Bernhard, pp. 29–33. Pergamon Press, London.

95. Pareti, F. I., Mannucci, P. M, D'Angelo, A., Smith, J. B., Sautebin, L., and Galli, G. (1980): Congenital deficiency of thromboxane and prostacyclin. *Lancet*, i:898–901.

96. Pickles, V. R., Hall, W. J., Best, F. A., and Smith, G. N. (1965): Prostaglandins in endometrium and menstrual fluid from normal and dysmenorrhoeic subjects. *J. Obstet. Gynaecol. Br. Commonw.*, 72:185–192.

97. Raz, A., Isakson, P. C., Minkes, M. S., and Needleman, P. (1977): Characterisation of a novel metabolic pathway of arachidonate in coronary arteries which generates a potent endogenous coronary vasodilator. *J. Biol. Chem.*, 252:1123–1126.

98. Raz, A., Minkes, M. S., and Needleman, P. (1977): Endoperoxides and thromboxanes. Structural determinants for platelet aggregation and vasoconstriction. *Biochim. Biophys. Acta*, 488:305–311.

99. Remuzzi, G., Livio, M., Cavenaghi, A. E., Marchesi, D., Mecca, G., Donati, M. B., and de Gaetano, G. (1978): Unbalanced prostaglandin synthesis and plasma factors in uraemic bleeding. A hypothesis. *Thromb. Res.*, 13:531–536.

100. Remuzzi, G., Marchesi, D., Livio, M., Cavenaghi, A. E., Mecca, G., de Gaetano, G., and Donati, M. B. (1978): Altered platelet and vascular prostaglandin-generation in patients with renal failure and prolonged bleeding time. *Thromb. Res.*, 13:1007–1015.

101. Remuzzi, G., Misiani, R., Marchesi, D., Livio, M., Mecca, G., de Gaetano, G., and Donati, M. B. (1978): Haemolytic-uremic syndrome: Deficiency of plasma factor(s) regulating prostacyclin activity? *Lancet*, ii:871–872.

102. Rittenhouse-Simmons, S. (1979): Production of diglyceride from phosphatidylinositol in activated human platelets. *J. Clin. Invest.*, 63:580–587.

103. Robinson, H. J., Phares, H. F., and Graessle, O. E. (1974): Prostaglandin synthetase inhibitors and infection. In: *Prostaglandin Synthetase Inhibitors*, edited by H. J. Robinson and J. R. Vane, pp. 327–342. Raven Press, New York.

104. Rosenblum, W. I., and El-Sabban, F. (1978): Enhancement of platelet aggregation by tranylcypromine in mouse cerebral microvessels. *Circ. Res.*, 43:238–241.

105. Rosenthale, M. E., Dervinis, A., Begany, A. J., Lapidus, M., and Gluckman, M. I. (1970): Bronchodilator activity of prostaglandin E_2 when administered by aerosol to three species. *Experientia*, 26:1119–1121.

106. Roth, G. J., and Majerus, P. W. (1975): The mechanism of the effect of aspirin on human platelets. 1. Acetylation of a particulate fraction protein. *J. Clin. Invest.*, 56:624–632.

107. Russell, F. A., and Deykin, D. (1976): The effect of thrombin on the uptake and transformation of arachidonic acid by human platelets. *Am. J. Hematol.*, 1:59–70.

108. Schafer, A. I., Cooper, B., O'Hara, D., and Hardin, R. I. (1979): Identification of platelet receptors for prostaglandins I_2 and D_2. *J. Biol. Chem.*, 254:2914–2917.

109. Sharpe, G. L., Larsson, K. S., and Thalme B. (1975): Studies on closure of the ductus arteriosus. XII. *In utero* effects of indomethacin and sodium salicylate in rats and rabbits. *Prostaglandins*, 9:585–596.

110. Sharpe, G. L., Thalme, B., and Larsson, K. S. (1974): Studies on closure of the ductus arteriosus. XI. Ductal closure in utero by a prostaglandin synthetase inhibitor. *Prostaglandins*, 8:363–368.

111. Siegel, M. I., McConnell, R. T., Abrahams, S. L., Porter, N. A., and Cuatrecasas, P. (1979): Regulation of arachidonate metabolism via lipoxygenase and cyclo-oxygenase by 12-HPETE, the product of human platelet lipoxygenase. *Biochem. Biophys. Res. Commun.*, 89:1273–1280.

112. Siegel, M. I., McConnell, R. T., and Cuatrecasas, P. (1979): Aspirin-like drugs interfere with arachidonate metabolism by inhibition of the 12-hydroperoxy-5,8,10,14-eicosatetraenoic acid peroxidase activity of the lipoxygenase pathway. *Proc. Natl. Acad. Sci. USA*, 76:3774–3778.

113. Siess, W., Roth, P., Scherer, B., Kurzmann, I., Böhlig, B., and Weber, P. C. (1980): Platelet-membrane fatty acids, platelet aggregation, and thromboxane formation during a mackerel diet. *Lancet*, i:441–444.

114. Silberbauer, K., Sinzinger, H., Winter, M., Feigl, W., and Ring, F. (1978): Prostacyclin-like activity of endothelium and subendothelium—important for atherosclerosis? *Experientia*, 34:1471–1472.

115. Simon, L. S., and Mills, J. A. (1980): Nonsteroidal anti-inflammatory drugs. *N. Engl. J. Med.*, 302:1179–1185.

116. Smith, E. F., III, Lefer, A. M., and Smith, J. B. (1980): Influence of thromboxane inhibition on the severity of myocardial ischemia in cats. *Can. J. Physiol. Pharmacol.*, 58:294–300.

117. Smith, J. B., Ingerman, C., Kocsis, J. J., and Silver, M. J. (1974): Formation of an intermediate in prostaglandin synthesis and its association with the platelet release reaction. *J. Clin. Invest.*, 53:1468–1472.

118. Smith, J. B., Silver, M. J., Ingerman, C. M., and Kocsis, J. J. (1974): Prostaglandin D_2 inhibits the aggregation of human platelets. *Thromb. Res.*, 5:291–299.

119. Smith, J. B., and Willis, A. L. (1971): Aspirin selectively inhibits prostaglandin production in human platelets. *Nature (New Biol.)*, 231:235–237.

120. Smith, M. J. H. (1975): Prostaglandins and aspirin; an alternative view (editorial). *Agents Actions*, 5:315–317.

121. Smith, M. J. H. (1978): Aspirin and prostaglandins: Some recent developments. *Agents Actions*, 8:427–429.

122. Smith, M. J. H., and Smith, P. (1966): *The Salicylates. A Critical Bibliographic Review.* John Wiley, New York.
123. Stoff, J. S., Stemerman, M., Steer, M. Salzman, E., and Brown, R. S. (1980): A defect in platelet aggregation in Bartter's Syndrome. *Am. J. Med.*, 68:171–180.
124. Svensson, J., and Fredholm, B. B. (1977): Vasoconstrictor effect of thromboxane A_2. *Acta Physiol. Scand.*, 101:366–368.
125. Szczeklik, A., and Gryglewski, R. J. (1978): Prostaglandins and aspirin-sensitive asthma. *Am. Rev. Resp. Dis.*, 118:799–800.
126. Tai, H-H., and Yuan, B. (1978): On the inhibitory potency of imidazole and its derivatives on thromboxane synthetase. *Biochem. Biophys. Res. Commun.*, 80:236–242.
127. Tateson, J. E., Moncada, S., and Vane, J. R. (1977): Effects of prostacyclin (PGX) on cyclic AMP concentrations in human platelets. *Prostaglandins*, 13:389–397.
128. Vane, J. R. (1971): Inhibition of prostaglandin synthesis as a mechanism of action for aspirin-like drugs. *Nature (New Biol.)* 231:232–235.
129. Vane, J. R. (1976): Prostaglandins as mediators of inflammation. In: *Advances in Prostaglandin and Thromboxane Research, Vol. 2,* edited by. B. Samuelsson and R. Paoletti, pp. 791–801. Raven Press, New York.
130. Vane, J. R., and McGiff, J. C. (1975): Possible contributions of endogenous prostaglandins to the control of blood pressure. *Circ. Res., (Suppl. 1),* 36:1-68–1-75.
131. Wasserman, M. A., DuCharme, D. W., Griffin, R. L., DeGraaf, G. L., and Robinson, F. G. (1977): Bronchopulmonary and cardiovascular effects of prostaglandin D_2 in the dog. *Prostaglandins*, 13:255–269.
132. Weber, R. W., Hoffman, M., Raine, D. A. Jr., and Nelson, H. S. (1979): Incidence of bronchoconstriction due to aspirin, azo dyes, non-azo dyes, and preservatives in a population of perennial asthmatics. *J. Allergy Clin. Immunol.*, 64:32–37.
133. Weiss, H. J., and Lages, B. A. (1977): Possible congenital defect in platelet thromboxane synthetase. *Lancet*, i:760–761.
134. Weiss, H. J., and Turitto, V.T. (1979): Prostacyclin (prostaglandin I_2, PGI_2) inhibits platelet adhesion and thrombus formation on subendothelium. *Blood*, 53: 244–250.
135. Weksler, B. B., Knapp, J. M., and Jaffe, E. A (1977): Prostacyclin (PGI_2) synthesized by cultured endothelial cells modulates polymorphonuclear leukocyte function. *Blood (Suppl. 1)*, 50:287.
136. Weksler, B. B., Ley, C. W., and Jaffe, E. A. (1978): Stimulation of endothelial cell prostacyclin production by thrombin, trypsin and the ionophore A 23187. *J. Clin. Invest.*, 62:923–930.
137. Whittle, B. J. R., Broughton-Smith, N. K., Moncada, S., and Vane, J. R. (1978): Actions of prostacyclia (PGI_2) and its product, 6-oxo-$PGF_{1\alpha}$, on the rat gastric mueosa *in vivo* and *in vitro*. *Prostaglandins*, 15: 955–967.
138. Woodbury, D. M., and Fingl, E. (1975): Analgesic-antipyretics, anti-inflammatory agents, and drugs employed in the therapy of gout. In: *The Pharmacological Basis of Therapeutics*, fifth edition, edited by L. S. Goodman and A. Gilman, pp. 325–358. Macmillan, New York.

Acetylsalicylic Acid: New Uses for an Old Drug,
edited by H. J. M. Barnett, J. Hirsh, and
J. F. Mustard. Raven Press, New York © 1982.

Prostaglandins as Mediators of Inflammation

Gerald Weissmann

Division of Rheumatology, Department of Medicine, New York University School of Medicine; and University Hospital and Bellevue Hospital, New York, New York 10016

It is generally appreciated that secretion of potentially inflammatory materials by neutrophils into tissues is accompanied by the generation of mediators of inflammation. Three major classes of mediators of inflammation are released from neutrophils in the course of phagocytosis: (a) neutral proteases released from lysosomes, (b) derivatives of molecular oxygen, and (c) products derived from membrane lipids, such as the thromboxanes and prostaglandins. The chief enzymes attacking tissue substrates are neutral proteases—collagenase, elastase, and cathepsin G. These do not act unopposed, however. Body fluids usually contain significant amounts of circulating antiproteases (α_1-antitrypsin and α_2-macroglobulin), and only when the inhibitory capacity of these serum constituents is overcome can the proteases act. The neutrophil also responds to phagocytosis by transforming molecular oxygen to highly reactive free radicals: superoxide anion (O_2^-), hydroxyl radical ($OH\cdot$), hydrogen peroxide (H_2O_2), and, possibly, singlet oxygen ($^1O_2^-$). Since these species, and especially H_2O_2, can kill bacteria and fungi, their action *inside* the phagocytic vacuole is beneficial to the host. Unfortunately, these products of molecular oxygen can also injure "bystander" cells or membranes, and can impair the integrity of connective tissue macromolecules, such as the hyaluronate of synovial fluid. The cytoplasm of the cell contains enzymes that protect intracellular structures against oxygen-derived products: superoxide anion is transformed to H_2O_2 by a dismutase and H_2O_2 to water by catalase. Again, serum carries a control protein, ceruloplasmin, that acts to dampen the extracellular toxicities of oxygen-derived free radicals. We have recently demonstrated that this copper protein is an efficient scavenger of O_2^-; perhaps ceruloplasmin is elaborated to protect us from the consequences of granulocyte-associated inflammation. The cell also utilizes molecular oxygen in the transformation of unsaturated fatty acids. Phagocytosis induces the neutrophil to transform arachidonate into biologically active compounds such as endoperoxides, stable prostaglandins, thromboxanes, mono- and dihydro(pero)xy acids, and the newly described leukotrienes. Here too, regulatory mechanisms are important: the rapid metabolism of "inflammatory" compounds (e. g., endoperoxides, thromboxane A_2) to stable prostaglandins (PGI_2) provides a negative feedback control of inflammation, since the latter act to *inhibit* secretion from neutrophils and therefore may be considered "anti-inflammatory."

17

It is generally accepted that some of the prostaglandins and/or their antecedents in the arachidonic acid cascade are in some manner involved in inflammation. However, it is not clear what role these derivatives of membrane lipids play in discrete processes of inflammation. To analyze whether derivatives of arachidonic acid mediate all, some, or none of the major signs of inflammation, it may be useful to define the criteria used to designate a substance as a mediator of inflammation.

In 1929, Sir Henry Dale (8) suggested three criteria for classification of a substance as a mediator of inflammation:

1. Induction by the putative mediator of some or all signs of inflammation
2. Release of the proposed mediator during an inflammatory reaction
3. Reduction in the release of the substance, or inactivation of the substance, by known anti-inflammatory drugs.

It may also be useful to outline the criteria of acute inflammation and to place these lipid products among the other recognized mediators of inflammation.

In the first century of the common era, Cornelius Celsus suggested that inflammation was *"rubor et tumor cum calore et dolore"* (redness and swelling with heat and pain). However, it was not until the 19th century that Rudolph Virchow (60) introduced the concept that tissue injury was associated with inflammation by adding the fifth cardinal sign, *"et functio laesa"* (and loss of function).

PROSTAGLANDINS AND THE CARDINAL SIGNS OF INFLAMMATION

The first of Dale's criteria, the induction by the putative mediator of some or all signs of inflammation, can be met by some of the derivatives of arachidonic acid, but not by all. Indeed, these derivatives appear to have either pro- or anti-inflammatory actions depending on the system studied. Consequently, it will be well to review the definitions of inflammation and to determine whether defined oxidation products or arachidonic acid can mimic these signs. We will examine each of the cardinal signs of inflammation and review the evidence that various oxidation products of arachidonic acid are involved in their mediation.

Rubor

Redness is due to vasodilatation, and it is clear that appropriate infusions of arachidonic acid are vasodilatory in a number of species (11). The metabolites of this fatty acid have distinctly different effects on the smooth muscles of blood vessels. Thus, PGG_2 and PGH_2 (the endoperoxides) appear to provoke vasoconstriction followed by secondary vasodilatation, but act only to constrict if inhibitors of their transformation to prostacyclin (PGI_2) are included in the experimental design (11,38). PGI_2 is a very potent vasodilator and, in this regard, it mimics the stable prostaglandins such as PGE_1, PGE_2, PGD_2, and PGA_2 (32,44,69). In contrast, the short-lived thromboxane A_2 (TXA_2) is a potent vasoconstrictor of most vascular smooth muscle (11). Turning to products of the lipoxygenase pathway, 12-L-hydroperoxy-5,8,10,14-eicosatetraenoic acid (HPETE) has been demonstrated to possess vasconstrictor activity (37). The effects on vasodilatation of the other metabolites have not been unequivocally established.

Tumor

Swelling, or edema, is usually the result of gaps in vascular endothelium that permit plasma protein to exude from the circulation into tissue spaces. Indeed, most of the products derived from arachidonic acid are not alone very potent inducers of edema; they appear, however, to enhance experimental edema provoked by other edema-causing substances. Thus, arachidonic acid has been shown to potentiate carrageenan edema (45). The prostaglandin endoperoxides PGG_2 and PGH_2 are weak potentiators of carrageenan edema as well as that provoked by injections of bradykinin or histamine (46,69). The work of Kuehl and his associates (36,37) has indicated that edema provoked by phorbol myristate acetate (PMA) is induced not by the endoperoxides themselves but by the free radical formed by the conversion of PGG_2 to PGH_2. In fact, specific scavengers of oxygen-derived free radicals (such as MK-447) enhance the formation of PGH_2 and of stable prostaglandins while at the same time exerting an anti-inflammatory effect in PMA-induced edema (36).

Prostacyclin, on the other hand, potentiates bradykinin and carrageenan edema, resembling in this respect the effects of PGE_2, PGI_2, and $PGF_{1\alpha}$, which at low doses potentiate edema provoked by croton oil, carrageenan, histamine, and bradykinin (2,18,35,69). However, high doses of the stable prostaglandins seem to inhibit carrageenan-induced edema in inflammation and have been shown to exert this effect by raising cyclic AMP levels in target tissues (2,45). Stable prostaglandins of the E and F series do not cause the edema in subcutaneous injury induced by carrageenan, because a study of the timing of their appearance in carrageenan-induced exudates indicates that it is attributable to earlier products (45,46). The effects of thromboxane have not been clearly established. Turning to products of the lipoxygenase pathway, Kuehl and his associates (36,37) have suggested that HPETE may be involved in PMA-induced edema, again by virtue of the generation of an oxygen-derived free radical. The role of HPETE has not been established.

Whether, indeed, arachidonic acid-derived products alone directly provoke edema at all has been rendered questionable by the careful studies of Williams and Peck (69). They suggest that the capacity of these products to provoke modest edema and to potentiate significantly edema induced by bradykinin or histamine simply reflects enhanced vasodilatation. These authors found that the rank order of different prostaglandins was the same for "exudation-potentiation potency" as for "blood flow-increasing potency," i.e., PGE > PGF > PGD. Secondly, they found that local injection of substances, other than prostaglandins, which increased skin blood flow (e.g., isoprenaline, ADP, and adenosine), also had "exudation-potentiating activity." Conversely, substances that reduced skin blood flow (e.g., noradrenaline and angiotensin II) reduced exudation and blood flow in parallel. From these results, the authors concluded that prostaglandins increased histamine- and bradykinin-induced plasma exudate *not* by increasing vascular permeability but by increasing vasodilatation.

Calore

The role of prostaglandins in fever is also unclear at the moment. Arachidonic acid, per se, when injected directly into the brain, provokes fever (7). In contrast, stable derivatives of the endoperoxides PGG_2 and PGH_2 do not provoke fever. There is no good evidence to indicate that prostacyclin is involved in febrile responses. With respect to the stable prostaglandins PGE_2 and PGE_2, the work of Feldenberg et al. (9,12,43) in the early 1970s clearly showed that prostaglandins were present in the cerebrospinal fluid of animals rendered febrile by endogenous and exogenous pyrogens and that PGE_1 and PGE_2 caused fever in experimental animals when injected either intrahypothalamically or intraventricularly. Moreover, Ziel and Krupp (71) found that endogenous pyrogens increased the activity of prostaglandin synthetase in cerebral tissue. However, the recent work of Cranston (7) has demonstrated that prostaglandin antagonists can inhibit fever induced by PGEs but not the fever provoked by endogenous pyrogen. Moreover, sodium salicylate inhibited the appearance of prostaglandins in cerebrospinal fluid of febrile rabbits, but did not abolish the temperature rise in response to pyrogen. Since arachidonic acid itself is pyrogenic and since almost all nonsteroidal anti-inflammatory agents are antipyretic agents, it may be inferred that as yet unknown metabolites derived from arachidonic acid are mediators of fever in the central nervous system.

Dolore

The role of arachidonic acid-derived metabolites in the provocation of pain is equally complex. In various experimental models, Ferreira (13) found that arachidonic acid per se provokes overt pain. In contrast, the prostaglandin endoperoxides provoke, at most, modest hyperalgesia (70). Ferreira has also indicated that prostacyclin does not provoke overt pain but appears to provoke hyperalgesia, which becomes overt pain after the subsequent addition of bradykinin or histamine (15). The hyperalgesia provoked by prostacyclin is short-lived (30 min), in contrast with the longer hyperalgesia (1–2 hr) provoked by PGE_1 and PGE_2 (15). These stable prostaglandins also exert their effects synergistically with bradykinin and histamine. Moreover, cyclic AMP and theophylline provoke hyperalgesia, the long-lasting effects of which are similar to those produced by PGE_2 (14). Finally, morphine and the enkephalins diminished PGE_2-induced hyperalgesia but not that induced by dibutyryl cyclic AMP (14). These studies suggested that agents that raised the intracellular level of cyclic GMP (e.g., morphine) antagonized those agents that raised the intracellular level of cyclic AMP, such as the stable prostaglandins. Since $PGF_{2\alpha}$ induces accumulation of intracellular cyclic GMP, it is not surprising that Ferreira found antagonism between the pain-provoking effects of PGE_2 and $PGF_{2\alpha}$. Although the role of thromboxanes in the provocation of pain or induction of hyperalgesia has not been established, Ferreira studied a series of hydroperoxides of fatty acids, including HPETE. He found that the hyperalgesia produced by these agents blended with the sensation of intense, immediate, overt pain and that these agents were far more effective than PGE_1, bradykinin, or histamine (13). These data remind us of the effects of various oxidation products of arachidonic acid on edema: Most of these products appear to potentiate pain induced by bradykinin or histamine rather than being themselves the cause of overt pain. The analgesic effects of various nonsteroidal anti-inflammatory agents would, however, suggest that the hyperalgesic action of stable prostaglandins may be important in the sensation of pain during inflammation in human diseases. The results of such experiments could equally well be interpreted as suggesting that products not yet identified may be more potent mediators of such pain.

Functio Laesa

The fifth sign of inflammation, loss of function, is perhaps the most important. Since *functio laesa* means tissue injury, and this implies cellular involvement, it is important to consider the effect of prostaglandins and their antecedents on the functions of inflammatory cells. Because of space limitations we will not consider the effects of prostaglandins on lymphocytes or macrophages, although these have been extensively described (21,26,61,62). We will limit this discussion to cells that are involved in acute inflammation: platelets and granulocytes.

Platelets exposed to various products of arachidonic oxidation first undergo reversible aggregation and, subsequently, "second wave" aggregation associated with release reaction. This involves release of materials such as serotonin and ADP. Arachidonic acid per se is a potent platelet aggregant (6,41). The role of endoperoxides is somewhat controversial, but it is clear that PGG_2 and PGH_2 are potent platelet aggregants (28,30,47,51). Although they may exert their effects only after transformation to the aggregant thromboxane A_2 (28), these agents certainly have the property of provoking decrements in intracellular cyclic AMP (40,42). In contrast, prostacyclin, which is not made in appreciable amounts by platelets, is the most potent inhibitor of platelet aggregation, far more potent, in fact, than PGE_1, PGE_2, or PGD_2 (27,44,48). These inhibitors of platelet aggregation appear to work by virtue of engaging platelet receptors that then couple to membrane adenylate cyclase. Exogenously added cyclic AMP or β-adrenergic agents (which raise endogenous levels of cyclic AMP) are also potent inhibitors of platelet aggregation (41,51). Thromboxane A_2 is a potent platelet aggregant (28,41), but it is not clear whether the platelet aggregation induced by arachidonic acid is directly attributable to thromboxane or to one of the intermediates in its formation (28 versus 47). The aggregant role of HPETE and HETE has not been completely established, although the lipoxygenase pathway is very active in the platelet (33,41,48).

For tissue damage to proceed to the stage of irreversibility, inflammatory cells are required. These produce hydrolytic enzymes, especially lysosomal enzymes, in response to inflammatory stimuli (65,66,74). Since the earliest response to acute injury is usually the influx of polymorphonuclear leukocytes (neutrophils), the chemotactic activity of arachidonic acid derivatives has attracted considerable attention. Purified arachidonate is chemotactic (49,56,57) when appropriate corrections are made for chemokinesis (increase in the random mobility of cells as opposed to directed migration). The chemotactic activity of pure arachidonate is significantly enhanced when this lipid is exposed to hydrogen peroxide or to ultraviolet light, suggesting that oxidation products are formed without enzymatic action from arachidonate (56). Recent experiments by Perez et al. (50) have shown that when arachidonic acid was acted on by a superoxide-anion generating system (xanthine oxidase plus acetaldehyde), a lipid product was formed that yielded a single peak of chemotactic activity on thin-layer radiochromatograms performed with radiolabeled [^{14}C]arachidonic acid as substrate. This material was chemotactic in nanogram quantities. Since human granulocytes exposed to most chemotactic stimuli also respond by generating O_2^- at the surface, this nonenzymatic generation of chemotactic material from arachidonate is another means whereby products of 20:4 fatty acids can produce influx of inflammatory cells to sites of injury.

The chemotactic activities of PGG_2 and PGH_2 have not been established. In contrast, PGI_2 (prostacyclin) has been shown to inhibit chemotaxis (67). PGE_1, PGE_2, and $PGF_{1\alpha}$ seem to have no direct effects on chemotaxis of human cells (10,22). Indeed, PGE_2 depresses chemokinesis whereas $PGF_{2\alpha}$ enhances chemokinesis (10). The stable prostaglandins provoke the appropriate changes in cyclic nucleotides: PGE_1 and PGE_2 tend to raise cyclic AMP levels in these cells; $PGF_{2\alpha}$ acts to raise cyclic GMP (74). Thromboxane A_2 has been shown to have chemotactic properties, though not as potent as 12-L-hydroxy-5,8,10-heptadecatrienoic acid (HHT) (10,22). The studies of Turner et al. (57) and Goetzl (22) have indicated that both HPETE and HETE are potent chemotactic substances for white cells from several species (49,57). There is some species difference, however, and earlier claims that prostaglandins of the E series were chemotactic for rabbit peritoneal neutrophils have not been confirmed for cells from peripheral blood of rabbits (10) or man (22).

It is important to appreciate that the major documented functions of the stable prostaglandins are to interact with specific membrane receptors of vasculature, connective tissue and, perhaps primarily, of those circulating cells that mediate acute and chronic inflammation: platelets, neutrophils, macrophages, and lymphocytes. In general, the stable prostaglandin and prostacyclin provoke their action by raising the intracellular level of cyclic AMP, and when cyclic AMP levels are raised in these cells of inflammation (see below), their major effect is to inhibit those parameters of cellular function that are proinflammatory. Thus, the products of the cyclo-oxygenase pathway appear to serve as "turn off" signals for the platelet, the granulocyte, the macrophage, and the lymphocyte. Save for the above-described effects on chemotaxis, the role of endoperoxides and products of the lipoxygenase pathway has not been adequately examined in models of acute and chronic inflammation.

RELEASE OF ARACHIDONIC ACID–DERIVED PRODUCTS BY THE CELLS OF INFLAMMATION

Each of the cells involved in acute and chronic inflammation (platelets, neutrophils, macrophages, and lymphocytes) has the capacity to transform arachidonic acid into its biologically active derivatives. Thus the second of Dale's criteria (release of the proposed mediator during inflammatory reaction) can be met. It is beyond the scope of this chapter to describe in detail the release of these products from platelets, macrophages, and lymphocytes. We focus instead on generation of these substances by human polymorphonuclear leukocytes, since these cells are the most important vectors of acute inflammation, and because activation of these cells antecedes the later influx of lymphocytes and macrophages, the vectors of chronic inflammation.

When human polymorphonuclear leukocytes are exposed to phagocytic stimuli or to soluble stimuli (e.g., chemotactic peptides), they respond with a carefully programmed sequence of secretory events that leads to the elaboration of three classes of mediators (63,64,72). Perhaps the best studies of these responses are those on the release from neutrophils of lysosomal hydrolases that are regurgitated inadvertently, so to speak, from human polymorphonuclear leukocytes on engagement by ligands present on opsonized particles. This secretion is ordinarily designed to insure that lysosomal hydrolases are introjected into the invaginated phagocytic vacuole. However, when the fungal metabolite cytochalasin B prevents closure of the phagocytic vacuole, a considerable portion of these hydrolases can be recovered on the outside of the cell. The agents that attack connective tissue substrates and interact with circulating mediators of inflammation are neutral proteases such as collagenase, elastase, and cathepsin G (63,65,72).

However, the cell also releases into the external milieu products derived from molecular oxygen, such as O_2^-, H_2O_2, $OH\cdot$, and $^1O_2^*$. These products of molecular oxygen are destined to act within the phagocytic vacuole, forming part of a microbicidal system (34). These products can then interact with neighboring cells and artificial biological membranes (25,39), causing injury both to proteins and to lipid substrates, acting further to injure the surrounding cellular environment of the white cell.

It had previously been established that the stable prostaglandins were elaborated from phagocytosing human polymorphonuclear leukocytes (73). Together with the Karolinska group, we were able to demonstrate that thromboxanes are also formed by human peripheral blood polymorphonuclear leukocytes (23,24). Polymorphonuclear leukocytes incubated for up to 60 sec in buffer alone generated minimal amounts of TXB_2 (15.7 $\pm$ 1.9 pg/10^6 polymorphonuclear leukocytes). However, when neutrophils were exposed to serum-treated zymosan, which they ingested avidly, up to 10-fold increments in thromboxane generation were observed (measured by a sensitive radioimmunoassay). The means $\pm$ SEM for 13 experiments were 65.8 $\pm$ 12.2 pg/10^6 granulocytes. This response varied with the particle-to-cell ratio and was time-dependent. Maximum thromboxane generation usually occurred before 15 min and an almost linear response was noted with concentrations of serum-treated zymosan between 0.5 and 5 mg/ml. To determine whether phagocytosis was a prerequisite for thromboxane generation, experiments were performed with cytochalasin B. Neutrophils treated with cytochalasin B and then exposed to serum-treated zymosan generated amounts of thromboxane that were comparable to amounts generated by normal cells. Generation of thromboxane B_2 by normal and cytochalasin B-treated leukocytes in response to stimulation was inhibited appropriately by the cyclo-oxygenase inhibitor indomethacin. Indomethacin interfered with neither particle-to-cell contact nor with other responses of these cells to surface stimulation (lysosomal enzyme release and superoxide anion generation). Furthermore, these concentrations of indomethacin did not influence the radioimmunoassay.

Appropriate control experiments demonstrated that generation of TXB_2 in these experiments could not be attributed to platelet contamination of the polymorphonuclear leukocyte suspensions.

Recent experiments by Borgeat et al. (3) and by Borgeat and Samuelsson (4) have demonstrated that the lipoxygenase pathway is very active in rabbit and human polymorphonuclear leukocytes. Products of the lipoxygenase pathway, as described recently (52), include not only monohydroperoxy acids (substitutions at 5 and 15) but also a novel dihydroxy fatty acid (4) recently designated as leukotriene B: (5S, 12R)-dihydroxy-6,8,10,14-icosatetraenoic acid). The precursor of this product, leukotriene A, also gives rise, in the presence of glutathione, to the slow-reactive substance of anaphylaxis (SRS-A). These pathways of arachidonate transformation via lipoxygenase are illustrated in Fig. 1.

Perez et al. (50) showed that when purified arachidonic acid is exposed to the superoxide-generating system (xanthine oxidase and acid aldehyde), a chemotactic lipid is formed *(see above)*. Thus, products formed both enzymatically and nonenzymatically from membrane arachidonic acid can be released from human polymorphonuclear leukocytes as they generate superoxide anion, a consequence of surface stimulation. These products include those formed via the lipoxygenase pathway as well as products of the cyclo-oxygenase pathway: stable prostaglandins and thromboxanes.

REDUCTION IN PROSTAGLANDIN RELEASE BY NONSTEROIDAL AND BY STEROIDAL ANTI-INFLAMMATORY AGENTS

Acetylsalicylic Acid and Nonsteroidal Anti-Inflammatory Agents

The third of Dale's criteria appears to be fulfilled for products derived from arachidonic acid, which is cleaved by cellular phospholipases from membrane phospholipids. The demonstration by Vane (58), since amply confirmed in innumerable studies, that nonsteroidal anti-inflammatory agents (especially acetylsalicylic acid and indomethacin) inhibit the transformation of arachidonic acid to the stable prostaglandins, provided the first evidence that this class of anti-inflammatory

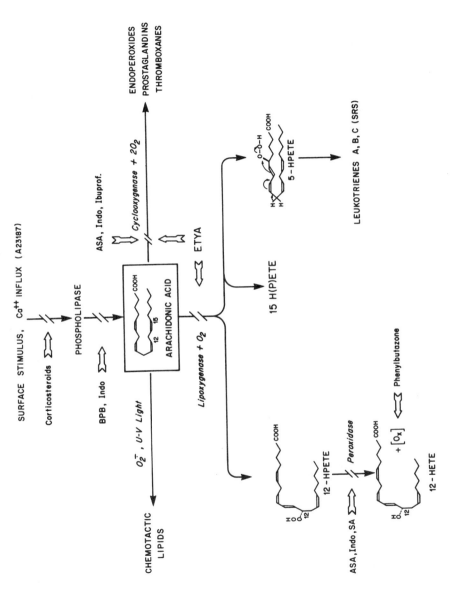

FIG. 1. Inhibitors of the arachidonic acid cascade.

agents had as its major locus of action this mediator system. Utilizing a cell-free enzyme system in guinea pig lung, Vane clearly demonstrated a dose-related inhibition of prostaglandin biosynthesis when indomethacin and acetylsalicylic acid were added. It was later found that the addition of indomethacin or acetylsalicylic acid to washed human platelets, which produce PGR and PGF when incubated with thrombin, substantially reduced prostaglandin formation in a dose-related manner. Moreover, prostaglandin production was abolished in platelets from three subjects 1 hr after they had ingested 10 grains of acetylsalicylic acid (54). Finally, it has been shown that the effects of ingested acetylsalicylic acid can persist for as long as 3 days and those of indomethacin more than 6 hr (20).

Thus, in both cell-free and single-cell systems, acetylsalicylic acid and indomethacin inhibited the synthesis of prostaglandins. Indomethacin and acetylsalicylic acid also abolished the release of prostaglandins normally observed when the perfused dog spleen was contracted by catecholamines or by nervous stimulation. Inhibition by indomethacin or acetylsalicylic acid of prostaglandin release has been shown in many other biological systems (16,18,59). Since tissues do not appear to store prostaglandins, release may very well be considered equivalent to synthesis. Since the early 1970s, it has become clear that most other nonsteroidal anti-inflammatory agents tested also inhibit prostaglandin biosynthesis (59). At present, most of the nonsteroidal agents used in clinical anti-arthritic therapy have the capacity both to inhibit experimental inflammation in animals and to inhibit prostaglandin biosynthesis (2). Prostaglandin biosynthesis, usually tested in a conventional system derived from sheep seminal vesicles, is now utilized in routine screening tests for possible new nonsteroidal anti-inflammatory compounds (16). Although there is no one-to-one relationship between the capacity of an agent to exert an anti-inflammatory effect in experimental animals and man and its capacity to inhibit prostaglandin biosynthesis, these differences are most probably due to pharmacokinetics. Thus, although differences exist between a drug's behavior in a clinical situation or in experimental animals and its behavior in specific enzyme systems, the fact remains that at the present time no clinically useful nonsteroidal anti-inflammatory drug is incapable of inhibiting prostaglandin biosynthesis.

Figure 1 indicates how other agents affect products of the arachidonic acid cascade. Corticosteroids (see below) block formation of all the products of membrane lipids. Inhibitors of phospholipase A_2 (indomethacin or p-bromophenacyl bromide) will also block generation of arachidonate and its metabolites (55). The classic nonsteroidal anti-inflammatory agents (acetylsalicylic acid, indomethacin, ibuprofen, etc.) will selectively block formation of products of the cyclo-oxygenase pathway. A useful agent, 5,8,11,14-eicosatetraynoic acid (ETYA), inhibits both the lipoxygenase and the cyclo-oxygenase pathways (55), and clinically useful drugs with this property are under development. The work of Kuehl has shown that phenylbutazone and some other nonsteroidal anti-inflammatory agents act to scavenge the free oxygen-derived radicals that form as a consequence of the transformation of 12- or 15-hydroperoxy fatty acids, HPETEs (or their endoperoxide analogues), to the corresponding 12- or 15-hydroxy fatty acids, HETEs (36,37). Finally, Cuatracasas (53) has shown that many of these compounds, now including salicylic acid, will inhibit the peroxidase(s) that transforms 12-HPETE to 12-HETE.

GLUCOCORTICOIDS AND PROSTAGLANDINS

Steroidal anti-inflammatory agents do not inhibit the activity of the "prostaglandin synthetase" system in microsomal fractions. In a series of experiments utilizing inflamed rat synovium, Floman and Zor (17) were unable to demonstrate marked suppression of prostaglandin release by incubation with corticosterone, dexamethasone, or prednisone. Noninflammatory steroids such as aldosterone and progesterone had no effect. In addition, the suppressive action of cortisone on PGR release could be reversed by the addition of arachidonic acid. By contrast, the inhibitory action of indomethacin was not affected by provision of exogenous substrate. Chang and co-workers (5) have recently demonstrated that glucocorticoids inhibit prostaglandin release from adipose tissue in an *in vitro* system, whereas Heraczynska-Cedro et al. (31), in an *in vivo* system utilizing whole-limb perfusion, have shown that hydrocortisone suppresses the release of PG-like substances. Gryglewski (29) has summarized various experimental systems in which glucocorticoids inhibit release of prostaglandins and thromboxanes. These now include:

(a) The isolated, perfused guinea-pig lung challenged by antigen or a releasing factor (RCS-RF).

(b) Blood vessels, which release prostacyclin after prolonged vasoconstriction induced by norepinephrine.

(c) The perfused cat spleen similarly stimulated with norepinephrine.

(d) Incubated slices of mesentery from ovalbumin-sensitized guinea pigs exposed to antigen.

(e) Inflamed ocular tissues, which release prostaglandins.

(f) Dogs or cats suffering from shock sufficient to raise myocardial prostaglandin levels.

(g) Human psoriatic skin which contains excessive amounts of HETE.

Moreover, Flower and co-workers (1,19) have shown that stimulated lung tissue failed to release free arachidonate from membrane phospholipids in the presence of glucocorticoids under circumstances in which both the cyclo-oxygenase and the lipoxygenase pathways were blocked by an appropriate inhibitor (ETYA). They were not able to show that steroids interfered with phospholipase activity in cell-free tissue homogenates. Finally, Goldstein and co-wokers (24) have shown that phagocytosing human leukocytes inhibit thromboxane generation, after preincubation of cells with hydrocortisone. Each of these findings strongly suggests that stabilization of the plasma membranes by cortisol has made arachidonic acid (the substrate) less accessible to phospholipases, presumably by packing phospholipid bilayers.

ACKNOWLEDGMENTS

This study was aided by grants from the National Institutes of Health (AM-11949, HL-19721), The National Foundation—March of Dimes, the National Science Foundation, and The Arthritis Foundation.

REFERENCES

1. Blackwell, G. J., Flower, R. J., Nijkamp, F. P., and Vane, J. R. (1978): Phospholipase A_2 activity of guinea-pig isolated perfused lungs: Stimulation, and inhibition of antiinflammatory steroids. *Br. J. Pharmacol.*, 62:79–89.
2. Bonta, I. L., and Parnham, M. J. (1978): Prostaglandins and chronic inflammation. *Biochem. Pharmacol.*, 27:1611–1623.
3. Borgeat, P., Hamberg, M., and Samuelsson, B. (1976): Transformation of arachidonic acid and homo-γ-linolenic acid by rabbit polymorphonuclear leukocytes. Monohydroxy acids from novel lipoxygenases. *J. Biol. Chem.*, 251:7816–7820.
4. Borgeat, P., and Samuelsson, B. (1979): Arachidonic acid metabolism in polymorphonuclear leukocytes: Effects of ionophore A23187. *Proc. Natl. Acad. Sci. USA*, 76:2148–2152.
5. Chang, J., Lewis, G. P., and Piper, P. J. (1977): Inhibition by glucocorticoids of prostaglandin release from adipose tissue *in vitro*. *Br. J. Pharmacol.*, 59:425–432.
6. Charo, I. F., Feinman, R. D., Detwiler, C., Smith, J. B., Ingerman, C. M., and Silver, J. J. (1977): Prostaglandin endoperoxides and thromboxane A_2 can induce platelet aggregation in the absence of secretion. *Nature*, 269:66–69.
7. Cranston, W. I. (1979): Central mechanisms of fever. *Fed. Proc.*, 38:49–51.
8. Dale, H. H. (1929): Some chemical factors in the control of the circulation. *Lancet*, i:1285–1289.
9. Dey, P. K., Feldberg, W., Gupta, K. P., Milton, A. S., and Wendlandt, S. (1974): Further studies on the role of prostaglandin in fever. *J. Physiol.*, 241:629–646.
10. Diaz-Perez, J. L., Goldyne, M. E., and Winkelman, R. K. (1976): Prostaglandins and chemotaxis: Enhancement of polymorphonuclear leukocyte chemotaxis by prostaglandin $F_{2\alpha}$. *J. Invest. Dermatol.*, 66:149–152.
11. Dusting, G. J., Moncada, S., and Vane, J. R. (1978): Vascular actions of arachidonic acid and its metabolites in perfused mesenteric and femoral beds of the dog. *Eur. J. Pharmacol.*, 49:65–72.
12. Feldberg, W., and Gupta, K. P. (1973): Pyrogen fever and prostaglandin-like activity in cerebrospinal fluid. *J. Physiol.*, 228:41–53.
13. Ferreira, S. H. (1972): Prostaglandins, aspirin-like drugs and analgesia. *Nature (New Biol.)*, 240:200–204.
14. Ferreira, S. H., and Nakamura, M. (1979): Humoral mediators of pain. In: *Advances in Inflammation Research, Vol. 1*, edited by G. Weissman, R. Paoletti, and B. Samuelsson, pp. 317–330. Raven Press, New York.
15. Ferreira, S. H., Nakamura, M., and de Abreu Castro, M. S. (1978): The hyperalgesic effects of prostacyclin and prostaglandin E_2. *Prostaglandins*, 16:31–37.
16. Ferreira, S. H., and Vane, J. R. (1974): New aspects of the mode of action of non-steroid antiinflammatory drugs. *Annu. Rev. Pharmacol.*, 14:57–82.
17. Floman, Y., and Zor, U. (1976): Mechanism of steroid action in inflammation: Inhibition of prostaglandin synthesis and release. *Prostaglandins*, 12:403–413.
18. Flower, R. J. (1974): Drugs which inhibit prostaglandin biosynthesis. *Pharmacol. Rev.*, 26:33–67.
19. Flower, R. J. (1978): Steroidal anti-inflammatory drugs as inhibitors of phospholipase A_2. In: *Advances in Prostaglandin and Thromboxane Research, Vol. 3*, edited by C. Galli, G. Galli, and G. Porcellati, pp. 105–111. Raven Press, New York.
20. Flower, R., Gryglewski, R., Kerbaczyńska-Cedro, K., and Vane, J. R. (1972): Effects of antiinflammatory drugs on prostaglandin biosynthesis. *Nature (New Biol.)*, 238:104–106.
21. Franks, D. J., MacManus, J. P., and Whitfield, J. P. (1971): The effect of prostaglandins on cyclic AMP production and cell proliferation in thymic lymphocytes. *Biochem. Biophys. Res. Commun.*, 44:1177–1183.

22. Goetzl, E. J., and Gorman, R. R. (1978): Chemotactic and chemokinetic stimulation of human eosinophil and neutrophil polymorphonuclear leukocytes by 12-L-hydroxy-5,8,10-heptadecatrienoic acid (HHT). *J. Immunol.*, 120:526–531.

23. Goldstein, I. M., Malsten, C. L., Kindahl, H., Kaplan, H. B., Rådmark, O., Samuelsson, B., and Weissman, G. (1978): Thromboxane generation by human peripheral blood polymorphonuclear leukocytes. *J. Exp. Med.*, 148:787–792.

24. Goldstein, I. M., Malmsten, C. L., Samuelsson, B., and Weissmann, G. (1977): Prostaglandins, thromboxanes, and polymorphonuclear leukocytes: Mediation and modulation of inflammation. *Inflammation*, 2:309–316.

25. Goldstein, I. M., and Weissmann, G. (1977): Effects of the generation of superoxide anion on permeability of liposomes. *Biochem. Biophys, Res. Commun.*, 75:604–609.

26. Goodwin, J. S., Bankhurst, A. D., and Messner, R. P. (1977): Suppression of human T-cell mitogenesis by prostaglandin. Existence of a prostaglandin-producing suppressor cell. *J. Exp. Med.*, 146:1719–1734.

27. Gorman, R. R. (1979): Modulation of human platelet function by prostacyclin and thromboxane A_2. *Fed. Proc.*, 38:83–88.

28. Gorman, R. R., Bundy, G. L., Peterson, D. C., Sun, F. F., Miller, O. V., and Fitzpatrick, F. A. (1977): Inhibition of human platelet thromboxane synthetase by 9,11-azoprosta 5,13-dienoic acid. *Proc. Natl. Acad. Sci. USA*, 74:4007–4011.

29. Gryglewski, R. J. (1979): Effects of anti-inflammatory steroids on the arachidonic acid cascade. In: *Advances in Inflammation Research, Vol. 1*, edited by G. Weissmann, R. Paoletti, and B. Samuelsson, p. 505. Raven Press, New York.

30. Hamberg, M., Svensson, J., and Samuelsson, B. (1974): Prostaglandin endoperoxides. A new concept concerning the mode of action and release of prostaglandins. *Proc. Natl. Acad. Sci. USA*, 71:3824–3829.

31. Heraczynska-Cedro, K., and Stasqewska-Barczak, J. (1977): Suppression of the release of PG-like substances by hydrocortisone in vivo. *Prostaglandins*, 13:517–521.

32. Higgs, G. A., Moncada, S., and Vane, J. R. (1978): Prostacyclin as a potent dilator of arterioles in the hamster cheek pouch (proceedings). *J. Physiol.*, 275:30P–31P.

33. Ho, P. P., Walters, C. P., and Sullivan, H. R. (1977): A particulate arachidonate lipoxygenase in human blood platelets. *Biochem. Biophys. Res. Commun.*, 76:398–405.

34. Klebanoff, S. J. (1975): Antimicrobial systems of the polymorphonuclear leukocyte. In: *The Phagocytic Cell in Host Resistance*, edited by J. A. Bellanti and D. H. Dayton, pp. 45–59. Raven Press, New York.

35. Komoriya, K., Ohmori, H., Azuma, A., Kurozumi, S., Hashimoto, Y., Nicolaou, K. C., Barnette, W. E., and Magolda, R. L. (1978): Prostaglandin I_2 as a potentiator of acute inflammation in rats. *Prostaglandins*, 15:557–564.

36. Kuehl, F. A., Jr., Humes, J. L., Egan, R. W., Ham, E. A., Beveridge, G. C., and Van Arman, C. G. (1977): Role of prostaglandin endoperoxide PGG_2 in inflammatory processes. *Nature*, 265:170–173.

37. Kuehl, F. A., Jr., Humes, J. L., Torchiana, M. L., Ham, E. A., and Egan, R. W. (1979): Oxygen-centered radicals in inflammatory processes. In: *Advances in Inflammation Research, Vol. 1*, edited by G. Weissmann, R. Paoletti, and B. Samuelsson, pp. 419–430. Raven Press, New York.

38. Lewis, G. P., Westwick, J., and Williams, T. J. (1977): Microvascular responses produced by the prostaglandin endoperoxide PGG_2 in vivo (proceedings). *Br. J. Pharmacol.*, 59:442P.

39. McCord, J. M., Stokes, S. H., and Wong, K. (1979): Superoxide radical as a phagocyte-produced chemical mediator of inflammation. In: *Advances in Inflammation Research, Vol. 1*, edited by G. Weissmann, R. Paoletti, and B. Samuelsson, pp. 273–291. Raven Press, New York.

40. Malmsten, C., Hamberg, M., Svensson, J., and Samuelsson, B. (1975): Physiological role of an endoperoxide in human platelets: Hemostatic defect due to platelet cyclooxygenase deficiency. *Proc. Natl. Acad. Sci. USA*, 72:1446–1450.

41. Marcus, A. J. (1978): The role of lipids in platelet function, with particular reference to the arachidonic acid pathway. *J. Lipid Res.*, 19:793–826.

42. Miller, O. V., Johnson, R. A., and Gorman, R. R. (1977): Inhibition of PGE_1-stimulated cAMP accumulation in human platelets by thromboxane A_2. *Prostaglandins*, 13:599–609.

43. Milton, A., and Wendlandt, S. (1970): A possible role for prostaglandin E as a modulator for temperature regulation in the central nervous system of the cat. *J. Physiol.*, 207:76P–77P.

44. Moncada, S., and Vane, J. S. (1979): The role of prostacyclin in vascular tissue. *Fed. Proc.*, 38:66–71.

45. Murota, S. -I., Chang, W. -C., Tsurufuji, S., and Morita, I. (1979): In: *Advances in Inflammation Research*, *Vol. 1*, edited by G. Weissmann, R. Paoletti, and B. Samuelsson, pp. 439–447. Raven Press, New York.
46. Murota, S. -I., and Morita, I. (1978): Effect of prostaglandin I_2 and related compounds on vascular permeability response in granuloma tissues. *Prostaglandins*, 15:297–301.
47. Needleman, P., Minkes, M., and Raz, A. (1976): Thromboxanes: Selective biosynthesis and distinct biological properties. *Science*, 193:163–165.
48. Nugteren, D. H. (1975): Arachidonate lipoxygenase in blood platelets. *Biochim. Biophys. Acta*, 380:299–307.
49. Penneys, N. S., Simon, P., Ziboh, V. A., and Schlossberg, J. (1977): *In vivo* chemotaxis induced by polyunsaturated fatty acids. *J. Invest. Dermatol.*, 69:435–438.
50. Perez, H. D., Weksler, B., and Goldstein, I. (1979): A new mechanism for the generation of biologically active products from arachidonic acid. *Clin. Res.*, 27:464A.
51. Salzman, E. W. (1977): Interrelation of prostaglandin endoperoxide (prostaglandin G2) and cyclic 3',5'-adenosine monophosphate in human blood platelets. *Biochim. Biophys. Acta*, 499:48–60.
52. Samuelsson, B. (1979): Oxidation and further transformation of polyunsaturated fatty acids. In: *Advances in Prostaglandin and Thromboxane Research*, edited by B. Samuelsson, P. W. Ramwell, and R. Paoletti. Raven Press, New York.
53. Siegel, M. I., McConnell, R. T., and Cuatracasas, P. (1979): Aspirin-like drugs interfere with arachidonate metabolism by inhibition of the 12-L-hydroperoxy, 5,8,10,14-eicosatetrainoic acid peroxidase pathway. *Proc. Natl. Acad. Sci. USA*, 76:3774–3779.
54. Smith, J. B., and Willis, A. L. (1971): Aspirin selectively inhibits prostaglandin production in human platelets. *Nature (New Biol.)*, 231:235–237.
55. Smolen, J. E., and Weissmann, G. (1980): Effects of indomethacin, 5,8,11,14-eicosatetraenoic acid, and p-promophenacyl bromide on lysosomal enzyme release and superoxide anion generation by human polymorphonuclear leukocytes. *Biochem. Pharmacol.*, 29:533–538.
56. Tainer, J. A., Turner, S. R., and Lynn, W. S. (1975): New aspects of chemotaxis. Specific target-cell attraction by lipid and lipoprotein fractions of *Escherichia coli* chemotactic factor. *Am. J. Pathol.*, 81:401–410.
57. Turner, S. R., Campbell, J. A., and Lynn, W. S. (1975): Polymorphonuclear leukocyte chemotaxis toward oxidized lipid components of cell membranes. *J. Exp. Med.*, 141:1437–1441.
58. Vane, J. R. (1971): Inhibition of prostanglandin synthesis as a mechanism of action for aspirin-like drugs. *Nature (New Biol.)*, 231:232–235.
59. Vane, J. R. (1978): The mode of action of aspirin-like drugs. *Agents Actions*, 8:430–431.
60. Virchow, R. (1882): Quoted in: Ryan, G. B., and Majno, G. (1977): Acute inflammation: A review. *Am. J. Pathol.*, 86:183–276.
61. Wahl, L. M., Olsen, C. E., Sandberg, A. L., and Mergenhagen, S. E. (1977): Prostaglandin regulation of macrophage collagenase production. *Proc. Natl. Acad. Sci. USA*, 74:4955–4958.
62. Weissmann, G., Dukor, P., and Zurier, R. B. (1971): Effect of cyclic AMP on release of lysosomal enzymes from phagocytes. *Nature (New Biol.)*, 231:131–135.
63. Weissmann, G., Korchak, H. M., Perez, H. D., Smolen, J. E., Goldstein, I. M., and Hoffstein, S. T. (1979): Leukocytes as secretory organs of inflammation. In: *Advances in Inflammation Research*, *Vol. 1*, edited by G. Weissmann, R. Paoletti, and B. Samuelsson, pp. 95–111. Raven Press, New York.
64. Weissmann, G., Korchak, H. M., Perez, H. D., Smolen, J. E., Goldstein, I. M., and Hoffstein, S. T. (1979): The secretory code of the neutrophil. *J. Reticuloendothel. Soc.*, 26:687–696.
65. Weissmann, G., Smolen, J. E., and Hoffstein, S. (1978): Polymorphonuclear leukocytes as secretory organs of inflammation. *J. Invest. Dermatol.*, 71:95–99.
66. Weissmann, G., Zurier, R. B., Spieler, P. J., and Goldstein, I. M. (1971): Mechanisms of lysosomal enzyme release from leukocytes exposed to immune complexes and other particles. *J. Exp. Med. (Suppl.)*, 134:149s–165s.
67. Weksler, B. B., Knapp, J. M., and Jaffe, E. A. (1977): Prostacyclin (PGI$_2$) synthesized by cultured endothelial cells modulates polymorphonuclear leukocyte functions. *Blood (Suppl. 1)*, 50:287.
68. Williams, T. J., and Morley, J. (1973): Prostaglandins as potentiators of increased vascular permeability in inflammation. *Nature*, 246:215–217.
69. Williams, T. J., and Peck, M. J. (1977): Role of prostaglandin-mediated vasodilatation in inflammation. *Nature*, 270:530–532.
70. Willis, A. L., and Cornelsen, M. (1973): Repeated injection of prostaglandin E$_2$ in rat paws induces chronic swelling and a marked decrease in pain threshold. *Prostaglandins*, 3:353–357.

71. Ziel, R., and Krupp, P. (1976): Influence of endogenous pyrogen on the cerebral prostaglandin synthetase system. *Experientia*, 32:1451–1452.
72. Zurier, R. B., Hoffstein, S., and Weissmann, G. (1973): Cytochalasin B: Effect on lysosomal enzyme release from human leukocytes. *Proc. Natl. Acad. Sci. USA*, 70:844–848.
73. Zurier, R. B., and Sayadoff, D. M. (1975): Release of prostaglandins from human polymorphonuclear leukocytes. *Inflammation*, 1:93–99.
74. Zurier, R. B., Weissmann, G., Hoffstein, S., Kammerman, S., and Tai, H. -H. (1974): Mechanisms of lysosomal enzyme release from human leukocytes. II. Effects of cAMP and cGMP, automatic agonists, and agents which affect microtubule function. *J. Clin. Invest.*, 53:297–309.

Acetylsalicylic Acid: New Uses for an Old Drug,
edited by H. J. M. Barnett, J. Hirsh, and
J. F. Mustard. Raven Press, New York © 1982.

Prostaglandins: Their Role in Hemostasis and Thrombosis

M. R. Buchanan and J. Hirsh

Department of Pathology, McMaster University, Hamilton, Ontario, Canada L8N 3Z5

Prostaglandin synthesis by platelets, vascular wall cells, and possibly other cells may be important in the regulation of hemostasis and in the pathogenesis of thrombosis. Activation of the prostaglandin synthetic pathway in platelets results in the formation of prostaglandin peroxides PGG_2 and PGH_2, which are then converted to thromboxane A_2 (TXA_2). Thromboxane A_2 induces platelet aggregation and causes vasoconstriction, and the endoperoxides may also contribute to platelet aggregation. Stimulation of the prostaglandin synthetic pathway in the vascular wall (including endothelial cells and smooth muscle cells) results in the synthesis of prostaglandin I_2, a powerful vasodilator and inhibitor of platelet aggregation. Thus, the principal products of prostaglandin synthesis in platelets have opposing actions on platelet aggregation and vessel wall contraction, two phenomena that are of fundamental importance in hemostasis and thrombosis. Prostaglandin synthesis by vascular wall cells and platelets has been investigated in experimental animals and in man by studying the effects of the inhibition of prostaglandin synthesis on hemostasis and thrombosis. Most studies have been performed with acetylsalicylic acid, a drug that irreversibly inactivates the enzyme cyclo-oxygenase and, therefore, inhibits the formation of TXA_2 by platelets and prostaglandin I_2 by vascular wall cells.

Other prostaglandin inhibitors, such as sulfinpyrazone and indomethacin, also inhibit cyclo-oxygenase, and corticosteroids inhibit either the activation or the activity of phospholipase A_2. The effect of acetylsalicylic acid on platelets and vascular wall cells differs, because platelet cyclo-oxygenase is more sensitive to acetylsalicylic acid than cyclo-oxygenase in vascular wall cells and because the effect of acetylsalicylic acid on vessel walls is relatively short-lived (presumably because, being nucleated, these cells can synthesize more of the enzyme), whereas its inhibitory effect on TXA_2 synthesis lasts throughout the life span of the platelet. In experimental animals and man, inhibition of thromboxane production by platelets prolongs the bleeding time and protects against experimental thrombosis induced by vascular wall injury. Results of studies exploring the antithrombotic effects of acetylsalicylic acid in man, although promising, have been less clear-cut. Inhibition of vascular wall PGI_2 production reduces bleeding and augments experimental arterial and venous thrombosis.

The synthesis of prostaglandins by platelets, vascular wall cells, and possibly other cells is thought to be important in the regulation of hemostasis and the

33

pathogenesis of thrombosis. Activation of prostaglandin synthesis in platelets results in the formation of products that aggregate platelets (21,22,27,28,57). In contrast, activation of prostaglandin synthesis in vascular wall cells results in the synthesis of a prostaglandin that inhibits platelet aggregation and causes vasodilatation (25,42). The effects of prostaglandins on hemostasis and thrombosis have been studied by observing (a) their effects on platelet function and vascular contractility *in vitro*; (b) their contribution to platelet aggregation, which is initiated by other aggregating agents such as thrombin and collagen; (c) the effect of infusion of prostaglandins and their products on hemostasis and thrombosis in experimental animals; (d) the effects of manipulating prostaglandin synthesis by drugs or diet in man and experimental animals; (e) the sensitivity of platelets to prostaglandins in thrombotic and hemorrhagic disorders; and (f) measurement of the levels of prostaglandins and their products in experimental atherosclerosis and in clinical disorders known to be associated with atherosclerosis.

IN VITRO STUDIES OF THE EFFECTS OF PROSTAGLANDINS ON PLATELET FUNCTION AND VASCULAR CONTRACTILITY

Platelet Prostaglandin Synthesis

Exposure of platelets to stimuli such as collagen and thrombin results in the activation of phospholipase A_2, which liberates arachidonic acid from membrane phospholipids. Arachidonic acid is asymmetrically distributed in the plasma membrane in human platelets (51) and is located primarily on the inside of the platelet, facilitating its conversion to prostaglandin metabolites. Arachidonic acid is oxidized to the endoperoxides PGG_2 and PGH_2 through an interaction with molecular oxygen that is catalyzed by the enzyme cyclo-oxygenase. PGH_2 is converted to stable prostaglandins PGD_2, PGE_2, and $PGF_{2\alpha}$ and the labile cyclo-ether thromboxane A_2 (TXA_2). TXA_2 has a number of effects on platelet function. It aggregates platelets directly (although this is probably a relatively weak effect), it enhances the effect of ADP on platelet aggregation, and it induces the platelet release reaction (including the release of ADP) and so contributes to platelet aggregation indirectly. PGD_2 inhibits platelet aggregation whereas PGE_2 and $PGF_{2\alpha}$ do not affect platelet function. PGG_2 and PGH_2 also induce platelet aggregation (46). In the platelet, TXA_2 is the major metabolite of prostaglandin synthesis and only small amounts of PGD_2 are formed (48,61). However, it is possible that, at very high concentrations of arachidonic acid, a sufficient amount is converted into PGD_2 to antagonize the platelet-aggregating effect of TXA_2. TXA_2 is very unstable, with a half-life of 3 to 5 min, whereas PGD_2 is relatively stable. Oelz et al. (48) have shown that, with appropriate stimulation, human platelets can produce sufficient amounts of PGD_2 during platelet aggregation to inhibit further aggregation and release. Recently, Linder et al. (37) reported that arachidonic acid stimulated the release of platelet growth factor (PGDF), whereas other fatty acids fail to do this. Interestingly, in this study there was a decrease in the amount of PGDF release with high concentrations of arachidonic acid, possibly as a result of the inhibitory effects of PGD_2.

Platelet Aggregation and Release that Occur Independently of Thromboxane A$_2$

A number of biologically important aggregating agents induce platelet aggregation independently of TXA$_2$ production and so are not inhibited by drugs that inhibit prostaglandin synthesis. Of these, the three most important are ADP, collagen, and thrombin. ADP induces platelet aggregation independently of TXA$_2$, although, when tested *in vitro*, the second wave of aggregation with ADP is associated with prostaglandin synthesis (45). Collagen produces platelet aggregation by at least two independent mechanisms (34). It stimulates prostaglandin (TXA$_2$) synthesis and it induces the release reaction independently of prostaglandin synthesis. At relatively weak concentrations, the aggregating effect of collagen can be accounted for almost entirely by TXA$_2$ production and, therefore, can be inhibited by drugs that inhibit prostaglandin synthesis. However, at higher collagen concentrations, ADP is released independently of TXA$_2$ production and induces aggregation despite inhibition of prostaglandin synthesis.

Thrombin induces platelet aggregation by activating prostaglandin synthesis, by stimulating the platelet release reaction (which occurs independently of prostaglandin synthesis), and by inducing aggregation by a mechanism that is independent of the above two reactions (35).

Thus, inhibitors of prostaglandin synthesis have no effect on primary aggregation by ADP, but only inhibit platelet aggregation induced by a relatively weak concentration of collagen, and have minimal effects on platelet aggregation induced by thrombin.

Prostaglandin Synthesis by Vascular Wall Cells

In contrast with the platelet, vascular wall cells (endothelial cells and smooth muscle cells) produce a prostaglandin, prostaglandin I$_2$ (PGI$_2$), that inhibits platelet aggregation and, therefore, has the potential of interfering with thrombosis and hemostasis (25,42). PGI$_2$ inhibits platelet shape change and pseudopod formation. It is also a powerful inhibitor of platelet aggregation and induces smooth muscle relaxation and, therefore, produces vasodilatation. PGI$_2$ is a more powerful inhibitor of platelet aggregation than PGE$_1$ or PGD$_2$ (42). Its effect on platelet adhesion is controversial. PGI$_2$ has been shown to inhibit platelet adhesion in a number of experimental models but at concentrations considerably higher than those required to inhibit platelet aggregation. Cazenave et al. (8) reported that PGI$_2$ did not completely prevent adhesion of ^{14}C-labeled platelets and ^{51}Cr-labeled platelets to collagen -coated or de-endothelialized aortic surfaces *in vitro*. Weiss and Turitto (64) reported that PGI$_2$ (10 nanamoles) inhibits platelet adhesion onto an everted de-endothelialized rabbit aorta in an annular perfusion chamber system with flow conditions equivalent to arterial flow. However, PGI$_2$ had no inhibitory effect on adhesion at shear stresses that simulated flow conditions in veins or capillaries. It is possible, therefore, that the effect of PGI$_2$ on adhesion is indirect and that it acts by preventing shape change and pseudopod formation which in turn reduces the capacity of platelets to effectively sustain adhesion to a de-endothelialized vessel wall at high rates of shear. The role of PGI_2 in preventing platelet adhesion to intact endothelium is uncertain. It has been suggested that plasma contains sufficient quantities of PGI_2 to prevent platelets from adhering to normal intact endothelium (18,24,26,43). However, there is considerable doubt that platelets ever adhere to intact endothelium.

It has been reported that platelets exposed to thrombin adhere to cultured endothelium cells when their synthesis of PGI_2 is inhibited by acetylsalicylic acid (13). However, it is possible that these experimental observations represent an inhibitory effect of PGI_2 on thrombin-induced platelet aggregation. Curwen et al. (12) studied the effects of platelet adhesion to normal cultured endothelial cells and to transformed endothelial cells (simian virus 40-treated) that do not produce PGI_2. More platelets adhered to the transformed cells than to normal cells. However, when both cell types were treated by acetylsalicylic acid to inhibit PGI_2 production by the normal cells, platelet adhesion to the normal cells was not altered, suggesting that PGI_2 may not be important in preventing platelet adhesion to endothelial cells.

Initially, it was suggested that endothelial cells were the major source of PGI_2 production by the vascular wall (26,43). However, it has since been demonstrated that cultured smooth muscle cells and fibroblasts also synthesize PGI_2. Quantitative studies indicate that endothelial cells produce about 10 times more PGI_2 than smooth muscle cells, which in turn produce more than four times the amount of PGI_2 produced by fibroblasts (1,5,56,65). Since smooth muscle cells are present in larger numbers than endothelial cells, the contribution of smooth muscle cells to PGI_2 production in the vessel wall could be considerable.

Metabolism of Prostaglandins

PGE_1, PGE_2, PGF_2, and TXA_2 are rapidly metabolized in the lung (18). In contrast, PGI_2 is not cleared from blood after passage through the lung (24). Wong et al. (66) and Dusting et al. (18) demonstrated that, after a single passage through the lung, less than 20% of the PGI_2 is metabolized.

There is controversy about whether or not PGI_2 circulates in plasma at concentrations sufficient to inhibit platelet adherence, aggregation, or release. Moncada et al. (43) have demonstrated the existence of circulating PGI_2-like activity; however, Haslam and McClenaghan (29), using a more sensitive system, failed to demonstrate this. McIntyre and associates, using a PGI_2 antibody, took citrated blood samples from volunteers and measured PGI_2-like activity within 3 min of collection (62). Concerning the amount of PGI_2 detected by bioassay, they were unable to detect differences between the blood samples collected into antibody and those collected into non-antibody containing anticoagulant. They concluded that the circulation did not contain sufficient PGI_2 to inhibit platelet aggregation.

Mechanism of Action of Prostaglandins on Platelet Aggregation

Prostaglandins that inhibit platelet aggregation (e.g., PGI_2 and PGD_2) activate adenylate cyclase and, therefore, raise platelet cyclic AMP levels. In contrast, prostaglandin products such as TXA_2, which induce or augment platelet aggregation, lower platelet cyclic AMP levels (28). Elevated levels of cyclic AMP inhibit platelet aggregation, possibly by reducing the mobility of cytoplasmic calcium by stimulating the cyclic AMP-dependent calcium pump.

Platelets have specific binding sites for PGD_2 that are separate from the platelet binding sites of PGE_2 and PGF_2 (41,54). Cooper (10) reported that the ability of PGD_2 to stimulate adenylate cyclase activity was decreased in a group of patients with acute thrombosis. In these patients, the platelet release reaction was not inhibited by PGD_2 while inhibition was obtained with PGI_2 and PGE_2, and these prostaglandins also increased adenylate cyclase activity.

Effects of Infusion of Prostaglandins into Experimental Animals

Silver et al. (58) reported that an intravenous infusion of arachidonic acid into rabbit ear veins produced sudden death which was associated with occlusion of the pulmonary microcirculation with platelet aggregates. Similarly, Furlow and Bass (23) demonstrated that the injection of arachidonic acid into the cerebral vascular system of rats produced occlusion of the cerebral microcirculation with platelet aggregates.

The effect of arachidonic acid infusions on the blood pressure of experimental animals is influenced by the relative amounts of thromboxane A_2 and PGI_2 formed. The intravenous injection of PGI_2 decreases systemic and pulmonary arterial blood pressure. Mullane et al. (44) reported that, in dogs, arachidonic acid infusion was associated with a fall in pulmonary arterial blood pressure whereas Kadowitz et al. (32) reported that the injection of arachidonic acid resulted in an increase in systemic vascular resistance.

EFFECTS OF MANIPULATING PROSTAGLANDIN SYNTHESIS BY DIET AND DRUGS

Diet

Arachidonic acid is the only fatty acid that is converted into TXA_2. Other fatty acids, such as eicosapentanoic acid (EAEA) and α-linoleic acid, are converted to TXA_3 (47,52). Unlike TXA_2, TXA_3 does not induce aggregation. Dyerberg and associates (19,20) suggested that the essential fatty acid composition of plasma and tissues might influence platelet function and thrombosis through their effects on thromboxane synthesis. These investigators reported that Eskimos in Greenland have a higher ratio of EAEA to arachidonic acid in their tissues than Europeans, and suggested that this might be responsible for the low incidence of myocardial infarction seen in Eskimos. Nordoy (47) fed rats linoleic acid and α-linoleic acid. Linoleic acid is converted to arachidonic acid and is, therefore, a substrate for TXA_2, whereas α-linoleic acid is a substrate for TXA_3. Rats fed α-linoleic acids produce PGI_3, which has an inhibitory activity on platelet aggregation similar to that of PGI_2. It is possible, therefore, to regulate the prostaglandin synthetic pathway by altering the fatty acid content of diet and so potentially to influence thrombo-genesis.

Other investigators have demonstrated that the production of PGI_2 by blood vessels is modified by feeding animals an atherogenic diet. Sinzinger et al. (60) reported that PGI_2 production was reduced in guinea pigs by a diet that induced hypercholesterolemia and atherosclerosis. They also noted that hypercholestero-lemic animals were able to generate significantly more PGI_2 from their pulmonary arteries than from their thoracic and abdominal aortas, and speculated that this might explain in part the distribution of diet-induced atherosclerosis. Dembinska-Kiec and associates (15,16) also demonstrated that isolated heart preparations from animals fed an atherosclerotic diet generated reduced amounts of PGI_2.

Drugs

The importance of TXA_2 and PGI_2 in hemostasis and thrombosis has also been studied by inhibiting their synthesis with drugs that selectively block certain steps in the prostaglandin synthetic pathway. Drugs that have been used include acetyl-salicylic acid, indomethacin, sulfinpyrazone, corticosteroids, and tranylcypromine. Acetylsalicylic acid, indomethacin, and sulfinpyrazone block the oxidation of ar-achidonic acid to the endoperoxide PGG_2 by inhibiting the enzyme cyclo-oxygenase. The inhibition of cyclo-oxygenase by acetylsalicylic acid is irreversible, whereas its inhibition by indomethacin and sulfinpyrazone is reversible. Indomethacin also has other effects on the prostaglandin synthetic pathway.

The effect of corticosteroids on prostaglandin synthesis has not been fully elu-cidated. There is evidence that corticosteroids inhibit the cleavage of arachidonic acid from membrane phospholipid of vascular wall cells by interfering with enzyme phospholipase A_2 (9) but corticosteroids do not inhibit platelet prostaglandin syn-thesis. Tranylcypromine inhibits the conversion of PGH_2 to PGI_2 (25), although its effect is not entirely specific. A number of newly described drugs inhibit the conversion of PGH_2 to TXA_2 in the platelet, but their effects on hemostasis and thrombosis have not been tested in the experimental animals.

There are quantitative differences in the effect of acetylsalicylic acid on pros-taglandin synthesis in platelets and vascular wall cells. These have been studied by using microsomal fractions obtained from platelets and vascular wall cells, by using cultured endothelial cells and comparing them with platelets, by comparing whole vessel-wall preparations with platelets, and by inhibiting either thromboxane pro-duction or PGI_2 production *in vivo* and studying the effects of this on experimental models of hemostasis and thrombosis.

The initial studies using subcellular fractions of platelets and vascular wall cells concluded that cyclo-oxygenase in platelets was many times more sensitive to inhibition by acetylsalicylic acid than cyclo-oxygenase of vascular wall cells, sug-gesting that a large dosage differential exists between inhibition of TXA_2 and PGI_2 by acetylsalicylic acid (7,53).

Using cultured endothelial cells, Jaffe and Weksler (30) reported that acetylsalicylic acid inhibited PGI_2 and TXA_2 formation at similar concentrations but that, in contrast to platelets, the effect on vascular wall cells was short-lived. Hoak and his group (13) also reported that the inhibitory effect of acetylsalicylic acid on PGI_2-like activity in cultured vascular wall cells was short-lived.

Using whole-vessel segments, Buchanan et al. (5,6) reported that the inhibitory effect of acetylsalicylic acid on PGI_2 formation was relatively short-lived in jugular veins of rabbits but lasted for up to 20 hr in carotid arteries of rabbits. Villa and associates (63) reported a similar prolonged inhibitory effect of acetylsalicylic acid on PGI_2 production in the rat. Buchanan et al. (6) also demonstrated that, in arteries, doses of acetylsalicylic acid of 10 mg/kg were sufficient to inhibit PGI_2 formation and to augment the adhesion of platelets to damaged cell endothelium.

A number of investigators have demonstrated that acetylsalicylic acid is thrombogenic when used in high doses. Kelton et al. (33) reported that high doses of acetylsalicylic acid (200 mg/kg) given to rabbits inhibited PGI_2 synthesis in jugular veins and that this was associated with enhanced fibrin deposition onto the injured veins. This thrombogenic effect was short-lived. Baumgartner (2) quantitated platelet adhesion and aggregation on the subendothelium of everted vessel wall segments in an annular perfusion chamber, using citrated flowing blood. Platelet adherence and aggregation was neither augmented nor inhibited by pre-treating either the platelets or the vessel wall with acetylsalicylic acid, suggesting that the roles of PGI_2 and TXA_2 were relatively unimportant in platelet adhesion. In contrast, Czervionke and associates (13) reported that thrombin-induced platelet aggregates adhere more readily to cultured endothelial cells that have been pre-treated with acetylsalicylic acid than to normal endothelial cells. Cazenave and associates (8) reported that PGI_2 inhibits platelet adhesion and the platelet release reaction to de-endothelialized aorta only in high concentrations that are unlikely to be achieved physiologically. They also demonstrated that pre-treatment of platelets with acetylsalicylic acid did not modify their adhesion to damaged aorta, suggesting that TXA_2 is not necessary for the platelet adhesion reaction (14). Zimmerman et al. (67) also found that acetylsalicylic acid in high doses enhances experimentally induced thrombosis in both arteries and veins, but reported that the thrombogenic effects of acetylsalicylic acid were not maintained when a second large dose (100 mg/kg) was given 12 hr after the first. The mechanism and significance of this interesting observation are uncertain.

Blajchman et al. (3) and Buchanan et al. (4) have examined the effects on bleeding of inhibiting vascular wall PGI_2 production in experimental animals. Both hydrocortisone and acetylsalicylic acid in doses that inhibit vascular wall PGI_2 production shorten the bleeding time in thrombocytopenic animals. These observations are consistent with the hypothesis that hydrocortisone and acetylsalicylic acid produce this effect by inhibiting PGI_2 formation and that the shortening of the bleeding time was due to a sustained vasoconstriction after vessel injury due to inhibition of the vasodilatory properties of PGI_2.

ABNORMAL PROSTAGLANDIN SYNTHESIS IN CLINICAL AND EXPERIMENTAL STATES

Deficiencies in platelet cyclo-oxygenase and TXA_2 and in platelet arachidonic acid metabolism have been reported in patients with mild hemorrhagic disorders (36,38). Altered arachidonic metabolism has also been found in platelets of patients with myeloproliferative disorders (50,55). Cooper (10) reported that the capacity of PGD_2 to stimulate adenylate cyclase activity was decreased in patients with acute thrombosis and suggested that there may be an association between the two phenomena. Cooper and associates (11) also demonstrated reduced sensitivity of PGD_2 in patients with myeloproliferative disorders.

Sinzinger et al. (59) measured PGI_2 production by fibrous plaques and fatty streaks obtained from human subjects and found that PGI_2 formation was decreased relative to normal controls. Dollery et al. (17) reported that the level of 6-oxo-PGF_1 was lower than normal in circulating plasma in six nondiabetic patients with proliferative vascular disease. Similar results were also seen in male diabetics with proliferative retinopathy. They suggested that the thromboembolic disorders associated with both the diabetic and nondiabetic patients in this study were a direct result of decreased PGI_2 production.

Other investigators have demonstrated that PGI_2 formation is reduced in experimental atherosclerotic lesions produced by dietary manipulation (47,60).

EFFECT OF ACETYLSALICYLIC ACID ON THE BLEEDING TIME

It is well recognized that acetylsalicylic acid, in therapeutic doses, prolongs the bleeding time in humans and that this effect may last for a number of days (39,40). The results of studies of the effects of high doses of acetylsalicylic acid on the bleeding time have been conflicting. O'Grady and Moncada (49) reported that, while low doses of acetylsalicylic acid prolonged the bleeding time, high doses had no effect, suggesting that this was due to inhibition of PGI_2 formation. Others have failed to demonstrate a dose-related effect in humans. Jorgensen et al. (31) reported that low doses of acetylsalicylic acid (1 mg/kg) prolonged the bleeding time in human volunteers between 18 and 70 years of age, whereas high doses (20 mg/kg) significantly decreased it in older patients.

REFERENCES

1. Baenziger, N. L., Becherer, P. R., and Majerus, P. W. (1979): Characterization of prostacyclin synthesis in cultured human arterial smooth muscle cells, venous endothelial cells and skin fibroblasts. *Cell*, 16:967–974.
2. Baumgartner, H. R. (1979): Effects of acetylsalicylic acid, sulfinpyrazone and dipyridamole on platelet adhesion and aggregation in flowing native and anticoagulated blood. *Haematosas.*, 8:340–352.
3. Blajchman, M. A., Senyi, A. F., Hirsh, J., Surya, Y., Buchanan, M., and Mustard, J. F. (1979): Shortening of the bleeding time in rabbits by hydrocortisone caused by inhibition of prostacyclin generation by the vessel wall. *J. Clin. Invest.*, 63:1026–1035.
4. Buchanan, M. R., Blajchman, M. A., Dejana, E., Mustard, J. F., Senyi, A. F., and Hirsh, J. (1979): Shortening of the bleeding time in thrombocytopenic rabbits after exposure of jugular vein to high aspirin concentrations. *Prostaglandins Med.*, 13:333–342.

5. Buchanan, M. R., Dejana, E., Cazenave, J. -P., Mustard, J. F., and Hirsh, J. (1979): PGI₂ production and effect of aspirin on endothelial and non-endothelial cells of the vessel wall. *Thromb. Haemost.*, 42:156.

6. Buchanan, M. R., Dejana, E., Mustard, J. F., and Hirsh, J. (1979): Prolonged inhibition of PGI₂ production and associated increased thrombogenic effect in arteries after aspirin administration. *Thromb. Haemost.*, 42:61.

7. Burch, J. W., Baenziger, N. L., Stanford, N., and Majerus, P. W. (1978): Sensitivity to fatty acid cyclo-oxygenase from human aorta to acetylation by aspirin. *Proc. Natl. Acad. Sci. USA*, 75:5181–5184.

8. Cazenave, J. -P., Dejana, E., Kinlough-Rathbone, R., Richardson, M., Packham, M. A., and Mustard, J. F. (1979): Prostaglandins I₂ and E₁ reduce rabbit and human platelet adherence without inhibiting serotonin release from adherent platelets. *Thromb. Res.*, 15:273–279.

9. Chandrabose, K. A., Lapetina, E. G., Schmitzer, C. J., Siegel, M. I., and Cuatrecasas, P. (1978): Action of corticosteroids in regulation of prostaglandin biosynthesis in cultured fibroblasts. *Proc. Natl. Acad. Sci. USA*, 75:214–217.

10. Cooper, B. (1979): Diminished platelet adenylate cyclase activation by prostaglandin D₂ in acute thrombosis. *Blood*, 54:684–693.

11. Cooper, B., Schafer, A. I., Puchalsky, D., and Haudin, R. I. (1978): Platelet resistance to prostaglandin D₂ in patients with myelo-proliferative disorders. *Blood*, 52:618–626.

12. Curwen, K. D., Gimbrone, M. A., and Hardin, R. I. (1980): In vitro studies of thromboresistance: The role of prostacyclin (PGI₂) in platelet adhesion to cultured normal and virally transformed human vascular endothelial cells. *Lab. Invest.*, 42:366–374.

13. Czervionke, R. L., Hoak, J. C., and Fry, G. L. (1978): Effect of aspirin on thrombin-induced adherence of platelets to cultured cells from blood vessel wall. *J. Clin. Invest.*, 62:847–856.

14. Dejana, E., Cazenave, J. -P., Groves, H. M., Kinlough-Rathbone, R. L., Richardson, M., Packham, M. A., and Mustard, J. F. (1980): The effect of aspirin inhibition of PGI₂ production on platelet adherence to normal and damaged rabbit aortae. *Thromb. Res.*, 17:453–464.

15. Dembinska-Kiec, A., Gryglewska, T., Zmuda, A., and Gryglewski, R. S. (1977): The generation of prostacyclin by arteries and by the coronary vascular bed is reduced in experimental atherosclerosis in rabbits. *Prostaglandins*, 14:1025–1034.

16. Dembinska-Kiec, A., Rucker, W., and Schonhofer, P. S. (1979): Effects of dipyridamole in experimental atherosclerosis. Action on PGI₂ platelet aggregation and atherosclerotic plaque formation. *Atherosclerosis*, 33:315–327.

17. Dollery, C. T., Friedman, L. A., Hensby, C. N., Kohner, E., Lewis, P. J., Porta, M., and Webster, J. (1979): Circulating prostacyclin may be reduced in diabetes (letter). *Lancet*, ii:1365.

18. Dusting, G. J., Moncada, S., and Vane, J. R. (1978): Recirculation of prostacyclin (PGI₂) in the dog. *Br. J. Pharmacol.*, 64:315–320.

19. Dyerberg, J., Bang, H. O., and Hjorne, N. (1975): Fatty acid composition of the plasma lipids in Greenland Eskimos. *Am. J. Clin. Nutr.*, 28:958–966.

20. Dyerberg, J., Bang, H. O., Stoffersen, E., Moncada, S., and Vane, J. R. (1978): Eicosapenaenoic acid and prevention of thrombosis and atherosclerosis. *Lancet*, ii:117–118.

21. Ellis, E. F., Oelz, O., Roberts, I. I., Payne, N., and Oates, J. (1976): Coronary arterial smooth muscle cell concentration by a substance released from platelets: Evidence that it is thromboxane A₂. *Science*, 193:1135–1137.

22. Furlow, T. W., and Bass, N. H. (1975): Stroke in rats produced by carotid injection of sodium arachidonate. *Science*, 187:658–660.

23. Furlow, T. W., and Bass, N. H. (1976): Arachidonate induced cerebrovascular occlusion in the rat. The role of platelets and aspirin in stroke. *Neurology*, 26:297–304.

24. Gryglewski, R. J. (1979): Prostacyclin as a circulatory hormone. *Biochem. Pharmacol.*, 28:3161–3166.

25. Gryglewski, R. J., Bunting, S., Moncada, S., Flower, R. J., and Vane, J. R. (1976): Arterial walls are protected against deposition of platelet thrombi by a substance (prostaglandin X) which they make from prostaglandin endoperoxides. *Prostaglandins*, 12:685–708.

26. Gryglewski, R. J., Korbut, R., Ocetkiewicz, A., Splawinski, J., Wojtaszek, B., and Swies, J. (1978): Lungs as a generator of prostacyclin—hypothesis on physiological significance. *Arch. Pharmacol.*, 304:45–50.

27. Hamberg, M., Svensson, J., and Samuelsson, B. (1974): Prostaglandin endoperoxides. A new concept concerning the mode of action and release of prostaglandins. *Proc. Natl. Acad. Sci. USA*, 71:3824–3828.

28. Hamberg, M., Svensson, J., and Samuelsson, B. (1975): Thromboxanes: A new group of biologically active compounds derived from prostaglandin endoperoxides. *Proc. Natl. Acad. Sci. USA*, 74:2994–2998.
29. Haslam, R. J., and McClenaghan, M. D. (1979): An assay for activators of platelet adenylate cyclase present in rabbit blood: Evidence that prostacyclin (PGI_2) is not a circulating hormone. (Poster presentations P6-080). *Thromb. Haemost.*, 42:117.
30. Jaffe, E. A., and Weksler, B. B. (1979): Recovery of endothelial cell prostacyclin production after inhibition by low dose aspirin. *J. Clin. Invest.*, 63:532–535.
31. Jorgensen, K. A., Olesen, A. S., Dyerberg, J., and Stoffersen, E. (1979): Aspirin and bleeding-time: Dependency of age (letter). *Lancet*, ii:302.
32. Kadowitz, P. J., Chapnick, B. M., Feigen, L. P., Hyman, A. L., Nelson, P. K., and Spannhake, E. W. (1978): Pulmonary and systemic vasodilator effects of the newly discovered prostaglandin, PGI_2. *J. Appl. Physiol.*, 45:408–413.
33. Kelton, J. G., Hirsh, J., Carter, C. J., and Buchanan, M. R. (1978): Thrombogenic effect of high dose aspirin in rabbits. Relationship to inhibition of vessel wall synthesis of prostaglandin I_2-like activity. *J. Clin. Invest.*, 62:892–895.
34. Kinlough-Rathbone, R. L., Mustard, J. F., Packham, M. A., Perry, D. W., Reimers, H. J., and Cazenave, J. -P. (1977): Properties of washed human platelets. *Thromb. Haemost.*, 37:291–308.
35. Kinlough-Rathbone, R. L., Perry, D. W., Packham, M. A., and Mustard, J. F. (1977): Pathways of thrombin-induced aggregation and release with human and rabbit platelets. *Thromb. Haemost.*, 38:124.
36. Lagarde, M., Byron, P. A., Vargaftig, B. B., and DeChevanne, M. (1979): Impairment of platelet thromboxane A_2 generation and of the platelet release reaction in two patients with a congenital deficiency of platelet cyclo-oxygenase. *Br. J. Haematol.*, 38:251–266.
37. Linder, B. L., Chernoff, A., Kaplan, K. L., and Goodman, D. S. (1979): Release of platelet-derived growth factor from human platelets by arachidonic acid. *Proc. Natl. Acad. Sci. USA*, 76:4107–4111.
38. Malmsten, C., Hamberg, M., Svensson, J., and Samuelsson, B. (1975): Physiological role of endoperoxides in human platelets: Hemostatic defect due to platelet cyclo-oxygenase deficiency. *Proc. Natl. Acad. Sci. USA*, 72:1446–1450.
39. Mielke, C. H., Kaneshiro, M. M., Maher, A., Werner, J. M., and Rapaport, S. I. (1969): The standardized normal Ivy bleeding time and its prolongation by aspirin. *Blood*, 34:204–215.
40. Mielke, C. H., Ramos, J. C., and Britton, A. F. H. (1973): Aspirin as an anti-platelet agent. Template bleeding time as a monitor of therapy. *Am. J. Clin. Pathol.*, 59:236–242.
41. Miller, O. V., and Gorman, R. R. (1979): Evidence for distinct prostaglandin I_2 and D_2 receptors in human platelets. *J. Pharmacol. Exp. Ther.*, 210:134–140.
42. Moncada, S., Herman, A. G., Higgs, E. A., and Vane, J. R. (1977): Differential formation of prostacyclin (PGX or PGI_2) by layers of the arterial wall. An explanation for the antithrombotic properties of vascular endothelium. *Thromb. Res.*, 11:323–344.
43. Moncada, S., Korbut, R., Bunting, S., and Vane, J. R. (1978): Prostacyclin is a circulating hormone. *Nature*, 273:767–768.
44. Mullane, K. M., Dusting, G. J., Salmen, J. A., Moncada, S., and Vane, J. R. (1979): Biotransformation and cardiovascular effects of arachidonic acid in the dog. *Eur. J. Pharmacol.*, 54:217–228.
45. Mustard, J. F., Perry, D. W., Kinlough-Rathbone, R. L., and Packham, M. A. (1975): Factors responsible for ADP-induced release reaction of human platelets. *Am. J. Physiol.*, 228:1757–1765.
46. Needleman, P., Wyche, A., and Raz, A. (1979): Platelet and blood vessel arachidonate metabolism and interaction. *J. Lab. Invest.*, 63:345–349.
47. Nordoy, A. (1979): Albumin-bound fatty acids, platelets and endothelial cells in thrombogenesis. *Haematosas.*, 8:193–202.
48. Oelz, O., Oelz, R., Knapp, H. R., Sweetnam, B. S., and Oates, J. A. (1978): Biosynthesis of prostaglandin D_2. 1. Formation of prostaglandin D_2 by human platelets. *Prostaglandins*, 12:225–234.
49. O'Grady, J., and Moncada, S. (1978): Aspirin: A paradoxical effect on bleeding time (letter). *Lancet*, ii:780.
50. Okuma, M., and Uchino, H. (1979): Altered arachidonic metabolism by platelets in patients with myeloproliferative disorders. *Blood*, 54:1258–1271.
51. Perret, B., Chap, H. J., and Douste-Blazy, L. (1979): Asymmetric distribution of arachidonic acid in the plasma membrane of human platelets. *Biochim. Biophys. Acta*, 556:434–446.

52. Raz, A., Minkes, M. S., and Needleman, P. (1977): Endoperoxides and thromboxanes structural determinants for platelet aggregation and vasoconstriction. *Biochim. Biophys. Acta*, 488:305–311.
53. Roth, G. J., and Majerus, P. W. (1975): The mechanism of the effect of aspirin on human platelets. 1. Acetylation of a particulate fraction protein. *J. Clin. Invest.*, 56:624–632.
54. Schafer, A. I., Cooper, B., O'Hara, D., and Hardin, R. I. (1979): Identification of platelet receptors for prostaglandin I_2 and D_2. *J. Biol. Chem.*, 254:2914–2917.
55. Siegel, M. I., McConnell, R. T., and Cuatrecasas, P. (1979): Aspirin-like drugs interfere with arachidonate metabolism by inhibition of the 12-hydroperoxy-5,8,10,14-eicosatetraenoic acid peroxidase activity of the lipoxygenase pathway. *Proc. Natl. Acad. Sci. USA*, 76:3774–3778.
56. Silberbauer, K., Sinzinger, H., and Winter, M. (1978): Prostacyclin production by vascular smooth muscle cells. *Lancet*, 2:1356.
57. Silver, M. J., Hoch, W., Kocsis, J. J., Ingerman, C. M., and Smith, J. B. (1974): Inhibition of PGE_1-stimulated cAMP accumulation in human platelets by thromboxane A_2. *Science*, 183:1085–1087
58. Silver, M. J., Hoch, W., Kocsis, J. J., Ingerman, C. M., and Smith, J. B. (1974): Arachidonic acid causes sudden death in rabbits. *Science*, 183:1085–1086.
59. Sinzinger, H., Silberbauer, K., Feigl, W., Wagner, O., Winter, M., and Auerswald, W. (1979): Prostacyclin activity is diminished in different types of morphologically controlled human atherosclerotic lesions. *Thromb. Haemost.*, 42:803–804.
60. Sinzinger, H., Silberbauer, K., Winter, M., and Clopath, P. (1979): Effects of experimental atherosclerosis on prostacyclin (PGI_2) generation in arteries of miniature swine. *Artery*, 5:448–462.
61. Smith, J. B., Silver, M. J., Ingerman, C. M., and Kocsis, J. J. (1974): Prostaglandin D_2 inhibits the aggregation of human platelets. *Thromb. Res.*, 5:291–299.
62. Steer, M. L., McIntyre, D. E., Levine, L., and Salzman, E. W. (1980): Is prostacyclin a physiologically important circulating anti-platelet agent? *Nature*, 283:194–195.
63. Villa, S., and de Gaetano, G. (1977): Prostacyclin-like activity in rat vascular tissues. Fast, long-lasting inhibition by treatment with lysine acetyl-salicylate. *Prostaglandins*, 14:1117–1126.
64. Weiss, H. J., and Turitto, V. T. (1979): Prostacyclin (prostaglandin I_2) inhibits platelet adhesion and thrombus formation on subendothelium. *Blood*, 53:244–250.
65. Weksler, B. B., Ley, C. W., and Jaffe, E. A. (1978): Stimulation of endothelial cell prostacyclin production by thrombin, trypsin and the ionophore A23187. *J. Clin. Invest.*, 62:923–930.
66. Wong, P. Y. -K., McGiff, J. C., Sun, F. F., and Malik, K. U. (1978): Pulmonary metabolism of prostacyclin (PGI_2) in the rabbit. *Biochem. Biophys. Res. Commun.*, 83:731–738.
67. Zimmerman, R., Thiessen, M., Morl, H., and Weckesser, G. (1979): The paradoxical thrombogenic effect of aspirin in experimental thrombosis. *Thromb. Res.*, 16:843–846.

Acetylsalicylic Acid: New Uses for an Old Drug,
edited by H. J. M. Barnett, J. Hirsh, and
J. F. Mustard. Raven Press, New York © 1982.

DISCUSSION

J. Hirsh: Dr. Weissmann, is there some obvious explanation of how the nonsteroidal anti-inflammatory drugs influence inflammation?

G. Weissmann: At present, each of our arthritis clinics has 110 to 120 patients with salicylate blood levels in the therapeutic range of 15 to 25 mg/dl. These patients are able to mount appropriate inflammatory responses to almost any stimulus they might encounter. They seem to have relatively little impairment of their clotting system, and the primary effect of treatment is on the inflammatory response in an affected joint, which is inflamed by some mechanism such as the one we use *in vitro* (immune complexes).

Articular erosion proceeds as in patients who are not treated with such high doses and this implies that the metabolites of arachidonic acid that have formed in the cyclo-oxygenase pathway, and have been held responsible for inflammation in man, contribute only modestly to this process—certainly to the inflammation we see in arthritis. These metabolites can produce effects as demonstrated in the laboratory, in that they enhance inflammation induced by other stimuli, but may not of themselves be the primary agents.

Paul Reilly: Does anyone know anything about the receptors through which prostaglandins mediate their cellular action? It is assumed that they probably act through receptors, because they work in the molar concentrations pharmacologically appropriate for receptor-type action.

Weissmann: The neutrophil has demonstrable receptors for stable prostaglandins of the "E" and "F" series and has prostacyclin receptors. These have not been isolated. As you know, the characteristics of a receptor are those of specificity, saturability, and appropriate affinity. These have been demonstrated for the stable prostaglandins and partially for prostacyclin and PGI_2. As Mälmsten and Goldstein have shown in our laboratory, the neutrophil ignores thromboxane for some reason: It does not have a thromboxane receptor. I do not know whether we can talk about hydroperoxyeicosatetraenoic acid receptors. The fact that cells respond to hydroxy and hydroperoxy fatty acids does not necessarily mean that they have a receptor. At the present time, only stable prostaglandin receptors have been identified in the neutrophil.

J. F. Mustard: It is essentially the same for the platelet. Receptors for PGI_2 and PGD_2 have been identified, but characterization is a long way from complete. Receptors for very unstable substances are difficult to study, but one can speculate that there are a variety of receptors. Indeed, such a variety would explain some of the differences we find in different tissues. Concerning cyclo-oxygenase and the action of acetylsalicylic acid, do we have any information about the turnover of cyclo-oxygenase in white blood cells? Do we have evidence concerning the duration of the acetylation effect in polymorphonuclear leukocytes and monocytes? This might have an important bearing on the duration of action of drugs and some of the reactions we have discussed.

Weissmann: Unless there is work from Charles Parker's laboratory that has not been published, I am not aware of any data on the half-life of cyclo-oxygenase inhibition in the neutrophil.

Mustard: Is there any evidence for the macrophage or about the prostaglandin pathway in the monocyte?

Weissmann: Philip Davies at Rahway has worked out the duration of inhibition. However, the monocyte and the macrophage are potent protein-synthesizing cells, whereas the neutrophil synthesizes only about three proteins avidly. They make plasminogen activator, a

45

pyrogen, and as we have recently demonstrated, fibrinectin. I do not think they synthesize cyclo-oxygenase. The neutrophil should be more like the platelet, but we have no direct evidence on this point. Monocyte data indicate only that they can regenerate cyclo-oxygenase.

F. Rosenberg: Both acetylsalicylic acid and sodium salicylate have been described as anti-inflammatory substances. Could Dr. Weissmann expand his comments on the differences between these two, in their action on the prostaglandin pathways? How might these relate to their inhibition of inflammation?

Weissmann: Ever since the "Vane hypothesis" about the action of acetylsalicylic acid in the early 1970s, the one exception has always been sodium salicylate—a drug once used quite frequently in the rheumatic diseases. Most investigators believe that sodium salicylate is not effective as a cyclo-oxygenase inhibitor, although it is an effective anti-inflammatory agent. It is not a very good antipyretic. We have only two pieces of evidence to explain this difference. First, according to Gryglewski, there is a differential susceptibility of brain cyclo-oxygenase to sodium salicylate and acetylsalicylic acid. Second, Cuatracasas indicates that sodium salicylate inhibits the peroxidase involved in taking 12-hydroperoxyeicosatetraenoic acid to 12-HETE. It shares this property with ASA and indomethacin.

Rosenberg: What is the relationship of the prostaglandins to lymphocyte stimulation and the inhibition of lymphocyte maturation by a variety of mitogens, as induced by the salicylates?

Weissmann: In 1969 and 1970, Rochelle Hirschhorn in our laboratories showed that any agent for which the lymphocyte has a receptor and stimulation of which raises its cyclic AMP will turn off or inhibit lymphocyte transformation. Thus, β-adrenergic agents, cholera enterotoxin and prostaglandins of the E and F series will inhibit transformation induced by appropriate plant lectins and mixed lymphocyte reactions. The story is much the same for the monocyte. All of the circulating cells of inflammation seem to be turned off by raising intracellular levels of cyclic AMP. There is controversy in the literature concerning agents that affect cyclic GMP. Most of the data, with respect to its action as an endogenous mediator of lymphocyte or leukocyte activation, are extremely questionable and some have been withdrawn. But the data are clear. Lymphocyte transformation is inhibited by stable prostaglandin such as PGE_2 or anything else that will raise intracellular cyclic AMP. Do you believe that salicylates turn on lymphocytes?

Rosenberg: Not that they turn them on, but they have been noted to turn them off. When ASA is given in anti-inflammatory doses producing blood salicylate levels in the 15 to 20 mg/dl range, lymphocytes from these patients were found to be resistant to phytohemagglutinin, pokeweed antigen, and a variety of other substances.

Weissmann: That work dates from the early and mid-1960s and the diminution was not particularly impressive. Parker's group, using inhibitors of both the cyclo-oxygenase and lipoxygenase pathways, has shown inhibition of lymphocyte transformation induced by various ligands, and that inhibition is related to the intracellular role of arachidonic acid metabolites in triggering. It is a very complicated story. There is good evidence that in a number of secretory and transformed cell types, products of the arachidonic acid cascade, formed by one or other of the pathways, are involved in mobilization of intracellular calcium. One of the problems with extrapolating from experiments in which high doses of salicylate are given, such as in humans with therapeutic levels of salicylate, is that the level of ionizable calcium in serum is enhanced by the modest metabolic acidosis. This is also true intracellularly. Metabolic changes secondary to the acidosis may influence lymphocyte function, and some of the effects on lymphocyte mitogenesis induced by drugs probably reflect changes in intracellular calcium as well as in cyclic AMP.

J. W. D. McDonald: Dr. Weissmann, could you comment on the relative concentrations of nonsteroidal anti-inflammatory drugs required to inhibit reactions other than those related to cyclo-oxygenase? Do these tend to be considerably higher than those required to inhibit cyclo-oxygenase?

Also, you showed that phenylbutazone specifically inhibited one of the reactions in the HPETE-HETE series, but did not show it as a cyclo-oxygenase inhibitor. Do you believe that this agent is really so specific?

Weissmann: Concerning the concentration of nonsteroidal anti-inflammatory agents, especially indomethacin, required to inhibit phospholipase relative to the cyclo-oxygenase, in the neutrophil there is only about a one log-order difference. Neutrophil cyclo-oxygenase is inhibited at about 10^{-6} M and phospholipase at 10^{-5} M. In monocytes, as Davies has shown, cyclo-oxygenase is inhibited by indomethacin at about 10^{-8} M. It is clear that the cyclo-oxygenase pathway is much more sensitive than the other pathways. This is not true for Cuatracasas' claims with respect to the HPETE-HETE transformation. The only reason I showed phenylbutazone in the hydroperoxy to the hydroxy fatty acid conversion of the lipoxygenase pathway was because it had previously been shown that the same oxygen-derived free radical is derived during the transformation of the endoperoxide, the 15-hydroxy-hydroperoxy-endoperoxide—the PGG_2 to PGH_2 transformation. This is the step at which Fred Kuehl, also at Rahway, believes phenylbutazone really acts. In other words, it is probably as inhibitory, if not even more inhibitory, to intermediate products of cyclo-oxygenase as to products of lipoxygenase. However, he believes that its major function is that of a free-radical scavenger, as with MK 447, which is the model compound in this regard.

McDonald: You showed data on the production of thromboxanes by leukocytes and, I believe, referred to it as "large amounts." How large are these in terms of picograms? Can you relate them, for example, to thromboxane formed in animal models where neutrophils are involved, and come up with a relationship that indicates the neutrophil might be the source?

Weissmann: Charles Parker's laboratory in St. Louis has indicated that thromboxane B_2 is a minor product of stimulated neutrophils, as we have found. The bulk of the products are stable prostaglandins. I would say that no more than 5–10% of arachidonate goes to thromboxane, relative to the 5-HPETEs, with the dihydroxy- and leukotrienes on the one hand and stable prostaglandins on the other. The neutrophil may make prostacyclin, but I am not certain that it is not due to mononuclear cells in the preparation. So you are correct in suggesting that the neutrophil is not a major source of thromboxane. The platelet is a far richer source.

W. R. Soller: Have clinical or laboratory conditions been described wherein the neutrophil receptors, and perhaps the platelet receptors, show phenomena akin to super- or subsensitivity? I am thinking of a situation analogous to dopamine-sensitive adenylate cyclase, and the super- and subsensitivity phenomena that have been shown in the brain.

Weissmann: First, there is no "up or down" regulation with respect to the neutrophil receptor. The neutrophil is a poorly synthetic cell and lives in the circulation for no more than about 6 hr. Hence, it does not need to generate new receptors. Second, maneuvers that enhance membrane fluidity will enhance coupling, and so you will not have supersensitivity, but enhanced or more tightly coupled receptor cyclase action. This results in enormous bursts of cyclic AMP from a stimulus which, without previously enhanced membrane fluidity, would have given only modest increments. And that is consistent with the Axelrod model for a number of systems. We have been through most of his "drills" in the neutrophil, and they correlate closely. If we give a ligand for which there is a receptor on the neutrophil, such as a chemotactic peptide, immunoglobulin, or complement, the neutrophil will respond by showing enhanced membrane fluidity. Following this, receptor cyclase coupling is significantly enhanced. To my knowledge, this is the only direct experiment that bears on your question.

E. Salzman: For the record, I would like to amplify Dr. Mustard's comment about Bartter's syndrome. You will remember that this is characterized by the increased urinary excretion of prostaglandins, particularly the E prostaglandins and prostaglandin 6-keto-$PGF_{1\alpha}$, and that this increase can be reduced by nonsteroidal anti-inflammatory agents. We found that there is a defect in platelet function in this syndrome, which is marked by an abnormality in both the first and second phases of platelet aggregation. This is associated with an increase in the platelet content of cyclic AMP. Some circulating plasma component seems to induce this defect in platelet function and this can be demonstrated by mixing the patient's plasma with normal platelets and vice versa. The plasma factor does not seem to be any of the conventional stable prostaglandins.

If one adds to the fresh, platelet-rich plasma of a patient with Bartter's syndrome an antibody that will neutralize the effects of PGI_2 (prostacyclin), it immediately corrects the defect in platelet function. The effect of this plasma factor can also be eliminated by treatment of the patient with indomethacin or other nonsteroidal anti-inflammatory agents. We do not think the circulating plasma factor is prostacyclin, because it is stable for hours on the bench at physiologic pH. It is probably a metabolite of prostacyclin or some other prostacyclin-like substance.

Mustard: I want to ask Dr. Weissmann to leave us with a clear message about the action of prostaglandins on the polymorphs. If I understand it correctly, he believes that although they can form thromboxane A_2, there is no evidence that thromboxane A_2 itself has an effect on them, but that prostaglandins, for which they have a receptor that increases cyclic AMP levels, will shut off their ability to secrete. Is that correct?

Weissmann: Absolutely correct.

Mustard: What about their ability to aggregate?

Weissmann: Neutrophil aggregation is less readily quantified. Several investigators have tested neutrophil suspensions in platelet aggregometers and the results are much the same for chemotaxis and secretion. Neutrophil aggregation is inhibited by agents that raise cyclic AMP levels.

Acetylsalicylic Acid: New Uses for an Old Drug,
edited by H. J. M. Barnett, J. Hirsh, and
J. F. Mustard. Raven Press, New York © 1982.

Pharmacokinetics of Salicylates

Jake James Thiessen

Faculty of Pharmacy, University of Toronto, Toronto, Ontario, Canada

Although acetylsalicylic acid (ASA) has been in use since the end of the 19th century, its fate in man was not elucidated until the last decade, and some aspects of its metabolism still remain unresolved. In the body, acetylsalicylic acid is rapidly hydrolyzed to salicylic acid (SA) by ubiquitous esterases. SA is removed from the body by five parallel and competing pathways: renal excretion; conjugation with glycine to form two glucuronides, SAG and SPG, and hydroxylation to yield salicyluric acid (SU); and conjugation of the carboxyl or hydroxyl group to form gentisic acid (GA). The biologic half-life of acetylsalicylic acid in man is only 15 to 20 min following an intravenous or rapidly absorbed oral preparation, whereas the apparent half-life of SA varies from 2.4 to 19 hr, because of two easily saturable SA biotransformation pathways. Acetylsalicylic acid must be prescribed with care, since the therapeutic concentration range of SA is quite narrow and a small change in dose may have a pronounced effect on steady-state blood drug levels.

Numerous past and present reports of drug levels in biologic fluids following acetylsalicylic acid administration, purporting to describe acetylsalicylic acid absorption and bioavailability, have employed analytical techniques that measure "total salicylate." These nonspecific procedures determine an assorted composite or total sum of acetylsalicylic acid, SA, SU, SAG, SPG, and GA. Consequently, there is little specific information on a particular salicylate, such as the presence of intact acetylsalicylic acid blood levels following administration of a selected product. Nevertheless, it is known that although acetylsalicylic acid is absorbed from the stomach after oral administration, the major site is in the upper portion of the small intestine. When a rapidly absorbed oral acetylsalicylic acid preparation is compared with an intravenous dose, it is found that about 30% of the oral dose is hydrolyzed to SA before systemic distribution. The acetylsalicylic acid in compressed tablets is generally all absorbed (as acetylsalicylic acid or SA), but the absorption of enteric-coated tablets may be delayed, slow, and/or incomplete. The observed absorption of rectal acetylsalicylic acid has been slow and the amount absorbed dependent on the time between insertion and defecation. On the basis of current knowledge, it is important that specific analytical methods be used to describe acetylsalicylic acid absorption, distribution, and elimination, thereby delineating more clearly the relationship between vascular or tissue levels and response.

The group of drugs known as the salicylates have in common the 2-hydroxybenzoate radical. They are drugs of great antiquity, having played a prominent role in herbal therapy. During the past century, the most important have been sodium salicylate, the methyl ester and amide of salicylic acid, and acetylsalicylic acid (Fig. 1). In this presentation I will not discuss salicylates other than acetylsalicylic acid, except where it will complete the pharmacokinetic profile of acetylsalicylic acid. The discipline of pharmacokinetics continues to explore quantitatively the metabolic fate and resultant actions of acetylsalicylic acid when administered in various dosage forms. The discussion will focus on (a) selected physical and chemical properties of acetylsalicylic acid, (b) its metabolic fate, (c) its pharmacokinetic profile, (d) methods for its chemical analysis, and (e) observations made after administering it in various dosage forms.

PHYSICAL AND CHEMICAL PROPERTIES OF ACETYLSALICYLIC ACID

Acetylsalicylic acid, a weak acid (pKa 3.5), exists primarily as the anion in the blood or body tissues. The aqueous solubility of acetylsalicylic acid increases with increased pH. At pH 2.25 its solubility is reported to be 3.4 g/liter, whereas at pH 7 it is 8220 g/liter (14). The instability of acetylsalicylic acid even in the powder state is evident when a bottle of tablets is opened. The odor is that of acetic acid, a product of hydrolysis caused by moist air. Edwards (10), investigating its aqueous hydrolysis at 17°C, found acetylsalicylic acid most stable at a pH close to 2.5, and saturated aqueous solutions exhibited such a pH. Increased hydrolysis was observed at pH values less than or greater than 2.5, becoming particularly exaggerated at a pH greater than 9. Thus, care must be taken in the preparation and use of acetyl-salicylic acid solutions. One would expect that a freshly prepared solution at pH

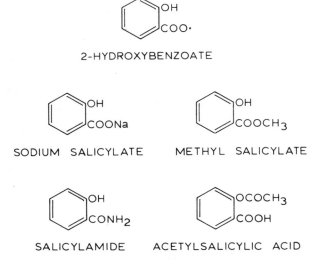

FIG. 1. Historically important salicylates.

7.4, stored at 17°C, would exhibit 10% hydrolysis to salicylic acid after 1 day, or less than 2% if stored for only 4 hr.

The acid- and base-catalyzed hydrolysis of acetylsalicylic acid can be explained by standard chemical mechanisms. The base-related process involves nucleophilic attack by OH⁻ A similar initial challenge by proteins accounts for the rapid hydrolysis of acetylsalicylic acid in the body (Fig. 2).

Metabolic Fate of Salicylates

In the body, acetylsalicylic acid is rapidly converted to salicylic acid, and its half-life is only 15 to 20 min (33). This hydrolysis is primarily a consequence of ubiquitous, perhaps nonspecific esterases found in many tissues. These proteins in turn may become acetylated, and it is this phenomenon that is purported to inactivate key enzymes such as prostaglandin synthetase (31). It is important to recognize, however, that many proteins are capable of being acetylated by acetylsalicylic acid (17,28,40). From a practical viewpoint, it is useful to compare the stability of acetylsalicylic acid in various biological fluids. The degradation half-lives at 37°C, relative to a buffer, are compared in Table 1 (16,34). These results demonstrate that gastrointestinal fluids contribute minimally to the degradation of acetylsalicylic acid during the rapid dissolution and absorption of acetylsalicylic acid from compressed tablets. However, during the absorption process, esterase activity in the membranes of the gastrointestinal tract (GIT) (19,37) leads to considerable hydrolysis of acetylsalicylic acid. The comparative activity of esterase in various segments of the GIT in man has been qualitatively examined and it has been demonstrated that it is greatest in the mucosal cells of the fundus of the stomach (9), whereas only moderate activity is found in the mucosal cells of the jejunum, ileum, and colon. Work in rabbits has shown that tissue (4 g) from the stomach,

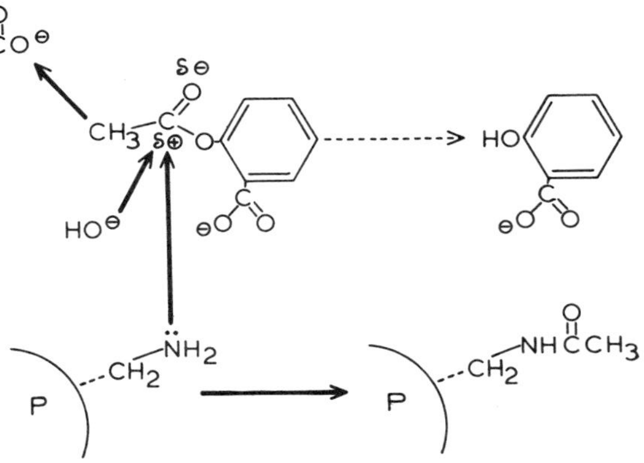

FIG. 2. A scheme depicting base-catalyzed hydrolysis of ASA to yield acetate and salicylate, or nucleophilic attack of ASA by a protein resulting in its acetylation accompanied by the liberation of salicylate.

TABLE 1. *Hydrolysis half-life of ASA at 37°C in various biological fluids compared with that in a pH 7.4 buffer*

Fluid	Initial ASA concentration (μg/ml)	ASA half-life (hr)
Krebs-Ringer bicarbonate	10	15.5
Human gastric	10	16
Human duodenal	10	17
Human blood[a]	13	0.5
Human plasma[a]	13	1.9

[a]Heparinized, diluted 9:10 (v/v) with saline.
Data from refs. 16, 34.

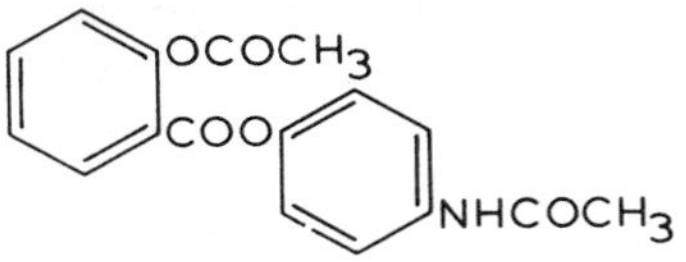

BENORYLATE

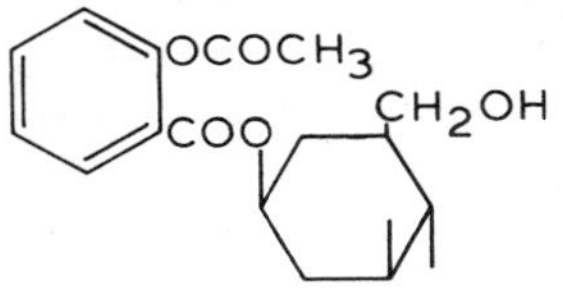

FIG. 3. Prodrugs of ASA synthesized to date. (From refs. 18,30.)

1-(2'-ACETOXYBENZOYL)-
2-DEOXY-ᗡ-D-GLUCOPYRANOSE

duodenum, middle ileum, lower ileum, and ascending colon will hydrolyze 11%, 39%, 38%, 29%, and 4% of acetylsalicylic acid, respectively, within 1 hr at 37°C (34). There appear to be clinically significant sex- and age-related differences in acetylsalicylic acid esterase activity in various tissues, because it has been observed that the blood of neonates, children, and adults exhibits different activity and the erythrocytes of adult females are less active than those of males (42).

Investigators have sought to take advantage of physiologic esterase activity by synthesizing "prodrugs" that would be hydrolyzed to acetylsalicylic acid after absorption and thus perhaps circumvent damage to the GIT (18,30). Two examples of such efforts are seen in Fig. 3. Benorylate, which is not available in Canada, is reported to produce less GIT blood loss than acetylsalicylic acid (8). A clinical evaluation of the glucopyranose analogue is currently not available.

Salicylic acid (SA) is removed from the body by five parallel and competing pathways (Fig. 4): renal excretion, conjugation with glycine to yield salicyluric acid (SU), conjugation of the carboxyl or phenolic group to form two glucuronides (SAG and SPG, respectively), and hydroxylation to form gentisic acid (GA). Two of these processes, the formation of SU and SPG, proceed by easily saturable Michaelis-Menten kinetics, whereas the others exhibit first-order kinetics (21,25). Because the V_{max} values of these processes are about 60 and 30 mg/hr, respectively, the steady-state amount of SA in the body increases more proportionately with increasing dose rates (24). For example, an increase in the daily acetylsalicylic acid dose from 2 to 4 g (as four divided doses per day) will raise the plateau level of salicylate in the body from 1.3 to 5.3 g, a fourfold increase. Also, the length of time required to reach the steady-state will increase as the daily dose is increased.

It is clear from the literature that pronounced intersubject differences are found in steady-state plasma or serum salicylate concentrations, even in normal subjects receiving the same daily dose of acetylsalicylic acid; these differences have been reviewed by Levy (22). With respect to the metabolic fate of SA, the V_{max} values may be genetically determined. Renal elimination of unchanged SA is exquisitely sensitive to urinary pH (36); as the pH is raised from 5 to 8, the amount of SA excreted increases more than twentyfold. This phenomenon has profound implications when doses approaching saturation of SU and SPG are ingested, and is a boon in the detoxification of patients overdosed with acetylsalicylic acid. It is also evident that excessive self-administration of antacids may lead to important plasma salicylate fluctuations in patients for whom large daily doses of acetylsalicylic acid are prescribed. Finally, a recent report has suggested that intrasubject variability

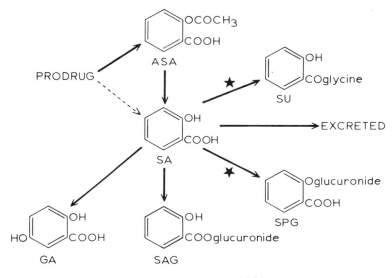

FIG. 4. Metabolic fate of ASA.

in the elimination of salicylate may be due to an induction of a metabolic pathway such as SU formation (35).

Pharmacokinetics of Acetylsalicylic Acid and Salicylic Acid

Rowland and Riegelman (33) provided the first definitive description of the compartmentalized pharmacokinetics of acetylsalicylic acid and SA based on plasma levels in man. Table 2 summarizes the pertinent mean parameters obtained after administering 650 mg or less of either agent intravenously. The fraction of each salicylate bound to plasma proteins (f_b) applies to total concentrations less than 10 mg/liter. SA is distributed in and is eliminated from the body more slowly than acetylsalicylic acid, and is more extensively bound to plasma proteins. It is important to recognize that, because of the rapid hydrolysis of acetylsalicylic acid to SA, the plasma acetylsalicylic acid levels are virtually nonexistent 90 min after intravenous acetylsalicylic acid. The "slow" elimination (low total body clearance) of SA is attributed to its high degree of plasma protein binding; i. e., excretion and metabolism are rate-limited by the unbound plasma concentration.

In the previous section it was noted that the amount of SA in the body increases disproportionately with the dose of acetylsalicylic acid. However, changes in plasma SA concentration with dose are complicated by the limited capacity of plasma proteins to bind SA. Thus the decreased plasma protein binding at increasing doses offsets the nonlinear SA elimination, so that the total body dose clearance of SA (based on total plasma levels) remains largely unchanged, and consequently the total plasma SA levels do not increase disproportionately in the manner anticipated (13). Yet, although total plasma SA levels are nearly directly related to the dosing rate, the unbound plasma SA levels increase disproportionately (11,13). By inference, unbound plasma SA levels should be monitored during high-dose chronic acetylsalicylic acid therapy, since they may influence the appearance of toxicity signs.

TABLE 2. *Summary of mean pharmacokinetic parameters obtained for acetylsalicylic acid and salicylic acid after administering 650 mg of each salicylate intravenously on separate occasions*

Pharmacokinetic parameter	Salicylate	
	ASA	SA
$t_{1/2}\alpha$ (min)	2.7	3.8
$t_{1/2}\beta$ (min)	14.9	238
V_p (1)	6.6	5.5
$V_{d_{ss}}$ (1)	11.3	9.4
TBC (ml/min)	680	27
f_b	~0.7	~0.9

The fraction bound to plasma proteins (f_b) applies to total concentrations less than 10 mg/liters.

When high-dose acetylsalicylic acid therapy is terminated, the apparent SA half-life will appear much longer than that stated in Table 1, because of the capacity-limited metabolic pathways. It may take as long as 10 days to reach steady-state conditions after high-dose acetylsalicylic acid administration is initiated.

Chemical Analysis of "Salicylates"

It is evident from Fig. 4 that plasma total salicylate should include the sum of all the molecules displayed. The same would be true for urine, although acetylsalicylic acid would not be present, since it is not excreted by the kidney.

Most laboratories that measure plasma, serum, or urinary salicylates use an adaptation of Trinder's method (38), which employs the chelation of iron by salicylic acid or its analogues to yield a colored complex whose absorbance is measured at 540 nm. This method is fraught with error, particularly when the salicylate levels are low. First, blanks from salicylate-free patients may give high (up to 50 μg/ml) and variably false salicylate values (6,38). Second, the reaction with salicyluric acid is poor. Third, the Trinder's reagent fails to react with acetylsalicylic acid and the glucuronide metabolites of SA (7). Consequently, to measure total salicylates, biological fluids must be hydrolyzed to convert all salicylates to SA before complexation. To quantitate specifically the urinary SA and individual metabolites, elaborate differential techniques have been developed (23).

The analysis of plasma acetylsalicylic acid has presented special challenges, and various methods, employing gas chromatography (41), gas chromatography/spectrofluorometry (32), or high-pressure liquid chromatography (1,27) have been developed. Of these, only the latter method avoids the use of "difference calculations" based on analysis before and after hydrolysis to ascertain the presence of acetylsalicylic acid, or the use of a derivatization procedure to quantitate the salicylates.

Considerable care must be taken in the collection and processing of biological fluids containing acetylsalicylic acid. Because of the rapid hydrolysis of acetylsalicylic acid in blood, samples should be collected with fluoride, the plasma harvested immediately, and the samples frozen quickly (32). Analysis should be completed as soon as possible, since acetylsalicylic acid stored even on dry ice has a hydrolysis half-life of 23.5 days (41).

Acetylsalicylic Acid Dosage Forms

In Canada, various tablets (compressed, effervescent, enteric-coated, sustained release), capsules, suppositories, and gum contain acetylsalicylic acid. It may be present as the only pharmacologically active ingredient or as one of a number of such ingredients. A commercial parenteral product is not available, but acetylsalicylic acid has been administered intravenously as the lysine (39) or N-methylglucamine salt (33). On the basis of information about solubility and stability (10,14), it is possible to prepare a satisfactory intravenous solution (pH 7.4) of the intact compound.

The importance of assessing vascular intact acetylsalicylic acid levels was not recognized until recently; earlier analytical efforts were directed primarily at SA or total salicylate. However, the situation has changed, and a literature search makes it obvious that there are few reports describing plasma acetylsalicylic acid levels after administration of the various products.

Before discussing available information, it may be helpful to consider several important criteria for evaluating product performance. Using the pharmacokinetic data established for acetylsalicylic acid and SA (33,34), it is possible to simulate plasma acetylsalicylic acid and SA levels after intravenous or oral acetylsalicylic acid (Fig. 5). The exhibited profiles would be those anticipated for intravenous (A), rapidly absorbing (B), and slowly absorbing (C) preparations. In generating the theoretical levels, it has been assumed that only about 70% of the oral dose reaches the systemic circulation as intact acetylsalicylic acid, the balance entering it as SA. The performance of different products can be assessed by comparing their maximum levels (C_{max}), the time needed to reach the maximum levels (t_{max}), or the area under the concentration (AUC) versus time profile, from time of administration until the drug completely disappears from the body. While this information is generally compiled for the administered intact drug, the comparison could be based on metabolite levels, provided all kinetic processes are first-order. On the basis of theoretical constraints, the oral products (B and C) would exhibit the same extent of intact acetylsalicylic acid absorption (identical acetylsalicylic acid AUC), but their C_{max} and t_{max} values would differ notably. Both products, however, would fail to deliver the acetylsalicylic acid equivalent of the intravenous product (acetylsalicylic acid AUCs for B and C are 70% of A), whereas the total salicylate absorbed would be equivalent to intravenous acetylsalicylic acid (SA AUCs for A, B, and C are identical). A short t_{max} is required if a rapid onset of action is desired. A further principle illustrated by the theoretical profiles is that the observed acetylsalicylic acid or SA half-life after the administration of a single dose of a product may not be as described earlier, but may reflect absorption rate limitations (product C). Generally, slow or delayed absorption will reduce the C_{max} and increase the t_{max}, and suggest a longer half-life for acetylsalicylic acid. Riegelman (29) observed this when he compared various acetylsalicylic acid preparations, as did Koch et al. (20) when they investigated the influence of food and fluid on acetylsalicylic acid bioavailability.

Alternatively, the performance of various products can be established by quantitating the recoverable urinary total salicylates (Fig. 4), since absorbed salicylate (acetylsalicylic acid or SA) can be recovered as the moieties displayed. Although it assesses the extent of absorption of total salicylate, this method fails to provide information about the presence of intact acetylsalicylic acid in the circulation.

Oral acetylsalicylic acid, when dissolved, is rapidly absorbed along the upper GI tract. The extent of a dose absorbed by the stomach or duodenum depends on gastric emptying and solubility of acetylsalicylic acid in the appropriate fluid. Enteric-coated products, which are designed to remain undissolved in the gastric fluid but release their contents in the intestinal fluid, are prone to erratic behavior.

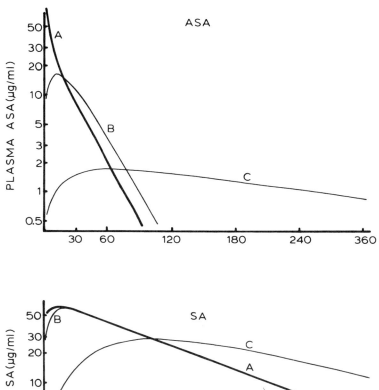

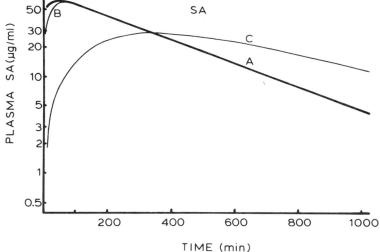

FIG. 5. A simulation of anticipated plasma ASA and SA levels following the administration of 650 mg intravenous ASA **(A)**, rapidly absorbed oral ASA **(B)**, or slowly absorbed oral ASA **(C)**. On the basis of published reports (33,34), common parameters used for the three preparations are as follows: ASA: V_1 = 6.6L, k_{21} = 0.119 min^{-1}, α = 0.24 min^{-1}, β = 0.047 min^{-1}. SA: V_1 = 5.5L, k_{21} = 0.11 min^{-1}, α = 0.19 min^{-1}, β = 0.0028 min^{-1}. Rate constant for conversion of ASA$_1$ to SA$_1$ = 0.103 min^{-1}. For the oral preparations the fraction of ASA reaching the systemic circulation intact (F) is 0.70; the remainder of the dose enters it as SA. The absorption rate constants (k_a) for ASA and SA are assumed to be identical, being 0.069 and 0.003 min^{-1} for preparations B and C, respectively.

Blythe et al. (3) have illustrated that some of these products may remain intact in the stomach up to 7 hr or longer after ingestion because they settle into the fundic portion, where there is little mixing or other motion. It has been suggested that enteric-coated products could be made statistically more reliable if they were formulated as enteric-coated granules. Bogentoft et al. (4) have demonstrated that such a preparation exhibits consistent absorption characteristics that are not influenced by food ingestion.

The number of products in Canada that contain acetylsalicylic acid is overwhelming (Tables 3 and 4). Often there is no information about their performance,

TABLE 3. *Summary of ASA –containing preparations available in Canada as compiled in the Canadian Drug Identification Code*

Number of products	Form	Total number of active ingredients	ASA content (mg)
39	TAB	1	81–15,600
25	EC TAB	1	300–975
1	SR TAB	1	650
5	SUPP	1	160–650
2	GUM	1	225
4	CAP	2	285–325
43	TAB	2	75–650
8	CAP	3	375–375
43	TAB	3	80–486
1	SR TAB	3	375
1	PDR	3	750
2	CAP	4	330
11	TAB	4	195–390
1	TAB	5	500
1	TAB	6	325
1	EFF TAB	6	330
1	TAB	7	225
189			

From ref. 5.

TABLE 4. *Over-the-counter (OTC) ASA–containing preparations available in Canada*

Number of products	Active ingredients	ASA content (mg)	Route
87	Single	75–975	Oral
6	Single	75–650	Rectal
209	Multiple	12.5–750	—
302			

From ref. 12.

and any that is supplied rarely describes intact circulating acetylsalicylic acid levels. Several of these limited reports were cited earlier (20,29,34,39), but some additional data are worthy of note. Riegelman, comparing the performance of buffered and unbuffered acetylsalicylic acid, observed a similar C_{max} but a prolonged t_{max} with unbuffered acetylsalicylic acid, indicative of slower absorption perhaps via delayed gastric emptying (29). Biggs et al. (2) measured plasma acetylsalicylic acid levels after administration of Aspirin®, Bufferin®, Ecotrin®, Entrophen®, and Novasen® as a 1.95 g dose to four subjects on separate occasions. In general, the three brands of enteric-coated acetylsalicylic acid yielded lower C_{max} and prolonged t_{max} values in agreement with the theoretical considerations presented earlier. Although one subject failed to exhibit measurable plasma acetylsalicylic acid levels with one of the products, their apparent absence may have been due to the blood sampling schedule. Finally, it is interesting to examine the performance of rectal acetylsalicylic acid products. Thus far I have found no reports describing circulating intact acetylsalicylic acid levels following their insertion. Nevertheless, it has been observed in children and adults that the absorption of drug (based on urinary excretion rate of total salicylate) is exceedingly slow and the amount absorbed is highly dependent upon the rectal retention time (time between insertion and defecation) (15,26).

CONCLUSIONS

This chapter has presented a number of salient features of the pharmacokinetics of salicylates. Despite the voluminous information available on acetylsalicylic acid and SA, several aspects are worthy of further research:

(a) The development of a specific and even more sensitive analytic procedure for acetylsalicylic acid.

(b) An evaluation of the relationship between plasma acetylsalicylic acid levels or the integral of such levels over time (an estimate of the amount of acetylsalicylic acid presented to the systemic circulation) and the effect. Such a comparison would be enlightening, since the effect of acetylsalicylic acid may be mediated by an irreversible acetylation in which equilibration considerations no longer apply.

(c) An evaluation of plasma acetylsalicylic acid levels achieved by the use of rectal preparations.

REFERENCES

1. Ali, M., McDonald, J. W. D., Thiessen, J. J., and Coates, P. E. (1980): Plasma acetylsalicylate and salicylate and platelet cyclooxygenase activity following plain and enteric-coated aspirin. *Stroke*, 2:9–13.
2. Biggs, D. F., Coutts, R. T., and Walter, L. J. (1977): A note on the bioavailability of five Canadian brands of acetylsalicylic acid. *Can. J. Pharm. Sci.*, 12:23–25.
3. Blythe, R. H., Grass, G. M., and MacDonnell, D. R. (1959): The formulation and evaluation of enteric coated aspirin tablets. *Am. J. Pharmacol.*, 131:206–216.
4. Bogentoft, C., Carlsson, I., Ekenved, G., and Magnusson, A. (1978): Influence of food on the absorption of acetylsalicylic acid from enteric coated dosage forms. *Eur. J. Clin. Pharmacol.*, 14:351–355.

5. Canadian Drug Identification Code, Section IV, 6th edit. Health and Welfare Canada, Ottawa, 1979.
6. Chiou, W. L., and Onyemelukwe, I. (1973): Possible errors and role of mercuric chloride in using Trinder's reagent for assay of salicylates in urine samples. *J. Pharm. Sci.*, 62:1742–1743.
7. Chiou, W. L., and Onyemeluke, I. (1974): Simple modified colorimetric method for total salicylate assay in urine after salicylate administration. *J. Pharm. Sci.*, 63:630–632.
8. Croft, D. N., Cuddigan, J.H. P., and Sweetland, C. (1972): Gastric bleeding and benorylate, a new aspirin. *Br. Med. J.*, 3:545–547.
9. Dawson, I., and Pryse-Davies, J. (1963): The distribution of certain enzyme systems in the normal human gastrointestinal tract. *Gastroenterology*, 44:745–760.
10. Edwards, L. J. (1950): The hydrolysis of aspirin. *Trans. Faraday Soc.*, 46:723–735.
11. Ekstrand, R., Alvan, G., and Borga, O. (1979): Concentration dependent plasma protein binding of salicylate in rheumatoid patients. *Clin. Pharmacokinet.*, 4:137–143.
12. Expert Committee on O.T.C. Analgesics, HPB, Ottawa, Canada.
13. Furst, D. E., Tozer, T. N., and Melmon, K. L. (1979): Salicylate clearance, the resultant of protein binding and metabolism. *Clin. Pharmacol. Ther.*, 26:380–389.
14. Garrett, E. R. (1957): Prediction of stability in pharmaceutical preparations. IV. The interdependence of solubility and rate in saturated solutions of acylsalicylates. *J. Am. Pharm. Assoc. Sci.*, 46:584–586.
15. Gibaldi, M., and Grundhofer, B. (1975): Bioavailability of aspirin from commercial suppositories. *J. Pharm. Sci.*, 64:1064–1066.
16. Harris, P. A., and Riegelman, S. (1967): Acetylsalicylic acid hydrolysis in human blood and plasma. I. Methodology and *in vitro* studies. *J. Pharm. Sci.*, 56:713–716.
17. Hawkins, D., Pinckard, R. N., and Farr, R. S. (1968): Acetylation of human serum albumin by acetylsalicylic acid. *Science*, 160:780–781.
18. Hussain, A., Truelove, J., and Kostenbauder, H. (1979): Kinetics and mechanism of hydrolysis of 1-(2'-acetoxybenzoyl)-2-deoxy-α-D glucopyranone, a novel aspirin prodrug. *J. Pharm. Sci.*, 68:299–301.
19. Inoue, M., Morikawa, M., Tsuboi, M., and Suajura, M. (1979): Hydrolysis of ester-type drugs by the purified esterase from human intestinal mucosa. *Jpn. J. Pharmacol.*, 29:17–25.
20. Koch, P. A., Schultz, C. A., Wills, R. J., Hallqvist, S. L., and Welling, P. G. (1978): Influence of food and fluid ingestion on aspirin bioavailability. *J. Pharm. Sci.*, 67:1533–1535.
21. Levy, G. (1965): Pharmacokinetics of salicylate elimination in man. *J. Pharm. Sci.*, 54:959–967.
22. Levy, G. (1979): Pharmacokinetics of salicylate in man. *Drug Metab. Rev.*, 9:3–19.
23. Levy, G., and Procknal, J. A. (1968): Drug biotransformation in man. I. Mutual inhibition in glucuronide formation of salicylic acid and salicylamide in man. *J. Pharm. Sci.*, 57:1330–1335.
24. Levy, G., and Tsuchiya, T. (1972): Salicylate accumulation kinetics in man. *N. Engl. J. Med.*, 287:430–432.
25. Levy, G., Tsuchiya, T., and Amsel, L. P. (1972): Limited capacity for salicyl phenolic glucuronide formation and its effect on the kinetics of salicylate elimination in man. *Clin. Pharmacol. Ther.*, 13:258–268.
26. Novak, M. M., Grundhofer, B., and Gibaldi, M. (1974): Rectal absorption from aspirin suppositories in children and adults. *Pediatrics*, 54:23–26.
27. Peng, G. W., Gadalla, A. F., Smith, V., Peng, A., and Chiou, W. L. (1978): Simple and rapid high-pressure liquid chromatographic simultaneous determination of aspirin, salicylic acid, and salicyluric acid in plasma. *J. Pharm. Sci.*, 67:710–712.
28. Pinckard, R. N., Hawkins, D., and Farr, R. S. (1968): In vitro acetylation of plasma proteins, enzymes and DNA by aspirin. *Nature*, 219:68–69.
29. Riegelman, S. (1971): The kinetic disposition of aspirin in the human. In: *Aspirin, Platelets and Stroke*, edited by W. S. Fields and W. K. Hass, pp. 105–114. Warren H. Green, St. Louis.
30. Robertson, A., Glynn, J. P., and Watson, A. K. (1972): The absorption and metabolism in man of 4-acetamidophenyl-2-acetoxybenzoate (Benorylate). *Xenobiotica*, 2:339–347.
31. Roth, G. J., and Chester, J. S. (1978): Acetylation of the NH2-terminal serine of prostaglandin synthetase by aspirin. *J. Biol. Chem.*, 253:3782–3784.
32. Rowland, M., and Riegelman, S. (1968): Determination of acetylsalicylic acid and salicylic acid in plasma. *J. Pharm. Sci.*, 56:717–720.
33. Rowland, M., and Riegelman, S. (1968): Pharmacokinetics of acetylsalicylic acid and salicylic acid after intravenous administration in man. *J. Pharm. Sci.*, 57:1313–1319.

34. Rowland, M., Riegelman, S., Harris, P. A., and Sholkoff, S. D. (1972): Absorption kinetics of aspirin in man following oral administration of an aqueous solution. *J. Pharm. Sci.*, 61:379–385.
35. Rumble, R. H., Brooks, P. M., and Roberts, M. S. (1980): Metabolism of salicylate during chronic aspirin therapy. *Br. J. Clin. Pharmacol.*, 9:41–45.
36. Smith, P. K., Gleason, H. L., Stoll, C. G., and Ogorzalek, S. (1946): Studies on the pharmacology of salicylates. *J. Pharmacol.*, 87:237–255.
37. Spenney, J. G. (1978): Acetylsalicylic acid hydrolase of gastric mucosa. *Am. J. Physiol.*, 234:606–610.
38. Trinder, P. (1954): Rapid determination of salicylate in biological fluids. *Biochem. J.*, 57:301–303.
39. van Voss, H., Göbel, U., Petrich, C., and Pütter, J. (1978): Pharmacokinetic investigations in adult humans after parenteral administration of the lysine salt of acetylsalicylic acid (authors' translation). *Klin. Wochenschr.*, 56:1119–1123.
40. Walker, J. E. (1976): Lysine residue 199 of human serum albumin is modified by acetylsalicylic acid. *FEBS Lett.*, 66:173–175.
41. Walter, L. J., Biggs, D. F., and Coutts, R. T. (1974): Simultaneous GLC estimation of salicylic acid and aspirin in plasma. *J. Pharm. Sci.*, 63:1754–1758.
42. Windorfer, A., Jr., Kuenzer, W., and Urbanêk, R. (1974): The influence of age on the activity of acetylsalicylic acid esterase and protein salicylate binding. *Eur. J. Pharmacol.*, 7:227–231.

Acetylsalicylic Acid: New Uses for an Old Drug,
edited by H.J.M. Barnett, J. Hirsh, and
J.F. Mustard. Raven Press, New York © 1982.

Mode of Action of Acetylsalicylic Acid

Marian A. Packham

*Department of Biochemistry, Faculty of Medicine, University of Toronto, Ontario,
Canada M5S1A8; and Department of Pathology, McMaster University, Hamilton, Ontario*

In addition to its inhibition of the synthesis of prostaglandins and related compounds, acetylsalicylic acid has other effects on cells. Some of these are caused by sodium salicylate, which is a weak inhibitor of cyclo-oxygenase but a strong anti-inflammatory agent. The stimulation of platelets or vessel walls activates phospholipases, which free arachidonate from membrane phospholipids. Arachidonate is converted by cyclo-oxygenase to the prostaglandin endoperoxides PGG_2 and PGH_2, which give rise to thromboxane A_2 (TXA_2) in platelets and to prostacyclin (PGI_2) in vessel walls. TXA_2 induces platelet aggregation and the release of platelet granule contents, whereas PGI_2 is a potent inhibitor of these reactions. Acetylsalicylic acid is unique among the nonsteroidal anti-inflammatory drugs that inhibit cyclo-oxygenase because it irreversibly acetylates this enzyme, thus blocking its action on arachidonate. Because it has been reported that less acetylsalicylic acid is required to inactivate platelet cyclo-oxygenase than the vessel wall enzyme, it has been suggested that low doses of acetylsalicylic acid should be used to inhibit platelet function while permitting the vessel wall to synthesize PGI_2. The effects of acetylsalicylic acid on platelets last for their lifetime, but its effects on the vessel wall are more transient because the vessel wall can resynthesize the enzyme. It is possible that acetylsalicylic acid, given once daily, may allow the vessel wall to regain its PGI_2-synthesizing ability.

The use of acetylsalicylic acid to prevent the clinical complications of atherosclerosis assumes that inhibition of TXA_2 formation would reduce the contribution of platelets to thrombosis and thromboembolism. This assumption must be reassessed, since acetylsalicylic acid does not consistently inhibit experimental thrombosis and has not conferred major benefit in clinical trials in patients who have had myocardial infarctions. Although thrombosis in which thromboxane A_2 plays a major role is likely to be inhibited by acetylsalicylic acid, thrombosis in which thrombin and ADP play dominant roles is not likely to be affected. Thromboxane A_2 may not be the main stimulus for platelet aggregation under some experimental conditions and in diseased coronary arteries.

Other effects of acetylsalicylic acid may result from acetylation of proteins other than cyclo-oxygenase and from the hydrolysis of acetylsalicylic acid to sodium salicylate. It has been reported that both acetylsalicylic acid and sodium salicylate inhibit the production of HETE (12-L-hydroxy-5,8,10,14-eicosatetraenoic acid) via the lipoxygenase pathway, inhibit glycolysis and oxidative phosphorylation, decrease the concentration of free fatty acids in plasma, enhance the fibrinolytic activity of whole blood, decrease cyclic AMP and cyclic GMP concentrations in some cells, decrease glycosaminoglycan synthesis, inhibit the synthesis of prothrombin and other vitamin K-dependent coagulation factors, suppress lymphocyte transformation, and reduce fever. The toxic effects of high concentrations of acetylsalicylic acid and sodium salicylate are unlikely to be mediated through inhibition of cyclo-oxygenase.

The actions of acetylsalicylic acid that result from acetylation of cyclo-oxygenase have received more attention recently than any of its other actions. It is apparent, however, that sodium salicylate and other nonsteroidal anti-inflammatory drugs do not exert all of their effects through inhibiting the synthesis of prostaglandins and related products.

In considering the mode of action of acetylsalicylic acid, we will summarize its effects on the synthesis of prostaglandins and related compounds, as well as its other effects not explained by this inhibition. Acetylsalicylic acid is rapidly converted to sodium salicylate (22), with as much as 50% of orally administered acetylsalicylic acid hydrolyzed before it enters the circulation. Further hydrolysis occurs rapidly (103). Therefore, the effects of both acetylsalicylic acid and sodium salicylate must be taken into account. Some of the effects of acetylsalicylic acid are related to its ability to acetylate proteins, particularly the enzyme cyclo-oxygenase that is responsible for prostaglandin synthesis. Other effects of acetylsalicylic acid are related to the salicylate formed from it.

The ability of acetylsalicylic acid to acetylate proteins has been recognized for some time. Acetylation of serum albumin and a number of other proteins by acetylsalicylic acid *in vitro* and *in vivo* was recognized in the 1960s (47,101). Since acetylated proteins may be handled differently from normal proteins, some of the as yet unexplained effects of acetylsalicylic acid may be attributable to acetylation of proteins other than cyclo-oxygenase. For example, it has been suggested (47) that acetylation of albumin may alter its antigenicity and result in the syndrome of "acetylsalicylic acid intolerance", characterized by asthma, rhinitis, and nasal polyps. Sodium salicylate does not cause this syndrome.

INHIBITION OF PROSTAGLANDIN SYNTHESIS

Enzymes responsible for the synthesis of prostaglandins and related products have been found in the microsomal fractions prepared from nearly all tissues that were examined (80). Among these enzymes is cyclo-oxygenase, which catalyzes the formation of prostaglandin endoperoxides from the long-chain unsaturated fatty acids (principally arachidonic acid) that are freed from membrane phospholipids upon stimulation of phospholipases (8,37,72,104). The acetylation of cyclo-oxygenase by acetylsalicylic acid results in irreversible inactivation of this enzyme (14,89,105). Other nonsteroidal anti-inflammatory drugs also inhibit cyclo-oxygenase, but most of them do not alter the enzyme irreversibly, and hence their effects do not persist after they and their active metabolites have been eliminated from the circulation (3,12,16,68,90). Sodium salicylate is a very weak inhibitor of cyclo-oxygenase (128), and its effects are not apparent at the concentrations usually achieved *in vivo* (89,129,135,141). Sodium salicylate is a noteworthy exception (117,119) to the strong correlation, noted by Moncada and Vane (82), between the ability of various nonsteroidal drugs to inhibit cyclo-oxygenase and their anti-inflammatory activity. In some types of inflammation, sodium salicylate is about as effective as acetylsalicylic acid (23,117).

PRODUCTS FORMED FROM ARACHIDONATE

Several products are formed from arachidonic acid following its conversion to prostaglandin G_2 under the influence of cyclo-oxygenase (Fig. 1). Thromboxane A_2, formed by platelets, and prostacyclin (prostaglandin I_2), formed by vessel walls, have attracted attention because of their effects on platelets and vessel wall tone (80). Thromboxane A_2 and PGI_2 are unstable, with half-lives under physiological conditions of about 30 sec and 2 to 3 min respectively, and break down into the relatively inactive, more stable products, thromboxane B_2 and 6-keto-$PGF_{1\alpha}$ (80). Thromboxane A_2 and PGI_2 have opposite effects on platelet aggregation and vessel wall tone. Thromboxane A_2 causes platelet aggregation and vessel contraction, whereas PGI_2 is a potent inhibitor of most platelet functions (adherence, shape change, aggregation, and release of granule contents) and causes vessel wall dilation (18,33,48,72,80,81,88).

Other products are also formed from arachidonate under the influence of cyclo-oxygenase (Fig. 1) (5,41,72,80). The first intermediate products are the prostaglandin endoperoxides PGG_2 and PGH_2. Both of these have short half-lives. PGE_2, PGD_2, and $PGF_{2\alpha}$ are relatively stable prostaglandins. HHT (12-L-hydroxy-5,8,10-heptadecatrienoic acid) and malondialdehyde (MDA) are also formed, and the colorimetric assay of MDA by a thiobarbituric acid reaction has frequently been used as an indication of the operation of this series of reactions (72,92,114,125). PGG_2, PGE_2, $PGF_{2\alpha}$, PGI_2, and 6-keto-$PGF_{1\alpha}$ have been implicated as mediators

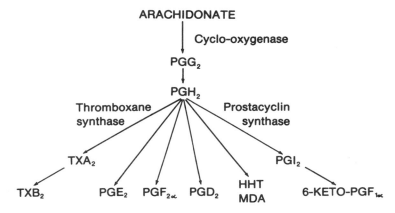

FIG. 1. Products formed from arachidonate in platelets and in the cells of the vessel wall. Platelets contain thromboxane synthase, whereas the cells of the vessel wall contain prostacyclin synthase. PG, prostaglandin; TXA_2, thromboxane A_2; TXB_2, thromboxane B_2; HHT, 12-L-hydroxy-5,8,10-heptadecatrienoic acid; MDA, malondialdehyde.

of inflammation (80). Acetylsalicylic acid inhibits the formation of all of these products and hence inhibits all of their effects.

PGI$_2$ differs from the prostaglandins and thromboxanes in that it does not have the typical hairpin configuration (5). Several groups of investigators have shown that the receptor for PGI$_2$ on platelets differs from that for PGD$_2$, although both of these prostaglandins stimulate adenylate cyclase and thus increase intracellular cyclic AMP concentrations (108,112). It is possible that cells in different tissues vary in the proportion of these receptors. In platelets, elevation of cAMP is associated with inhibition of many functions (18,33,48,81,85) and acceleration of platelet deaggregation (43,77). Thus, acetylsalicylic acid-induced inhibition of PGI$_2$ formation by the vessel wall would remove any potential effect of PGI$_2$ on the cAMP levels of platelets adjacent to the wall.

ACETYLATION OF CYCLO-OXYGENASE BY ACETYLSALICYLIC ACID

Although acetylsalicylic acid can acetylate other proteins besides the cyclo-oxygenase in platelets, it has been shown that such acetylation occurs over hours rather than minutes and requires millimolar concentrations (14). Since acetylsalicylic acid is rapidly hydrolyzed, it may not persist in the circulation long enough to acetylate other proteins to an extent that alters their function. It is also likely that the concentration of acetylsalicylic acid that reaches cells not directly exposed to blood may be much less than the initial concentration in the circulation.

Acetylation of platelet cyclo-oxygenase occurs within minutes even at micromolar concentrations of acetylsalicylic acid (T$_{1/2}$ at 10 μM is approximately 3 min) (14). Roth and Siok (107) demonstrated that the enzyme was covalently modified by acetylation of a serine at its NH$_2$ terminus. A single oral dose of acetylsalicylic acid as low as 160 mg results in 82% acetylation of the enzyme at 24 hr (15).

Irreversible acetylation of cyclo-oxygenase by acetylsalicylic acid is demonstrated by its effects on platelets, which are unable to synthesize new enzyme molecules (14). The effect of acetylsalicylic acid on platelets persists for their life-span. As new platelets enter the circulation, this inhibitory effect is gradually lost (15,60,89,125,135). If as few as 10% of the platelet population has not been exposed to acetylsalicylic acid, platelet function is largely restored (19,89,127). The extent to which circulating platelets recover the ability to synthesize malondialdehyde has been used as a measure of platelet survival (actually platelet production, which equals platelet destruction when the platelet count remains constant). This technique is useful in subjects to whom radioisotopes may not be administered (110,125).

Acetylsalicylic acid has been shown to acetylate the cyclo-oxygenase in isolated megakaryocytes (28), and it has been proposed that the platelets derived from megakaryocytes of subjects who have ingested acetylsalicylic acid may be affected for several days (14,89). The lag observed by some investigators before the platelets from such subjects begin to regain their ability to synthesize malondialdehyde (60,64) or to be acetylated *in vitro* with radiolabeled acetylsalicylic acid (15) has been cited as evidence for this theory. However, other investigators have not noted this delay (125), and it seems probable that megakaryocytes, like the cells of the vessel wall, can replace the acetylated cyclo-oxygenase by synthesizing new enzyme molecules. When the cyclo-oxygenase has been replaced, platelets that are subsequently formed should function normally. Nevertheless, Burch and Majerus (14) have proposed that since acetylsalicylic acid can acetylate megakaryocyte cyclooxygenase, alternate-day therapy with low-dose acetylsalicylic acid should prevent platelet prostaglandin (and thromboxane A_2) production.

The cells of the vessel wall can recover their ability to synthesize prostaglandins (notably PGI_2) within hours after acetylsalicylic acid administration or treatment (Table 1) (10,24,54,57,134). The time required for recovery is not well established, nor is the question of whether veins or arteries more rapidly regain their synthetic capacity (Table 1). It seems likely that most cells capable of protein synthesis can eventually replace the acetylated enzyme after acetylsalicylic acid administration.

Tissues appear to differ in the sensitivity of their cyclo-oxygenase to inhibition by acetylsalicylic acid. Ferreira and Vale (34) have put forward the theory that the enzyme may exist in multiple molecular forms or isozymes that differ in their sensitivity to acetylsalicylic acid-like drugs. This could account for the apparent differences in sensitivity of the cyclo-oxygenase to acetylsalicylic acid inhibition from tissue to tissue and could be responsible for the differences among the effects of the various nonsteroidal anti-inflammatory drugs in different tissues. The question of how much unhydrolyzed acetylsalicylic acid reaches the tissues must also be considered.

The enzyme in human aorta microsomes has been reported to be much more resistant to acetylation by acetylsalicylic acid than the enzyme in platelets (13,73). This has led to the suggestion that acetylsalicylic acid should be administered in doses high enough to inhibit platelet cyclo-oxygenase but too low to inhibit PGI_2 production by the arterial wall (13,72). Jaffe and Weksler (54), however, have

TABLE 1. *Recovery of the ability of the cells of the vessel wall to synthesize PGI_2 after exposure to ASA*

System studied	Time to recover ability to synthesize PGI_2	Investigators
Rabbit jugular vein	2.5 hr	Kelton et al. (57)
Rabbit carotid artery	20 hr (56%)	Buchanan et al. (10)
Rabbit jugular vein	3 hr (60%)	Buchanan et al. (10)
Rat aorta	24–72 hr	Villa et al. (134)
Rat inferior vena cava	< 24 hr	Villa et al. (134)
Cultured venous endothelial cells	26 hr	Jaffe and Weksler (54)
Cultured venous endothelial cells	2 hr	Czervionke et al. (24)

reported that the cyclo-oxygenase enzymes in platelets and cultured endothelial cells are inhibited to the same extent by low doses of acetylsalicylic acid. Villa and his co-workers (134) have observed that 1 hr after intraperitoneal injection into rats, doses of acetylsalicylic acid that inhibit platelet malondialdehyde production by 95% inhibit vessel wall synthesis of PGI_2 by 38 to 66%. Thus, the question of whether it is possible to find a dose of acetylsalicylic acid that inhibits the cyclo-oxygenase in platelets but not that in vessel wall remains to be settled.

Some of the other nonsteroidal anti-inflammatory drugs have been shown to compete with acetylsalicylic acid for the active site on cyclo-oxygenase and thus protect the enzyme from acetylation. These drugs include indomethacin (121), diflunisal (71), sulfinpyrazone (2), and salicylic acid (75,130).

Although low doses of acetylsalicylic acid prolong bleeding times (49,102,135), probably by inhibiting thromboxane A_2 formation, high doses of acetylsalicylic acid have been reported to shorten the bleeding time, possibly by inhibiting PGI_2 formation and hence removing its vasodilation effect (4,91).

Interest has recently been focused on the possibility that acetylsalicylic acid, particularly in high doses, may actually be thrombogenic, because it inhibits the synthesis of PGI_2 by acetylating cyclo-oxygenase in the cells of the vessel wall (57,91).

Although acetylsalicylic acid can be shown to promote thrombus formation under some circumstances (57), it does not cause increased platelet adherence to the endothelium or subendothelium of large arteries (27), where flow is rapid and laminar. This observation indicates that PGI_2 is unlikely to be responsible for the nonthrombogenic nature of vascular endothelium, as has been suggested (76), or for the rapid development of a nonthrombogenic surface following removal of the endothelium. Controversy exists concerning the possibility that circulating PGI_2 levels may be high enough to affect platelet function, particularly in the presence of a phosphodiesterase inhibitor such as dipyridamole, which enhances the ability of PGI_2 to raise the cAMP concentration in platelets (43,56,78). In studies using 15-hydroperoxy-arachidonic acid, an inhibitor of PGI_2 synthetase, or antibodies directed at a stable PGI_2 analogue, Gryglewski et al. (42) and Moncada et al. (79) obtained evidence causing them to suggest that PGI_2 is a circulating hormone, generated in the lungs, that inhibits platelet aggregation *in vivo*. However, Smith et al. (115) and Steer et al. (122) could find no evidence that addition of the antibody to depress circulating PGI_2 levels affected blood pressure in the absence of exogenous PGI_2 or changed the response of platelets to ADP. In the study by Steer et al. (122), attention was paid to the problem that PGI_2 levels in blood decline rapidly after the blood is drawn, and the aggregation tests were done with platelet-rich plasma prepared within 3 min of venous or arterial puncture.

If PGI_2 were responsible for the nonthrombogenic characteristics of endothelium and circulating PGI_2 acted as an inhibitor of platelet aggregation, patients receiving high doses of acetylsalicylic acid over prolonged periods would be expected to show an enhanced incidence of arterial thrombosis and its complications. Evidence that this is not the case comes from the 10-year study of 473 patients with rheumatoid arthritis in Rochester, Minnesota, by investigators at the Mayo Clinic (66). The incidence of myocardial infarction, angina pectoris, sudden death, or cerebral infarction in these patients receiving high doses of acetylsalicylic acid was not significantly different from that of age- and sex-specific incidence rates in the general population of Rochester. Although a control group of untreated rheumatoid arthritis patients cannot be included in such a study, it does indicate that high doses of acetylsalicylic acid over a 10-year period do not promote thrombosis despite the likelihood that they inhibit PGI production. Earlier studies also support this conclusion (25,138). Davis and Engleman (25) found that at autopsy 62 patients with rheumatoid arthritis showed significantly lower morbidity and mortality from myocardial infarction than 62 matched control patients.

Platelet hypersensitivity to aggregating agents has been observed in conjunction with a number of disease states, including those of a thromboembolic nature, diabetes, and hyperbetalipoproteinemia (95). In many cases this hypersensitivity appears to result from increased production of thromboxane A_2 in response to stimulation, and hence administration of acetylsalicylic acid prevents the platelet manifestations of hypersensitivity. Although this observation has been used to support the theory that platelet hypersensitivity leads to an enhanced tendency for arterial thrombosis, which should be lessened by acetylsalicylic acid, it may be that platelet hypersensitivity is the result of the disorder rather than its cause, in which case acetylsalicylic acid could not be expected to be beneficial.

Many studies have been done in experimental animals in attempts to determine whether or not acetylsalicylic acid inhibits arterial thrombosis (29,85,86,98). Results have varied from inhibition to no inhibition to potentiation. It seems likely that the method used to induce thrombus formation, the site of vessel wall injury, and possibly the species of animal have all affected the results. Thrombosis in which thromboxane A_2 formation by platelets plays a major role is likely to be inhibited by acetylsalicylic acid. In contrast, thrombus formation resulting from platelet reactions in which thromboxane A_2 plays only a minor or no role, such as aggregation induced by thrombin or ADP, is not likely to be affected by acetylsalicylic acid.

Although much of the current interest in the inhibitory effects of acetylsalicylic acid has been directed at thromboxane A_2 formation by platelets and PGI_2 formation by the vessel wall, several other effects of acetylsalicylic acid mediated through inhibition of prostaglandin synthesis will be discussed by other contributors to this volume.

EFFECTS NOT EXPLAINED BY PROSTAGLANDIN INHIBITION

It seems likely that these other effects of acetylsalicylic acid result from, first, the acetylation of proteins other than cyclo-oxygenase, and second, the actions of sodium salicylate, which apparently has little effect on cyclo-oxygenase (128,129) but nevertheless has strong anti-inflammatory properties (23,117). It seems likely that most of the effects of sodium salicylate are not mediated through inhibition of prostaglandin synthesis. When acetylsalicylic acid and sodium salicylate have similar inhibitory effects, it is unlikely that acetylsalicylic acid is acting through its acetylation action but is more probably acting after its conversion to sodium salicylate or in the same fashion as sodium salicylate. Although it has been suggested that sodium salicylate must be converted to gentisic acid before becoming active as an inhibitor of prostaglandin synthesis (35), recent experiments do not support this suggestion (119). In addition, only small amounts (7%) of sodium salicylate are converted to gentisic acid in man (22).

The list of physiologic reactions that are inhibited by acetylsalicylic acid and sodium salicylate is long (22,80,82,139). In many cases, the effects can be attributed to acetylsalicylic acid inhibition of the cyclo-oxygenase in cells, but in other cases, particularly if sodium salicylate is strongly inhibitory, other explanations must be sought. Many reports describe inhibitory effects, but little attempt has been made to determine the mechanisms.

LIPOXYGENASE PATHWAY

Cyclo-oxygenase is only one of two enzymes that act on arachidonate after it has been liberated from membrane phospholipids. The other enzyme is a lipoxygenase that converts arachidonate to 12-L-hydroperoxy-5,8,10,14-eicosatetraenoic acid (HPETE), which is in turn acted on by a putative peroxidase to form 12-L-hydroxy-5,8,10,14-eicosatetraenoic acid (HETE) (44). The latter has been reported to be chemotactic for PMN leukocytes (40,126). Most investigators have found that the lipoxygenase is not inhibited by acetylsalicylic acid or other nonsteroidal anti-inflammatory drugs (45,62,63) but that inhibiting cyclo-oxygenase diverts more arachidonate into the lipoxygenase pathway, resulting in increased HPETE and HETE formation (45,113). Siegel et al. (113) have recently reported that acetylsalicylic acid, sodium salicylate, and indomethacin block conversion of HPETE to HETE and that their inhibitory effect on this reaction is reversible. These investigators speculate that at least some of the common pharmacological actions of these drugs may be related to their ability to influence arachidonate metabolism via the lipoxygenase pathway. They point out that inhibition of HETE production would block its chemotactic effect and thus prevent its inflammatory activity related to the recruitment of phagocytic cells. However, little is known of the effects of HPETE or HETE on cells, so one can only speculate on other consequences of interference with the peroxidase responsible for conversion of HPETE to HETE. In earlier reports of increased HETE formation in the presence of acetylsalicylic acid or indomethacin, it seems likely that HPETE and HETE, which co-chromatograph in most systems, were measured together and designated as HETE.

EFFECT ON CONCENTRATIONS AND ACTIONS OF OTHER DRUGS AND ENDOGENOUS SUBSTANCES

At concentrations that are clinically achieved, 50 to 90% of the salicylate ion is bound to plasma protein, mainly to albumin; the free hydroxyl group is required for protein binding (22). Salicylate binds more strongly to plasma proteins than many other drugs and thus enhances the pharmacological effects of some drugs by displacing them from their binding sites. This has been shown for penicillin analogues, sulfonamides, methotrexate, tolbutamide, thiopental, phenytoin, sulfinpyrazone, naproxen, and coumarin anticoagulants (22,139). Endogenous substances that are displaced include thyroxine, bilirubin, uric acid, tryptophan, some peptides, and possibly steroids (139). Salicylates have been shown to reduce fatty acid binding to albumin *in vitro* (26). Acetylsalicylic acid as such is bound to plasma protein to only a limited extent; however, it acetylates plasma albumin by reacting with the ϵ-amino group of lysine (47,139). The acetylated protein has an increased affinity for phenylbutazone, decreased affinity for flufenamic acid, and unchanged affinity for dicumarol (20). Acetylsalicylic acid or sodium salicylate increases plasma levels of dipyridamole when administered concurrently and prolongs its effect (11). This may result from saturation of the glucuronide pathway, the major route of clearance of dipyridamole from the circulation.

Small doses of salicylate antagonize the action of probenecid and other uricosuric agents that act by decreasing the tubular reabsorption of uric acid (139).

EFFECTS ON GLYCOLYSIS AND OXIDATIVE PHOSPHORYLATION

The concentrations of acetylsalicylic acid or sodium salicylate required to inhibit glycolysis in platelets are far greater than therapeutic levels, although an acetylsalicylic acid concentration of 50 μM was shown to have some inhibitory effect on glucose uptake (31). It now seems unlikely that this is responsible for the actions of acetylsalicylic acid.

The suggestion that salicylates may act by uncoupling oxidative phosphorylation was made by Adams and Cobb (1) long before the effects of acetylsalicylic acid on prostaglandin synthesis were recognized. Whitehouse (137) also considered this possibility. High concentrations (0.2 to 2 mM) of salicylate are required to uncouple oxidative phosphorylation *in vitro* (118,140), but these concentrations of unbound drug do occur with the doses of salicylate used to treat rheumatoid arthritis (139). Uncoupling of oxidative phosphorylation would result in inhibiting many ATP-dependent reactions, but under normal physiological conditions the process is not proceeding at a maximum rate and could increase to compensate if oxidative phosphorylation were impaired. An uncoupling effect cannot be shown in the whole animal (118). However, uncoupling may account for the salicylate-induced increases in oxygen consumption and CO_2 production. Depletion of hepatic glycogen and the pyretic effect of high doses of salicylates may also be attributed to this uncoupling action.

EFFECT ON PLASMA CONCENTRATIONS OF FREE FATTY ACIDS

In dogs, sodium salicylate reduced plasma concentration of free fatty acids (9,17), apparently through a non-insulin-dependent inhibition of free fatty acid mobilization (131). The reduction in mobilization seems to be caused both by inhibition of adipose tissue lipolysis and by enhanced reesterification of free fatty acid within the same tissue (133). Inhibition of fatty acid synthesis and increased oxidation in muscle (22) may also diminish plasma levels. The lowering of plasma free fatty acids caused by salicylate administration is not likely to be related to inhibition of prostaglandin synthesis, since indomethacin has no antilipolytic effect *in vitro* (38).

Although salicylates raise plasma insulin levels in man (36), they reduce insulin levels in dogs and rats (131). It appears that changes in insulin concentration may be a consequence of the alterations in plasma concentrations of free fatty acids rather than their cause (131). In addition, salicylates inhibit catecholamine-induced lipolysis *in vitro* where an insulin effect cannot be responsible (109,123). It has been suggested that a rise in free fatty acids increases the incidence of arrhythmia (61), and Moschos et al. (84) have postulated that the antiarrhythmic effect of acetylsalicylic acid during nonthrombotic coronary occlusion in dogs may in part be related to its ability to block the increment in free fatty acids that they observed in untreated animals. They also point out that indomethacin enhances injury during myocardial ischemia (59), indicating that this effect of acetylsalicylic acid is unlikely to be mediated through inhibition of prostaglandin synthesis. Vik-Mo and Mjøs (132) have also suggested that acetylsalicylic acid and sodium salicylate reduce epicardial ST-segment elevation and myocardial ischemia during coronary occlusion in dogs by reducing the utilization of free fatty acids by the myocardium.

PROTECTION OF THE ENDOTHELIUM

Hladovec (50) has proposed that acetylsalicylic acid may have a stabilizing effect on the endothelium, on the basis of experiments in rats in which intravenous injections of trisodium citrate were used to damage the endothelium. However, Harker (46) did not observe a protective effect of acetylsalicylic acid on the endothelium of primates receiving continuous infusions of homocysteine.

Jamieson et al. (55) observed that sodium salicylate in combination with azathioprine prolonged the survival of heart allografts in rats. These investigators point out that the mode of action of the sodium salicylate is not clear and suggest that it may lessen endothelial damage by interfering with the formation of antigen-antibody complexes and possibly subsequent platelet interactions. However, Di Minno et al. (30) did not find a significant effect of acetylsalicylic acid on the time of rejection of heart allografts in mice. Their experiments differed from those of Jamieson et al. (55) in two ways: azathioprine was not administered and acetylsalicylic acid was used instead of sodium salicylate. Di Minno and his colleagues concluded that the beneficial effect of sodium salicylate in the experiments of Jamieson et al. (55) was unlikely to be caused by an effect on platelets and suggested that enhancement of blood fibrinolysis might be involved, since sodium salicylate increases fibrinolytic activity to as great an extent as acetylsalicylic acid (83).

In animal experiments involving removal or injury of the endothelium of arteries, acetylsalicylic acid has been found to have no effect on the resulting smooth muscle cell proliferation (7,21). This is not surprising, since acetylsalicylic acid does not block release of granule contents [including the mitogen for smooth muscle cells (106)] from platelets adherent to constituents of the subendothelium (58,136).

There have been several studies of the effect of acetylsalicylic acid on cholesterol-induced atherosclerosis in animals. Bailey and Butler (6) found acetylsalicylic acid to have no effect on the development of atherosclerotic plaques in rabbits fed cholesterol-rich diets, although other nonsteroidal anti-inflammatory drugs, such as phenylbutazone, flufenamic acid, and mefenamic acid, were protective. Höpker et al. (52) also observed that acetylsalicylic acid had no effect on cholesterol-induced atherosclerosis in the aorta of rabbits, but Hollander et al. (51) found that although acetylsalicylic acid did not decrease the size of aortic plaques in rabbits, it did change the nature of the lesions by reducing the amount of fibrous material in them. Pick and her colleagues (99) have recently reported that administration of acetylsalicylic acid to monkeys fed a diet enriched with cholesterol and butter fat decreased the number of coronary vessels with atherosclerotic involvement, although no effect on aortic atherosclerosis was observed. On the basis of these data, no conclusions could be reached concerning the mechanisms that were inhibited by acetylsalicylic acid. It is also difficult to postulate a mechanism to account for inhibitory effects in coronary arteries but not in the aorta.

EFFECT OF SALICYLATES ON ENZYMES

Acetylsalicylic acid and sodium salicylate may affect the function of many enzymes, particularly when the drugs are at toxic levels (0.6 to 5 mM) (101,118). In the 1950s and 1960s, many cellular enzyme systems were investigated in an attempt to determine which enzymes were modified by these drugs. Fewer studies of this type have been done since discovery of the action of acetylsalicylic acid and other nonsteroidal anti-inflammatory drugs on prostaglandin synthesis. However, it should be kept in mind that these drugs may exert some of their effects by inhibiting enzymes other than cyclo-oxygenase.

In 1971, Smith and Dawkins (118) reviewed evidence concerning the effects of salicylates on enzymes. Activities that had been shown to be inhibited *in vitro* by high concentrations of these drugs include those involving enzymes in oxidative-phosphorylation dehydrogenases, decarboxylases, aminotransferases, aminoacyl-tRNA synthetases and nucleic acid polymerases. Only two *in vitro* interactions with enzyme systems occurring in the 0.15 to 0.6 mM range had been established at that time—namely, the uncoupling effect on oxidative phosphorylation and the inhibition of protein synthesis, although inhibition of prostaglandin synthesis by 0.005 to 0.02 mM acetylsalicylic acid had also been observed (116,128). It seems quite possible that salicylates may act on several sites, rather than interfering with a single enzyme system. A recent report records acetylsalicylic acid inhibition of exogenous sialyl-transferase activity in platelets from cancer patients (111). Platelets from these patients had higher levels of enzyme than platelets from normal controls, and acetylsalicylic acid reduced the level of this enzyme to control values. The reason for this effect of acetylsalicylic acid was not explored.

EFFECT OF ACETYLSALICYLIC ACID AND SODIUM SALICYLATE ON CYCLIC NUCLEOTIDES

The effect of acetylsalicylic acid inhibition on the formation of PGI_2 and PGD_2, the prostaglandins that normally raise cAMP concentrations in cells, has already been outlined. Acetylsalicylic acid has been shown to decrease cAMP in lymphocytes and inhibit its rise in response to isoproterenol and prostaglandin (120). Bradykinin elevates both cAMP and cGMP in guinea pig lung, probably by stimulating PGI_2 synthesis, and inhibition of prostaglandin synthesis with acetylsalicylic acid prevents this rise in cAMP (87,124). Many other examples can be found in which acetylsalicylic acid affects the response of cells by preventing the prostaglandin-stimulated increase in cAMP.

However, some of the effects of acetylsalicylic acid on cyclic nucleotide levels are shared by sodium salicylate, indicating that they are not mediated through inhibition of cyclo-oxygenase. Peters et al. (97) found that sodium salicylate decreased cAMP levels in embryonic mouse fibroblasts in both the presence and absence of PGE_1. The dose-dependent decrease in cAMP in the presence of PGE_1 correlated with a dose-dependent decrease in glycosaminoglycan secretion. Pickett et al. (100) concluded that acetylsalicylic acid inhibition of the ascorbate-induced elevations of platelet cGMP that they observed is probably not mediated through inhibition of cyclo-oxygenase, since ascorbate does not activate the phospholipase responsible for freeing arachidonate and the effect of ascorbate is fully manifest under anaerobic conditions.

EFFECT ON GLYCOSAMINOGLYCAN FORMATION

Sodium salicylate decreases glycosaminoglycan synthesis in canine (96) and human (70) articular cartilage and in mouse fibroblasts (97). It has been suggested (97) that sodium salicylate exerts this effect by interfering with cAMP formation or function. This has not been thoroughly explored, and although the observation that sodium salicylate decreases glycosaminoglycan synthesis seems to be well established, the mechanism by which sodium salicylate exerts this effect is not.

INCREASED FIBRINOLYTIC ACTIVITY

In 1970, Menon (74) observed that acetylsalicylic acid enhanced the euglobulin lysis time in man, although various effects, including inhibition of fibrinolysis, have been reported in vitro (53). Moroz (83) found that similar doses (1.8 g) of acetylsalicylic acid and sodium salicylate increased human whole blood fibrinolytic activity. Sodium salicylate also increased in vitro whole blood fibrinolytic activity but not that of cell-free plasma. This was attributed to an enhancing effect of sodium salicylate on the membrane-associated fibrinolytic activity of polymorphonuclear leukocytes. Other cells may be similarly affected in vivo. Because sodium salicylate is as effective as acetylsalicylic acid, it seems unlikely that inhibition of prostaglandin synthesis is responsible for the increased fibrinolytic activity.

Bleeding time and the healing of peptic ulcers may be influenced by this en-hancement of fibrinolysis. The report by McKenna and her colleagues (69) of a reduction in the incidence of deep vein thrombosis by high dosages of acetylsalicylic acid (1.3 g t.i.d.) in patients (mainly female) undergoing total knee replacement could be related to enhancement of fibrinolytic activity caused by acetylsalicylic acid and sodium salicylate. A lower dosage of acetylsalicylic acid (325 mg t.i.d.) did not reduce the incidence of deep vein thrombosis in this study.

EFFECT OF SODIUM SALICYLATE ON COAGULATION FACTORS

In the 1940s, Link and his group (65) showed that sodium salicylate inhibited the synthesis of prothrombin and other vitamin K-dependent coagulation factors. They investigated this inhibitory effect because sodium salicylate is a metabolic product formed from dicumarol. The effect was found to be slight, and prolongation of the bleeding time was reported to be very minor.

EFFECTS OF SODIUM SALICYLATE ON WHITE BLOOD CELLS

Sodium salicylate has some effects on white blood cells that are not related to inhibition of prostaglandin synthesis by these cells. Acetylsalicylic acid and sodium salicylate suppress lymphocyte transformation *in vitro* and *in vivo* (67,93,94). Since the drugs are equally effective, they probably do not act by inhibiting cyclo-oxy-genase. Sodium salicylate inhibits the generation of granulocyte and macrophage colonies in *in vitro* cultures (39). Since E-type prostaglandins also suppress this proliferation, it is unlikely that the salicylate effect is mediated through inhibition of prostaglandin synthesis.

The overall effect of inhibition of these cellular functions in the whole animal is not understood, since many other systems are influenced simultaneously.

EFFECTS OF SALICYLATES ON TUMORS

Anti-inflammatory drugs have been shown to affect tumor growth, particularly in experimental animals (32). However, there is no evidence of beneficial effects in man, and most of the observations from animal experiments are confusing and contradictory, with different effects at different doses. Some of the changes caused by these drugs may involve the immunological system. The author of a recent editorial in *Lancet* could not come to a firm conclusion on this topic (32).

ANTIPYRETIC EFFECT OF SODIUM SALICYLATE

Sodium salicylate has an antipyretic effect, and the suggestion has been made that it may act directly on neuronal membranes. This topic is covered in another chapter in this volume.

TOXIC EFFECTS OF SALICYLATES

High doses of salicylates are associated with a number of toxic effects (Table 2) (22,139), but there seems to be little or no information concerning which biochem-

TABLE 2. *Toxic effects of high doses of salicylates (22,139)*

Neurological effects: convulsions, confusion, dizziness, tinnitus, high-tone deafness, delirium, psychosis, stupor, coma
Nausea and vomiting
Hyperventilation and, initially, respiratory alkalosis
Changes in acid-base balance, electrolytes, and water balance

---

ical reactions are affected. Since extremely high concentrations of salicylates are required to produce toxic symptoms and inhibition of cyclo-oxygenase by acetylsalicylic acid occurs at very low concentrations, it seems likely that the toxic effects are not related to inhibition of prostaglandin synthesis.

CONCLUSIONS

In the last decade, the effects of acetylsalicylic acid resulting from the acetylation of cyclo-oxygenase have received far more attention than any of its other actions. Other nonsteroidal anti-inflammatory drugs have also been extensively studied in relation to their ability to inhibit this enzyme. Sodium salicylate is a very weak inhibitor of cyclo-oxygenase, although it has many of the beneficial effects of the nonsteroidal anti-inflammatory drugs. Among the noteworthy effects of sodium salicylate are its anti-inflammatory properties, its ability to increase fibrinolysis, its inhibition of glycosaminoglycan synthesis, and its effects on white blood cells. It seems likely that sodium salicylate and other nonsteroidal anti-inflammatory drugs do not exert all of their actions through inhibition of prostaglandin synthesis.

REFERENCES

1. Adams, S. S., and Cobb, R. (1958): A possible basis for anti-inflammatory activity of salicylates and other non-hormonal anti-rheumatic drugs. *Nature*, 181:773–744
2. Ali, M., and McDonald, J. W. D. (1977): Effects of sulfinpyrazone on platelet prostaglandin synthesis and platelet release of serotonin. *J. Lab. Clin. Med.*, 89:868–875.
3. Ali, M., and McDonald, J. W. D. (1978): Reversible and irreversible inhibition of platelet cyclooxygenase and serotonin release by non-steroidal anti-inflammatory drugs. *Thromb. Res.*, 13:1057–1066.
4. Amezcua, J. L., Parsons, M., and Moncada, S. (1978): Unstable metabolites of arachidonic acid, aspirin, and the formation of the haemostatic plug. *Thromb. Res.*, 13:477–488.
5. Armstrong, J. M., Dusting, G. J., Moncada, S., and Vane, J. R. (1978): Cardiovascular actions of prostacyclin (PGI_2), a metabolite of arachidonic acid which is synthesized by blood vessels. *Circ. Res.* (Suppl. 1), 43:112–119.
6. Bailey, J. M., and Butler, J. (1973): Anti-inflammatory drugs in experimental atherosclerosis. Part 1, Relative potencies for inhibiting plaque formation. *Atherosclerosis*, 17:515–522.
7. Baumgartner, H. R., and Studer, A. (1977): Platelet factors and the proliferation of vascular smooth muscle cells. In: *Atherosclerosis IV*, edited by G. Schettler, Y. Goto, Y. Hata, and G. Klose, pp. 605–609. Springer-Verlag, Berlin.
8. Bell, R. L., Kennerly, D. A., Stanford,N., and Majerus, P. W. (1979): Diglyceride lipase: A pathway for arachidonate release from human platelets. *Proc. Natl. Acad. Sci. U.S.A.*, 76:3238–3241.
9. Bizzi, A., Garattini, S., and Veneroni, E. (1965): The action of salicylate in reducing plasma free fatty acids and its pharmacological consequences. *Br. J. Pharmacol.*, 25:187–196.

10. Buchanan, M. R., Dejana, E., Mustard, J. F., and Hirsh, J. (1979): Prolonged inhibition of PGI_2 production and associated increased thrombogenic effect in arteries after aspirin administration. *Thromb. Haemost.*, 42:61.

11. Buchanan, M. R., Rosenfeld, J., Gent, M., Lawrence, W., and Hirsh, J. (1979): Increased dipyridamole plasma concentrations associated with salicylate administration. Relationship to effects on platelet aggregation in vivo. *Thromb. Res.*, 15:813–820.

12. Buchanan, M. R., Rosenfeld, J., and Hirsh, J. (1978): The prolonged effect of sulfinpyrazone on collagen-induced platelet aggregation in vivo. *Thromb, Res.*, 13:883–892.

13. Burch, J. W., Baenziger, N. L., Stanford, N., and Majerus, P. W. (1978): Sensitivity of fatty acid cyclooxygenase from human aorta to acetylation by aspirin. *Proc. Natl. Acad. Sci. U.S.A.*, 75:5181–5184.

14. Burch, J. W., and Majerus, P. W. (1979): The role of prostaglandins in platelet function. *Semin. Hematol.*, 16:196–207.

15. Burch, J. W., Stanford, N., and Majerus, P. W. (1978): Inhibition of platelet prostaglandin synthetase by oral aspirin. *J. Clin. Invest.*, 61:314–319.

16. Butler, K. D., Dieterle, W., Maguire, E. D., Pay, G. F., Wallis, R. B., and White, A. M. (1980): Sustained effects of sulfinpyrazone. In: *Cardiovascular Actions of Sulfinpyrazone: Basic and Clinical Research*, edited by M. McGregor, J. F. Mustard, M. F. Oliver, and S. Sherry, pp. 19–35. Symposia Specialists, Miami.

17. Carlson, L. A., and Østman, J. (1961): Effect of salicylates on plasma-free fatty acid in normal and diabetic subjects. *Metabolism*, 10:781–787.

18. Cazenave, J.-P., Dejana, E., Kinlough-Rathbone, R. L., Richardson, M., Packham, M. A., and Mustard, J. F. (1979): Prostaglandins I_2 and E_1 reduce rabbit and human platelet adherence without inhibiting serotonin release from adherent platelets. *Thromb. Res.*, 15:273–279.

19. Cerskus, A. L., Ali, M., Davies, B. J., and McDonald, J. W. D. (1980): Possible significance of small numbers of functional platelets in a population of aspirin-treated platelets in vitro and in vivo. *Thromb. Res.*, 18:389–397.

20. Chignell, C. F., and Starkweather, D. K. (1971): Optical studies of drug-protein complexes. V. The interaction of phenylbutazone, flufenamic acid, and dicoumarol with acetylsalicylic acid-treated human serum albumin. *Mol. Pharmacol.*, 7:229–237.

21. Clowes, A. W., and Karnovsky, M. J. (1977): Failure of certain antiplatelet drugs to affect myointimal thickening following arterial endothelial injury in the rat. *Lab. Invest.*, 36:452–464.

22. Cohen, L. S. (1976): Clinical pharmacology of acetylsalicylic acid. *Semin. Thromb. Hemostas.*, 2:146–175.

23. Collier, H. O. J. (1969): A pharmacological analysis of aspirin. In: *Advances in Pharmacology and Chemotherapy*, edited by S. Garattini, A. Goldin, F. Hawking, and I. J. Kopin, pp. 333–405. Academic Press, New York.

24. Czervionke, R. L., Smith, J. B., Fry, G. L., Hoak, J. C., and Haycraft, D. L. (1979): Inhibition of prostacyclin by treatment of endothelium with aspirin. Correlation with platelet adherence. *J. Clin. Invest.*, 63:1089–1092.

25. Davis, R. F., and Engleman, E. G. (1974): Incidence of myocardial infarction in patients with rheumatoid arthritis. *Arthritis Rheum.*, 17:527–533.

26. Dawkins, P. D., McArthur, J. N., and Smith, M. J. H. (1970): The effect of sodium salicylate on the binding of long-chain fatty acids to plasma proteins. *J. Pharm. Pharmacol.*, 22:405–410.

27. Dejana, E., Cazenave, J-P., Groves, H. M., Kinlough-Rathbone, R. L., Richardson, M., Packham, M. A., and Mustard, J. F. (1980): The effect of aspirin inhibition of PGI_2 production on platelet adherence to normal and damaged rabbit aortae. *Thromb. Res.*, 17:453–464.

28. Demers, L. M., Budin, R., and Shaikh, B. (1977): The effects of aspirin on megakaryocyte prostaglandin production. *Blood* (Suppl. 1), 50:239.

29. Didisheim, P., and Fuster, V. (1978): Actions and clinical status of platelet-suppressive agents. *Semin. Hematol.*, 15:55–72.

30. Di Minno, G., Reyers, I., Donati, M. B., and de Gaetano, G. (1979): Salicylates and survival of heart allografts in rats (letter). *Lancet*, 1:731.

31. Doery, J. C. G., and Hirsh, J. (1971): Divergent effects of aspirin and salicylate on glucose and glycogen metabolism in human platelets. *Experientia*, 27:533–534.

32. Editorial. (1979): Anti-inflammatory drugs and tumour growth. *Lancet*, 1:420–421.

33. Ehrman, M., Jaffe, E. A., and Weksler, B. B. (1979): Prostacyclin (PGI_2) inhibits the development in platelets of ADP and arachidonate-mediated shape change and procoagulant activity. *Clin. Res.*, 27:293A.

34. Ferreira, S. H., and Vane, J. R. (1974): New aspects of the mode of action of nonsteroid anti-inflammatory drugs. *Annu. Rev. Pharmacol.*, 14:57–73.
35. Ferreira, S. H., and Vane, J. R. (1979): Mode of action of anti-inflammatory agents which are prostaglandin synthetase inhibitors. In: *Handbook of Experimental Pathology 50/II, Anti-Inflammatory Drugs*, edited by J. R. Vane and S. H. Ferreira, pp. 348–398. Springer-Verlag, Berlin.
36. Field, J. B., Boyle, C., and Remer, A. (1967): Effect of salicylate infusion on plasma-insulin and glucose tolerance in healthy persons and mild diabetics. *Lancet*, 1:1191–1194.
37. Flower, R. J., and Blackwell, G. J. (1976): The importance of phospholipase A_2 in prostaglandin biosynthesis. *Biochem. Pharmacol.*, 25:285–291.
38. Fredholm, B. B., and Hedqvist, P. (1975): Indomethacin and the role of prostaglandins in adipose tissue. *Biochem. Pharmacol.*, 24:61–66.
39. Gabourel, J. D., Moore, M. A. S., Bagby, Jr., G. C., and Davies, G. H. (1977): Effect of sodium salicylate on human and mouse granulopoesis in vitro. *Arthritis Rheum.*, 20:59–64.
40. Goetzl, E. J., Woods, J. M., and Gorman, R. R. (1977): Stimulation of human eosinophil and neutrophil polymorphonuclear leukocyte chemotaxis and random migration by 12-L-hydroxy-5,8,10,14-eicosatetraenoic acid. *J. Clin. Invest.*, 59:179–183.
41. Gorman, R. R. (1979): Modulation of human platelet function by prostacyclin and thromboxane A_2. *Fed. Proc.*, 38:83–88.
42. Gryglewski, R. J., Korbut, R., and Ocetkiewicz, A. (1978): Generation of prostacyclin by lungs *in vivo* and its release into the arterial circulation. *Nature*, 273:765–767.
43. Gryglewski, R. J., Korbut, R., and Ocetkiewicz, A. (1978): De-aggregatory action of prostacyclin *in vivo* and its enhancement by theophylline. *Prostaglandins*, 15:637–644.
44. Hamberg, M., and Samuelsson, B. (1974): Prostaglandin endoperoxides. Novel transformations of arachidonic acid in human platelets. *Proc. Natl. Acad. Sci. U.S.A.*, 75: 5181–5184.
45. Hamberg, M., Svensson, J., and Samuelsson, B. (1974): Prostaglandin endoperoxides. A new concept concerning the mode of action and release of prostaglandins. *Proc. Natl. Acad. Sci. U.S.A.*, 71:3824–3828.
46. Harker, L. A: Sulfinpyrazone in primate models of vascular disease. In: *Cardiovascular Actions of Sulfinpyrazone: Basic and Clinical Research*, edited by M. McGregor, J. F. Mustard, M. F. Oliver, and S. Sherry, pp. 81–98. Proceedings of an International Symposium, Hamilton, Bermuda. Symposia Specialists, Inc., Miami, Fla.
47. Hawkins, D., Pinckard, R. N., Crawford, I. P., and Farr, R. S. (1969): Structural changes in human serum albumin induced by ingestion of acetylsalicylic acid. *J. Clin. Invest.*, 48:536–542.
48. Higgs, E. A., Moncada, S., Vane, J. R., Caen, J. P., Michel, H., and Tobelem, G. (1978): Effect of prostacyclin (PGI_2) on platelet adhesion to rabbit arterial subendothelium. *Prostaglandins*, 16:17–22.
49. Hirsh, J., Street, D., Cade, J. F., and Amy, H. (1973): Relation between bleeding time and platelet connective tissue reaction after aspirin. *Blood*, 41:369–377.
50. Hladovec, J. (1979): Is the antithrombotic activity of "antiplatelet" drugs based on protection of endothelium. *Thromb. Haemos.*, 41:774–778.
51. Hollander, W., Kramsch, D. M., Franzblau, C., Paddock, J., and Colombo, M. A. (1974): Suppression of atheromatous fibrous plaque formation by anti-proliferative and anti-inflammatory drugs. *Circ. Res.*, 34/35 (Suppl. 1):131–141.
52. Höpker, W.-W., Hofmann, W., Weib, J., Zimmerman, R., Walter, E., Dittmar, H.-A., and Weizel, A. (1975): The effect of acetylsalicylic acid, extremely restricted movement and a cholesterol-rich diet on atheromatosis of the rabbit aorta: Comparative investigations. *Virchows Arch. (Pathol. Anat.)*, 367:307–323.
53. Iatridis, P. G., Iatridis, S. G., Markidou, S. G., and Ragatz, B. H. (1974): In vitro effects of aspirin in fibrinolysis. *Haemostas.*, 3:55–64.
54. Jaffe, E. A., and Weksler, B. B. (1979): Recovery of endothelial cell prostacyclin production after inhibition by low doses of aspirin. *J. Clin. Invest.*, 63:532–535.
55. Jamieson, S. W., Burton, N. A., Reitz, B. A., and Stinson, E. B. (1979): Survival of heart allografts in rats treated with azathioprine and sodium salicylate. *Lancet*, 1:130–131.
56. Jørgensen, K. A., Dyerberg, J., and Stoffersen, E. (1979): Prostacyclin (PGI_2) and the effect of phosphodiesterase inhibitors on platelet aggregation. *Pharmacol. Res. Commun.*, 2:605–612.
57. Kelton, J. G., Hirsh, J., Carter, C. J., and Buchanan, M. R. (1978) Thrombogenic effect of high-dose aspirin in rabbits. Relationship to inhibition of vessel wall synthesis of prostaglandin I_2-like activity. *J. Clin. Invest.*, 62:892–895.

58. Kinlough-Rathbone, R. L., Cazenave, J.-P., Packham, M. A., and Mustard, J. F. (1980): Effect of inhibitors of the arachidonate pathway on the release of granule contents from platelets adherent to collagen. *Lab. Invest.*, 42:28–34.

59. Kirmser, R., Berger, H. J., Cohen, L. S., and Wolfson, S. (1976): Effect of indomethacin, a prostaglandin inhibitor, on epicardial ST elevation and myocardial flow after coronary occlusion. *Circulation*, (Suppl. II), 54:194.

60. Kocsis, J. J., Hernandovich, J., Silver, M. J., Smith, J. B., and Ingerman, C. (1973): Duration of inhibition of platelet prostaglandin formation and aggregation by ingested aspirin or indomethacin. *Prostaglandins*, 3:141–144.

61. Kurien, V. A., and Oliver, M. F. (1971): Free fatty acids during acute myocardial infarction. *Prog. Cardiovasc. Dis.*, 13:361–373.

62. Lapetina, E. G., Chandrabose, K. A., and Cuatrecasas, P. (1978): Ionophore A23187- and thrombin-induced platelet aggregation: Independence from cyclo-oxygenase products. *Proc. Natl. Acad. Sci. U.S.A.*, 75:818–822.

63. Lapetina, E. G., Schmitges, C. J., Chandrabose, K., and Cuatrecasas, P. (1977): Cyclic adenosine 3',5'-monophosphate and prostacyclin inhibit membrane phospholipase activity in platelets. *Biochem. Biophys. Res. Commun.*, 76:828–835.

64. Leone, G., Agostini, A., DeCrescenzo, A., and Bizzi, B. (1979): Platelet heterogeneity. Relationship between buoyant density, size, lipid peroxidation and platelet age. *Scand. J. Haematol.*, 23:204–210.

65. Link, K. P., Overman, R. S., Sullivan, W. R., Huebner, C. F., and Scheel, L. D. (1943): Studies on the hemorrhagic sweet clover disease. XI. Hypoprothrombinemia in the rat induced by salicylic acid. *J. Biol. Chem.*, 147:463–474.

66. Linos, A., Worthington, J. W., O'Fallon, W., Fuster, V., Whisnant, J. P., and Kurland, L. T. (1978): Effect of aspirin on prevention of coronary and cerebrovascular disease in patients with rheumatoid arthritis. A long-term follow-up study. *Mayo Clin. Proc.*, 53:581–586.

67. Loveday, C., and Eisen, V. (1973): Suppression of lymphocyte transformation by salicylates. *Lancet*, 2:676.

68. McIntyre, B. A., Philp, R. B., and Inwood, M. J. (1978): Effect of ibuprofen on platelet function in normal subjects and hemophiliac patients. *Clin. Pharmacol. Ther.*, 24:616–621.

69. McKenna, R., Galante, J., Bachmann, F., Wallace, D. L., Kaushal, S. P., and Meredith, P. (1980): Prevention of venous thromboembolism after total knee replacement by high-dose aspirin or intermittent calf and thigh compression. *Br. Med. J.*, 1:514–517.

70. McKenzie, L. S., Horsburgh, B. A., Ghosh, P., and Taylor, T. K. F. (1976): Effect of anti-inflammatory drugs on sulphated glycosaminoglycan synthesis in aged human articular cartilage. *Ann. Rheum. Dis.*, 35:487–497.

71. Majerus, P. W., and Stanford, N. (1977): Comparative effects of aspirin and diflunisal on prostaglandin synthetase from human platelets and sheep seminal vesicles. *Br. J. Clin. Pharmacol.*, 4:15S–18S.

72. Marcus, A. J. (1978): The role of lipids in platelet function. *J. Lipid Res.*, 19:793–826.

73. Masotti, G., Galanti, G., Poggesi, L., Abbate, R., and Neri Serneri, G. G. (1979): Differential inhibition of prostacyclin production and platelet aggregation by aspirin. *Lancet*, 2:1213–1216.

74. Menon, S. I. (1970): Aspirin and blood fibrinolysis. *Lancet*, 1:364.

75. Merino, J., Livio, M., Rajtar, G., and de Gaetano, G. (1980): Salicylate reverses in vitro aspirin inhibition of rat platelet and vascular prostaglandin generation. *Biochem. Pharmacol.*, 29:1093–1096.

76. Moncada, S., Gryglewski, R., Bunting, S., and Vane, J. R. (1976):An enzyme isolated from arteries transforms prostaglandin endoperoxides to an unstable substance that inhibits platelet aggregation. *Nature*, 263:663–665.

77. Moncada, S., Gryglewski, R. J., Bunting, S., and Vane, J. R. (1976): A lipid peroxide inhibits the enzyme in blood vessel microsomes that generates from prostaglandin endoperoxides the substance (prostaglandin X) which prevents platelet aggregation. *Prostaglandins*, 12:715–736.

78. Moncada, S., and Korbut, R. (1978): Dipyridamole and other phosphodiesterase inhibitors act as antithrombotic agents by potentiating endogenous prostacyclin. *Lancet*, 1:1286–1289.

79. Moncada, S., Korbut, R., Bunting, S., and Vane, J. R. (1978): Prostacyclin is a circulating hormone. *Nature*, 273:767–768.

80. Moncada, S., and Vane, J. R. (1978): Pharmacology and endogenous roles of prostaglandin endoperoxides, thromboxane A_2 and prostacyclin. *Pharmacol. Rev.*, 30:293–331.

81. Moncada, S., and Vane, J. R. (1979): The role of prostacyclin in vascular tissue. *Fed. Proc.*, 38:66–71, 1979.
82. Moncada, S., and Vane, J. R. (1979): Mode of action of aspirin-like drugs. In: *Advances in Internal Medicine*, vol. 24, edited by G. H. Stollerman, pp. 1–22. Year Book Medical Publishers, Chicago.
83. Moroz, L. A. (1977): Increased blood fibrinolytic activity after aspirin ingestion. *N. Engl. J. Med.*, 296:525–529.
84. Moschos, C. B., Haider, B., De La Cruz, Jr., C., Lyons, M. M., and Regan, T. J. (1978). Antiarrhythmic effects of aspirin during nonthrombotic coronary occlusion. *Circulation*, 57:681–684.
85. Mustard, J. F., and Packham, M. A. (1978): Platelets, thrombosis and drugs. In: *Cardiovascular Drugs*, vol. 3, *Antithrombotic Drugs*, edited by G. S. Avery, pp. 1–83. Adis Press, New York.
86. Mustard, J. F., and Packham, M. A. (1980): Are aspirin and sulfinpyrazone useful in the prevention of myocardial infarction, strokes or venous thromboembolism? In: *Controversies in Therapeutics*, edited by L. Lasagna, pp. 319–332. W. B. Saunders, Philadelphia.
87. Nasjletti, A., and Malik, K. U. (1979): Relationships between the kallikrein-kinin and prostaglandin systems. *Life Sci.*, 25:99–110.
88. Needleman, P., Kulkarni, P. S., and Raz, A. (1977): Coronary tone modulation: Formation and actions of prostaglandins, endoperoxides, and thromboxanes. *Science*, 195:409–412.
89. O'Brien, J. R. (1968): Effects of salicylates on human platelets. *Lancet*, 1:779–783.
90. O'Brien, J. R., Finch, W., and Clark, E. (1970): A comparison of an effect of different anti-inflammatory drugs on human platelets. *J. Clin. Pathol.*, 23:522–525.
91. O'Grady, J., and Moncada, S. (1978): Aspirin: A paradoxical effect on bleeding time. *Lancet*, 2:780.
92. Okuma, M., Steiner, M., and Baldini, M. (1971): Studies on lipid peroxides in platelets. II. Effect of aggregating agents and platelet antibody. *J. Lab. Clin. Med.*, 77:728–742.
93. Opelz, G., Terasaki, P. I., and Hirata, A. A. (1973): Suppression of lymphocyte transformation by aspirin. *Lancet*, 2:478–480.
94. Pachman, L. M., Esterly, N. B., and Giacomoni, D. (1973): Suppression of lymphocyte transformation by aspirin. *Lancet*, 2:1212–1213.
95. Packham, M. A. (1978): Methods for detection of hyper-sensitive platelets. *Thromb. Haemost.*, 40:175–195.
96. Palmoski, M. J., and Brandt, K. D. (1979): Effect of salicylate on proteoglycan metabolism in normal canine articular cartilage in vitro. *Arthritis Rheum.*, 22:746–754.
97. Peters, H. D., Dinnendahl, V., and Schönhöfer, P. S. (1975): Mode of action of antirheumatic drugs on the cyclic 3',5'-AMP regulated glycosaminoglycan secretion in fibroblasts. *Naunyn. Schmiedebergs Arch. Pharmacol.*, 289:29–40.
98. Philp, R. B. (1979): Experimental animal models of arterial thrombosis and the screening of platelet-inhibiting, anti-thrombotic drugs: A review. *Methods Findings Exp. Clin. Pharmacol.*, 1:197–224.
99. Pick, R., Chediak, J., and Glick, G. (1979): Aspirin inhibits development of coronary atherosclerosis in cynomolgus monkeys (Macaca fascicularis) fed an atherogenic diet. *J. Clin. Invest.*, 63:158–162.
100. Pickett, W. C., Austen, K. F., and Goetzl, E. J. (1979): Inhibition by non-steroidal anti-inflammatory agents of the ascorbate-induced elevations of platelet cyclic GMP levels. *J. Cyclic Nucleotide Res.*, 5:197–209.
101. Pinckard, R. N., Hawkins, D., and Farr, R. S. (1968): In vitro acetylation of plasma proteins, enzymes and DNA by aspirin. *Nature*, 219:68–69.
102. Quick, A. J. (1966): Salicylates and bleeding: The aspirin tolerance test. *Am. J. Med. Sci.*, 252:265–269.
103. Riegelman, S. (1971): The kinetic disposition of aspirin in human. In: *Aspirin, Platelets and Stroke. Background for a Clinical Trial*, edited by W. S. Fields and W. K. Hass, pp. 105–114. W. H. Green, St. Louis.
104. Rittenhouse-Simmons, S. (1979): Production of diglyceride from phosphatidylinositol in activated human platelets. *J. Clin. Invest.*, 63:580–587.
105. Rome, L. H., Lands, W. E. M., Roth, G. J., and Majerus, P. W. (1976): Aspirin as a quantitative acetylating reagent for the fatty acid oxygenase that forms prostaglandins. *Prostaglandins*, 11:23–30.
106. Ross, R., and Vogel, A. (1978): The platelet-derived growth factor. *Cell*, 14:203–210.

107. Roth, G. J., and Siok, C. J. (1978): Acetylation of the NH_2-terminal serine of prostaglandin synthetase by aspirin. *J. Biol. Chem.*, 253:3782–3784.
108. Schafer, A. I., Cooper, B., O'Hara, D., and Handin. R. I. (1979): Identification of platelet receptors for prostaglandin I_2 and D_2. *J. Biol. Chem.*, 254:2914–2917.
109. Schönhöffer, P. S., Sohn, J., Peters, H. D., and Dinnendahl, V. (1973): Effects of sodium salicylate and acetylsalicylic acid on the lipolytic system. *Biochem. Pharmacol.*, 22:629–637.
110. Schwartz, A. D. (1974): A method for demonstrating shortened platelet survival utilizing recovery from aspirin effect. *J. Pediatr.*, 84:350–354.
111. Scialla, S. J., Speckart, S. F., Haut, M. J., and Kimball, D. B. (1979): Alterations in platelet surface sialyltransferase activity and platelet aggregation in a group of cancer patients with a high incidence of thrombosis. *Cancer Res.*, 39:2031–2035.
112. Siegl, A. M., Smith, J. B., and Silver, M. J. (1979): Selective binding site for [^{3}H] prostacyclin on platelets. *J. Clin. Invest.*, 63:215–220.
113. Siegel, M. I., McConnell, R. T., and Cuatrecasas, P. (1979): Aspirin-like drugs interfere with arachidonate metabolism by inhibition of the 12-hydroperoxy-5,8,10,14-eicosatetraenoic acid peroxidase activity of the lipoxygenase pathway. *Proc. Natl. Acad. Sci. U.S.A.*, 76:3774–3778.
114. Smith, J. B., Ingerman, C. M., and Silver, M. J. (1976): Malondialdehyde formation as an indicator of prostaglandin production by human platelets. *J. Lab. Clin. Med.*, 88:167–172.
115. Smith, J. B., Ogletree, M. L., Lefer, A. M., and Nicolaou, K. C. (1978): Antibodies which antagonise the effects of prostacyclin. *Nature*, 274:64–65.
116. Smith, J. B., and Willis, A. L. (1971): Aspirin selectively inhibits prostaglandin production in human platelets. *Nature (New Biol.)*, 231:235–237.
117. Smith, M. J. H. (1975): Prostaglandins and aspirin: An alternative view. *Agents Actions*, 5:315–317.
118. Smith, M. J. H., and Dawkins, P. D. (1971): Salicylate and enzymes. *J. Pharm. Pharmacol.*, 23:729–744.
119. Smith, M. J. H., Ford-Hutchinson, A. W., Walker, J. R., and Slack, J. A. (1979): Aspirin, salicylate, and prostaglandins. *Agents Actions*, 9:483–487.
120. Snider, D. E., and Parker, C. W. (1976): Aspirin effects on lymphocyte cyclic AMP levels in normal human subjects. *J. Clin. Invest.*, 58:524–527.
121. Stanford, N., Roth, G. J., Shen, T. Y., and Majerus, P. W. (1977): Lack of covalent modification of prostaglandin synthetase (cyclo-oxygenase) by indomethacin. *Prostaglandins*, 13:669–675.
122. Steer, M. L., MacIntyre, D. E., Levine, L., and Salzman, E. W. (1980): Is prostacyclin a physiologically important circulating anti-platelet agent? *Nature*, 283:194–195.
123. Stone, D. B., Brown, J. D., and Steele, A. A. (1969): Effect of sodium salicylate on induced lipolysis in isolated fat cells of the rat. *Metabolism*, 18:620–624.
124. Stoner, J., Manganiello, V. C., and Vaughan, M. (1973): Effects of bradykinin and indomethacin on cyclic GMP and cyclic AMP in lung slices. *Proc. Natl. Acad. Sci. U.S.A.*, 70:3830–3833.
125. Stuart, M. J., Murphy, S., and Oski, F. A. (1975): Simple nonradioisotope technique for the determination of platelet life-span. *N. Engl. J. Med.*, 292:1310–1313.
126. Turner, S. R., Tainer, J. A., and Lynn, W. S. (1975): Biogenesis of chemotactic molecules by the arachidonate lipoxygenase system of platelets. *Nature*, 257:680–681.
127. Valeri, C. R., and Feingold, H. (1974): Hemostatic effectiveness of liquid-preserved platelets stored at 4°C or 22°C and freeze-preserved platelets stored with 5 percent DMSO at − 150°C or stored with 6 percent DMSO at − 80°C. In: *Platelets: Production, Function, Transfusion, and Storage*, edited by M. G. Baldini and S. Ebbe, pp. 377–391. Grune and Stratton, New York.
128. Vane, J. R. (1971): Inhibition of prostaglandin synthesis as a mechanism of action of aspirin-like drugs. *Nature (New Biol.)*, 231:232–235.
129. Vargaftig, B. B. (1978): Salicylic acid fails to inhibit generation of thromboxane A_2 activity in platelets after in vivo administration to the rat. *J. Pharm. Pharmacol.*, 30:101–104.
130. Vargaftig, B. B. (1978): The inhibition of cyclo-oxygenase of rabbit platelets by aspirin is prevented by salicylic acid and by phenanthrolines. *Eur. J. Pharmacol.*, 50:231–241.
131. Vik-Mo, H., Hove, K., and Mjøs, O. D. (1978): Effects of sodium salicylate on plasma insulin concentration and fatty acid turnover in dogs. *Acta Physiol. Scand.*, 103:113–119.
132. Vik-Mo, H., and Mjøs, O. D. (1977): Effect of sodium salicylate and acetylsalicylic acid on epicardial ST-segment elevation during coronary artery occlusion in dogs. *Scand. J. Clin. Lab. Invest.*, 37:287–294.
133. Vik-Mo, H., and Mjøs, O. D. (1978): Mechanisms for inhibition of free fatty acid mobilization by nicotinic acid and sodium salicylate in canine subcutaneous adipose tissue in situ. *Scand. J. Clin. Lab. Med.*, 38:209–216.

134. Villa, S., Livio, M., and de Gaetano, G. (1979): The inhibitory effect of aspirin on platelet and vascular prostaglandins cannot be completely dissociated. *Br. J. Haematol.*, 42:425–431.
135. Weiss, H. J., Aledort, L. M., and Kochwa, S. (1968): The effect of salicylates on the hemostatic properties of platelets in man. *J. Clin. Invest.*, 47:2169–2180.
136. Weiss, H. J., Tschopp, T. B., and Baumgartner, H. R. (1975): Impaired interaction (adhesion-aggregation) of platelets with the subendothelium in storage-pool disease and after aspirin ingestion. A comparison with von Willebrand's disease. *N. Engl. J. Med.*, 293:619–623.
137. Whitehouse, M. W. (1965): Some biochemical and pharmacological properties of anti-inflammatory drugs.*Prog. Drug Res.*, 8:321–429.
138. Wood, L. (1972): Aspirin and myocardial infarction. *Lancet*, 2:1021–1022.
139. Woodbury, D. M., and Fingl, E. (1975): Analgesic-antipyretics, anti-inflammatory agents, and drugs employed in the therapy of gout. In: *The Pharmacological Basis of Therapeutics*, edited by L. S. Goodman and A. Gilman, pp. 325–343. Macmillan, New York.
140. Yue, K. T. N., Davis, J. W., and Aldridge, E. G. (1973): Effect of aspirin and benadryl on human platelet oxidative phosphorylation and aggregation. *Thromb, Diath. Haemorrh.*, 30:577–585.
141. Zucker, M. B., and Peterson, J. (1970): Effect of acetylsalicylic acid, other nonsteroidal anti-inflammatory agents, and dipyridamole on human blood platelets. *J. Lab. Clin. Med.*, 76:66–75.

Acetylsalicylic Acid: New Uses for an Old Drug,
edited by H. J. M. Barnett, J. Hirsh, and
J. F. Mustard. Raven Press, New York © 1982.

DISCUSSION

J. Hirsh: Is there any good evidence that patients who take enteric-coated acetylsalicylic acid tablets are less likely to experience gastrointestinal side effects? Also, do patients absorb acetylsalicylic acid or just salicylate if they take enteric-coated products?

J. J. Thiessen: Studies have suggested that enteric-coated products are less harmful to the gastrointestinal tract, but a number of these are open to question. A prodrug, benorylate, has been demonstrated to have less adverse effects, and it has been suggested that as one increases lipid solubility of the agent, gastrointestinal bleeding may decrease. The benorylate study was published by Croft in the *British Medical Journal* in 1972.

The performance of enteric-coated acetylsalicylic acid preparations is still in doubt, and we await the results of large-scale evaluations. The matter has been further confused because many of the enteric-coated products have been reformulated in recent years to ensure that they dissolve in the intestinal contents. However, in our experience, failures in absorption are not uncommon even after reformulation, and it also appears that certain individuals just do not absorb enteric-coated products well. It has recently been suggested that a patient who is a poor absorber of one enteric-coated preparation will probably be a poor absorber of the others.

J. W. D. McDonald: I will be reviewing some of the evidence for the differential effect of enteric-coated and compressed acetylsalicylic acid tablets a little later, and I expect that Dr. Jick will comment as well.

T. Yaksh: Could Drs. Thiessen or Packham comment on the kinetics of passage of salicylates into the brain, as measured in the cerebrospinal fluid? Because acetylsalicylic acid has a central antipyretic action, how much gets into the brain? Also, relative to the differential effects of salicylates and acetylsalicylic acid, could they comment on central versus peripheral prostaglandin synthetase?

M. Packham: The tissues that seem to be most affected by acetylsalicylic acid are those directly bathed by the blood, namely platelets and the cells of the vessel walls.

Thiessen: Work to date suggests that cerebrospinal fluid levels, like saliva levels, relate to the free concentration of salicylic acid found in plasma. Gary Graham in Australia has shown that patients can be monitored by measuring drug levels in saliva. I am not aware of any study that demonstrates the same relationship for cerebrospinal fluid, but I suspect it is so.

Yaksh: In terms of the blood-brain barrier, does it not seem probable that acetylsalicylic acid is largely ionized at the pH of blood and for this reason would have difficulty in crossing the barrier?

Thiessen: No, I don't think so. The same thing is true for the penicillins, which do cross the blood-brain barrier.

K. E. Cooper: In the early 1960s, Grundman gave rabbits intravenous sodium salicylate and estimated the amount of salicylate in the brain. Blood levels of 35 to 55 mg/100 μl plasma salicylate, concentrations of 1 to 7 mg/100 μl, and brain tissue concentrations of 0.67 to 3.2 mg/100 g were found.

Weissmann: The salicylates are organic anions, and almost all cells have facilitated organic anion transport systems that are inhibited by SITS (4-acetamido-4'-iso-thiocyanos-tilbene-2,2'-disulfonate), DIDS (4,4'-diisothiocyano-2,2'-stilbene disulfonate), pyridoxal phosphate, and probenecid. This explains the way they are handled by renal tubular cells and how they compete with urate for transport sites. Thus, mass-action solubility laws do not apply because the membranes of most cells, including those of the neurons and endothelial cells, possess facilitated transport mechanisms.

McDonald: Dr. Weissmann gave us a good deal of information about the synthesis of prostaglandins by polymorphonuclear leukocytes and the effects of various drugs on them. Dr. Packham has pointed out that sodium salicylate, which appears to be anti-inflammatory in some respects, is a weak inhibitor. Is it possible that another cell line is involved, which salicylate inhibits effectively? Is it possible that cells other than the polymorph are inhibited by all of the nonsteroidal anti-inflammatory drugs, including sodium salicylate?

Weissmann: In each cell of the peripheral blood—macrophages, monocytes, the various polymorphonuclear leukocytes, platelets and lymphocytes—sodium salicylate appears to have a weak effect on cyclo-oxygenase. However, we do not know what putative mediators of inflammation they may release that could be inhibited by sodium salicylate.

McDonald: Do you know of any clinical evidence that sodium salicylate may inhibit the effect of acetylsalicylic acid or of the other nonsteroidal anti-inflammatory drugs? Is it possible that it has an antagonistic rather than additive action to acetylsalicylic acid, in patients with rheumatoid disease, for example?

Weissmann: In the last 8 years, I have visited many of the rheumatology centers in the United States, Canada, and Europe. Most of the physicians treating patients for rheumatoid arthritis seem to treat them with mixtures of anti-inflammatory agents. Whether this is good or not is hard to determine, but it seems to work clinically. Controlled studies of such *ad lib.* mixtures have not been carried out. Most patients who have had rheumatoid arthritis or osteoarthritis for many years have mixed their drugs and have taken a wide variety of drugs.

Hirsh: For what length of time does acetylsalicylic acid in therapeutic doses turn off thromboxane synthesis in platelets? The literature is confusing and difficult to interpret.

McDonald: Measurement of malondialdehyde formation has shown that some of the suppressed activity has returned in 24 hours, and this has been confirmed by other groups measuring the return of platelet function following a single acetylsalicylic acid tablet. We have studied the return of cyclo-oxygenase activity in washed platelets following a single ingestion of acetylsalicylic acid, and have found a similar pattern; that is, 24 hours after ingestion, 10% of the activity has returned. This is the figure that one might expect based on the turnover time for platelets, if megakaryocytes are not affected or if the platelets they produce after having been acetylated regenerate their cyclo-oxygenase enzyme activity. J. Bryan Smith in Philadelphia has found similar results. Dr. Majerus's group obtained conflicting results by measuring the ability of washed platelets to accept radioactive acetate from radioactive acetylsalicylic acid *in vitro*, following a dose of acetylsalicylic acid—and presuming that enzyme is completely acetylated, it cannot accept radioactive acetate. This result is sometimes described as a measurement of enzyme activity, but it is not. In most circumstances it can relate very closely to enzyme activity, but may not in all. But the controversy does not end there. If the synthesis of thromboxane by platelets is studied in plasma, as opposed to a buffer system, 24 hours after the dose of acetylsalicylic acid, one does not find the 10% increase in thromboxane B_2 detectable by radioimmunoassay. There appears to be a difference between the results in the washed platelet system and in platelets in platelet-rich plasma.

There are a number of possible explanations. First, Dr. Majerus has suggested that our platelet suspensions contain contaminating leukocytes, which synthesize thromboxane and either recover quickly or turn over very quickly. We do not believe this to be the case, because we have studied concentrated suspensions of leukocytes and have not been able to detect much thromboxane formation. It has something to do with the effect of plasma albumin on the cyclic endoperoxides and the pathway they follow after formation by cyclo-oxygenase. Thus, if we are measuring the correct products, we may be able to show that they are formed in plasma at 24 hours.

Packham: It is important to point out that the presence of only 10% of platelets that have not been exposed to acetylsalicylic acid will restore the aggregating ability of the remainder to normal levels. Megakaryocytes should be able to resynthesize cyclo-oxygenase, and that is why the lag phase in the experiments done by Dr. Majerus's group is surprising.

McDonald: The testing of acetylation may create a problem. Those samples in which there was only 2% or 5% activity are based on a small number of counts—and I am not certain one can differentiate between zero and 10%.

Mustard: Another problem we face relates to the separation of platelets from blood. New platelets have a slightly different density and we may be sampling different platelet populations—and it is difficult to get 100% recovery. While Dr. Weissmann has convinced us that prostaglandins do not tell the whole story of inflammation, I am convinced that acetylation of cyclo-oxygenase, in those tissues reached by acetylsalicylic acid, explains some of these effects.

Returning to my first question, what is the tissue distribution of acetylsalicylic acid following a single dose? Obviously the blood cells are affected. Does acetylsalicylic acid penetrate the whole wall of the blood vessel? Does it reach muscle? Do we get a gradient of acetylation in tissues, depending on the degree and rate of diffusion and rate of acetyl-salicylic acid hydrolysis? It seems reasonable to expect that other pathways are involved in inflammation and that these agents, particularly salicylate, are affecting some of these. To what extent are they influenced?

Thiessen: Concerning tissue distribution, the information is just not available, primarily because we have only recently developed the analytical procedures for such measurements.

McDonald: What evidence do we have for any other pathway that may be affected by these agents, other than the two described?

Weissmann: Acetylsalicylic acid does not seem to affect the peripheral action and release of histamine, serotonin, or other vasoactive amines. It has no effect on the release of platelet-activating factor or the eosinophil chemotactic factor of anaphylaxis. It has no effect on the transformation of prekallekrein to kallekrein and activation of the kinins. It has no effect on leucokinin action on leucokininogen, in the formation of acid kinins. It has no reproducible effect on any of the known complement components or on activation of the complement systems, in the fluid phase compartment.

Of the materials released from cells, it has no effect on lysosomal hydrolases, although indomethacin, which is a cyclo-oxygenase and phospholipase inhibitor, does have such an action. It has no effect on the generation of superoxide anion or the free radicals derived therefrom.

It also has no effect on release of the mediators of delayed hypersensitivity from lymphocytes—lymphokine liberation.

Of all the effects that have been studied with respect to release of the mediators of inflammation, the only ones that appear to be affected and of which I am aware, involve the cyclo-oxygenase pathway and the newly described one of Cuatracasas. I cannot name a new mediator of inflammation that is inhibited by either sodium salicylate or acetylsalicylic acid.

McDonald: With respect to the role of platelets as mediators of some aspects of inflammation and immunologic reaction, is there any possibility that nonsteroidal anti-inflammatory drugs, acetylsalicylic acid in particular, exert their effects by inhibiting platelet function rather than by influencing polymorph function?

Weissmann: In blood, the two chief actors in the events that follow injury are platelets and neutrophils. Neutrophils cannot migrate unless vascular "gaps" have been formed in the endothelium, either by histamine or by materials released from platelets and basophils.

Consequently, even though this effect on platelets may be part of the explanation, it does not explain it in terms of chemotaxis. Most of the effects on neutrophils that have been described relate to neutrophil movement, and just getting a neutrophil to the site does not guarantee that it is going to dump its hydrolases or do damage. I believe prostaglandins and the whole group of arachidonic acid-derived metabolites make only a modest contribution to the drama of inflammation—no more than 5 to 12%.

Reilly: Concerning volume of distribution, I believe Dr. Thiessen's figure was somewhere between 7 and 15 liters. This does not approach extracellular fluid volume. If salicylic acid were distributed into total body water, as are the barbiturates, it would be about 1 liter/kg. However, this is much lower and indicates they may not go much beyond the systemic circulation.

Thiessen: You are correct. The apparent volume of distribution is quite low. This is generally attributed to the fact that these compounds are highly plasma-protein bound, restricting their distribution throughout the body. However, this is misleading, because the unbound molecule may still distribute throughout the total body water.

Reilly: A computer simulation of the dose-dependent kinetics of acetylsalicylic acid shows a dramatic difference between dosages of 1 g/day and 3 g/day. This could have a great effect on the pharmacological action of the drug in certain diseases, specifically thrombosis and hemostasis. What is it that is increasing? Why is it increasing and is it pharmacologically active?

Thiessen: The computer simulation of which you speak demonstrates the accumulation of salicylic acid in the body as the dose is increased from 0.5 g every 8 hours to 1.0 g every 8 hours. It is salicylic acid that is increasing and this is caused by saturation of the two pathways—the formation of salicyluric acid and phenolic-like glycuronide. These are the primary pathways responsible for this accumulation. The role of plasma protein displacement is also crucial, simply because salicylic acid can displace acetylsalicylic acid and thus prevent it from exerting its acetylating effect. Vargaftig has investigated the acetylation, not only of platelets (The inhibition of cyclo-oxygenase of rabbit platelets by aspirin is prevented by salicylic acid and by phenanthrolines. *Eur. J. Pharmacol.*, 50:231–241, 1978), but also of isolated proteins. He has demonstrated that if one begins with a high concentration of salicylic acid relative to acetylsalicylic acid used as the challenge, and then adds acetylsalicylic acid, one does not get nearly the acetylation obtained if only acetylsalicylic acid is added. The danger in extrapolating low-dose to high-dose studies arises because of the displacement or inhibition of the activity of the acetyl moiety.

Wassenaar: Could someone briefly comment on the metabolites of salicylate and their activities?

Packham: I have examined the literature concerning the effects of gentisic acid. Much of this work has been done in rats, which convert a great deal of salicylate to gentisic acid. Humans convert much less salicylate to gentisic acid.

Thiessen: In short, it is highly unlikely that metabolites contribute much to the drug effect. Levels are exceedingly low—especially those of glucuronide and gentisic acid—relative to the salicylic acid and tend to be low even relative to acetylsalicylic acid. Remember, gentisic acid is excreted as only 2 or 3% of the original dose.

Acetylsalicylic Acid: New Uses for an Old Drug,
edited by H. J. M. Barnett, J. Hirsh, and
J. F. Mustard. Raven Press, New York © 1982.

Effects of Acetylsalicylic Acid on Gastric Mucosa

John W. D. McDonald

Department of Medicine, University of Western Ontario, London, Ontario, Canada N6A 5A5

Epidemiological studies show a strong association between regular, heavy acetylsalicylic acid intake and both benign gastric ulcer and major upper gastrointestinal hemorrhage but no link between acetylsalicylic acid use and duodenal ulcer. Direct endoscopic studies have demonstrated that acetylsalicylic acid produces mucosal lesions (erythema) in approximately 80% of patients with rheumatic diseases; the incidence of erosions and gastric ulcer was approximately 40% and 15%, respectively. In 30 to 50% of patients with gastric mucosal lesions, including ulcer, there were no accompanying gastrointestinal symptoms. Therefore, the incidence of gastric mucosal lesions in regular acetylsalicylic acid users is high and is not accurately reflected by symptoms.

The mechanism of the acetylsalicylic acid effect on gastric mucosa is not fully elucidated. Although topically applied acetylsalicylic acid induces changes in gastric mucosa and permits back diffusion of H^+ ions, parenterally administered acetylsalicylic acid is also ulcerogenic. There is evidence that the inhibition of synthesis of prostaglandins is an essential component of the acetylsalicylic acid effect. Gastric acid is also required, since cimetidine protects against acetylsalicylic acid-induced lesions in experimental animals. Gastric mucosal preparations actively synthesize prostaglandins from arachidonic acid. Synthesis is blocked by acetylsalicylic acid and other nonsteroidal anti-inflammatory drugs (NSAID). NSAID can produce gastric ulceration in experimental animals. Treatment with PGE_2, synthetic PGE_2 analogs, and other prostaglandins protects against ulcer formation. A protective effect against acetylsalicylic acid-induced "micro bleeding" has also been demonstrated in humans.

Various efforts to protect against the adverse acetylsalicylic acid effect include the use of cimetidine to block acid production or antacids to neutralize acids. The use of enteric-coated acetylsalicylic acid is based on the assumption that the topical effect of acetylsalicylic acid is very important. One clinical study has shown a reduced incidence of gastric erosions with an enteric-coated preparation.

Mailing address: Dr. J.W.D. McDonald, University of Western Ontario, University Hospital, P.O. Box 5339, "A", London, Ontario, Canada N6A 5A5

It has long been recognized by clinicians and patients that acetylsalicylic acid may produce gastrointestinal symptoms. Probably the best known objective evidence of an association between acetylsalicylic acid use and gastric ulcer is provided by an epidemiological study whose results are summarized below. More recently, the importance of endoscopic assessment in defining the true extent and frequency of lesions induced by acetylsalicylic acid has come to be appreciated. However, because of the difficulties of performing endoscopies on large numbers of patients, clinical investigations have also relied on "microbleeding" studies, which measure the loss of small volumes of radioactively labeled red cells from the gastrointestinal tract. These studies have contributed important information, and animal research has also provided some information about the mechanisms of acetylsalicylic acid damage.

EPIDEMIOLOGIC STUDIES

The purpose of the Boston Collaborative Drug Surveillance Program (10) was to evaluate the relationship between a number of drugs, taken regularly before hospital admission, and a variety of diseases. This study, which embraced 25,000 consecutive medical and surgical admissions to 24 Boston hospitals, showed that heavy regular use of acetylsalicylic acid (at least 4 days/week for at least 3 months) was associated with major upper gastrointestinal bleeding and with uncomplicated benign gastric ulcer. No definite association with either uncomplicated or bleeding duodenal ulcer was demonstrated. Several previous case control studies had suggested a relationship between acetylsalicylic acid use and bleeding, but the data in all were inconclusive because of two defects. First, the studies evaluated the acetylsalicylic acid intake only for periods immediately before admission. It was impossible to know whether the patients were taking acetylsalicylic acid for disorders that had caused the bleeding. Also, the controls were inadequate for other factors that might relate both to acetylsalicylic acid use and to bleeding, such as cancer and cirrhosis.

ENDOSCOPIC STUDIES IN PATIENTS WITH RHEUMATOID ARTHRITIS

More recently, the wider use of endoscopy has demonstrated a high frequency of gastric lesions in patients on chronic acetylsalicylic acid therapy. The prospective study of Silvoso and colleagues (19) was particularly informative. Endoscopic studies were performed on 82 patients with rheumatoid arthritis and other rheumatic disorders who had been taking at least 2,600 mg of acetylsalicylic acid/day for 3 or more months, and the findings were compared with those in 45 normal subjects who did not have arthritis and were not taking acetylsalicylic acid. None of the patients had a history of peptic ulcer disease, had consulted a physician about major gastrointestinal symptoms, or had had an upper GI series; 24 of the 82 were taking an additional nonsteroidal anti-inflammatory drug. Whereas only 2 of 45 controls showed gastric erythema and none had erosions or ulcer, a majority of acetylsalicylic acid users had gastric lesions (Table 1). Of these, 62 (76%) had erythema, 33 (40%) had erosions, and 14 (17%) had gastric ulcers. Erosions, ulcers, or both were present in over 50%. Of the 14 patients with ulcer, 4 were completely asymp-

TABLE 1. *Endoscopically defined lesions in arthritic patients after receiving ASA*

	Type of ASA preparation		
	Regular	Buffered	Enteric-coated
Erythema	24/30	13/16	25/36
Erosions	13/30	11/16	9/36
Ulcer	7/30	5/16	2/36

From Silvoso, G.R. et al. (19), with permission.

tomatic, 3 admitted to symptoms retrospectively (after having been told that they had an ulcer), and 7 described burning or gnawing epigastric pain relieved by antacids. The high incidence of lesions and low incidence of symptoms were quite striking. This relationship has been confirmed in other studies in which endoscopy was performed. Other clinical studies have shown that the high incidence of ulcer is related to acetylsalicylic acid use rather than to the underlying rheumatoid disease. These studies emphasize that in clinical trials the physician can place little reliance on symptoms in his assessment of the frequency of gastrointestinal side effects in patients receiving acetylsalicylic acid. Radiographic studies, which underestimate the evidence of ulcer, show that 3 to 7% of patients with rheumatoid arthritis who are receiving acetylsalicylic acid have gastric ulcer; the incidence in controls is less than 1%.

INFLUENCE OF BUFFERED AND ENTERIC-COATED PREPARATIONS

Various attempts have been made to reduce the damaging effect of acetylsalicylic acid on gastric mucosa. For example, it has been shown that the ingestion of amounts of alkali sufficient to neutralize hydrochloric acid is effective. Approximately 18 mmoles of $NaHCO_3$ are required to neutralize the effects of 650 mg of acetylsalicylic acid (2). Unfortunately, the usual buffered preparations of acetylsalicylic acid contain only 3 mmoles of $NaHCO_3$. Silvoso's study (Table 1) showed that gastritis and ulcer were as common in rheumatoid subjects taking buffered acetylsalicylic acid as in those taking regular acetylsalicylic acid. However, erosions and ulcers were much less frequent in patients taking equivalent doses of enteric-coated acetylsalicylic acid; the difference was statistically significant. It should be emphasized, however, that the superiority of enteric-coated preparations has not been established in a randomized double-blind trial.

BIOCHEMICAL PATHOLOGY

There is no doubt that direct contact of acetylsalicylic acid with the gastric mucosa, as occurs following ingestion of acetylsalicylic acid tablets or after the instillation of acetylsalicylic acid solutions directly into the stomach of animals, causes damage. There is also some evidence that acetylsalicylic acid may cause damage after it reaches the mucosa through its blood supply, as occurs after parenteral administration of acetylsalicylic acid or ingestion of enteric-coated acetylsalicylic acid.

Topical Effects of Acetylsalicylic Acid

Davenport (5) has proposed that acetylsalicylic acid denatures mucus and breaks the mucosal barrier that protects the gastric mucosa against back diffusion of H^+. Various workers have shown that topically applied acetylsalicylic acid decreases the potential difference that exists between tissue and gastric lumen. This change occurs within 10 min of acetylsalicylic acid ingestion and persists for approximately 1 hr, so that it appears and subsides too quickly to have a systemic effect. Rainsford (13) has proposed that the following series of events occurs when acetylsalicylic acid comes in contact with gastric mucosa. Particles form as acetylsalicylic acid tablets disintegrate and disperse, and drug molecules cause aggregation and sloughing of the protective mucus layer. This change permits the molecules to penetrate the barrier and induce direct denaturation of underlying mucus-secreting cells. The cells then become susceptible to additional destruction through the action of HCl. Acetylsalicylic acid accumulates in large quantities inside parietal cells, and these cells become disrupted. Capillaries also become disrupted, and the inhibitory effect of acetylsalicylic acid on platelet function may contribute to focal hemorrhage.

Importance of HCl: Effects of Anticholinergics and Cimetidine

The absorption of acetylsalicylic acid is favored by the low pH of the gastric contents, and there is evidence that the acetylsalicylic acid effect requires HCl. Hydrochloric acid favors absorption of acetylsalicylic acid. A pH of less than 3 depresses ionization of the acetylsalicylate ion, and the nonionized form more rapidly crosses the cell membrane. Inside the cell, ionization occurs again.

MacKercher (11) studied the effects of acetylsalicylic acid on the potential difference across gastric mucosa and on mucosal histology as observed in suction biopsies before and during cimetidine therapy. In control subjects who did not receive cimetidine, gastric pH fell slowly, and after acetylsalicylic acid the mean potential difference fell from −49 to −39 mV. After treatment with 300 mg of cimetidine, the mean potential difference rose to −63 V as pH rose to 6.9. Acetylsalicylic acid induced a drop in potential difference, but not to a value less than the basal level. Brodie (3) had previously shown that anticholinergic drugs that inhibit HCl secretion protect against the effect of acetylsalicylic acid.

Baseline biopsies of normal gastric mucosa taken before acetylsalicylic acid administration showed only 2.4% of abnormal surface epithelial cells. Damage was defined as apical membrane disruption associated with nuclear destruction. Ten minutes after administration of acetylsalicylic acid, at the time of peak change in potential difference, this damage increased to 19% of surface cells; within an hour this value fell to 9%. Pretreatment with cimetidine reduced the cell damage caused by acetylsalicylic acid to only 4.4% of surface cells. The interpretation of some of these results is confounded by the observation that cimetidine may protect against acetylsalicylic acid-induced lesions even when HC1 is perfused directly into the stomach, suggesting that this drug may exert an undefined effect in addition to its antisecretory action.

SYSTEMIC EFFECTS OF ACETYLSALICYLIC ACID

A number of observations suggest that acetylsalicylic acid reaching the mucosa through the circulation is also capable of causing damage. For example, Kauffman (8) has shown that in rats the i.v. infusion of acetylsalicylic acid in a large dose (40 mg/kg) produces gastric ulceration. The serum salicylate levels achieved in these experiments were extremely high, in the range of .3 to .4 mg/ml, and it may be that only such high acetylsalicylic acid levels produce mucosal damage by this route.

Gastric Mucosal Prostaglandin Synthesis

There is evidence that one mechanism by which acetylsalicylic acid damages the mucosa is the inhibition of cyclo-oxygenase activity in cells of the gastric mucosa, with resulting inhibition of prostaglandin synthesis. This removes from the gastric luminal surface a prostaglandin that may protect the mucosa against the effects of HC1. A number of animal and human studies show that prostaglandin E_2 and analogs of this compound and other prostaglandins (17,18,20) exert such a protective effect. Cohen (4) showed that the oral administration of PGE_2 to normal human volunteers prevented the microbleeding induced by acetylsalicylic acid. Blood loss in control subjects increased from approximately 1 ml/day to a mean of 8 ml/day after ingestion of acetylsalicylic acid in a dosage of 600 mg q.i.d. No such increase occurred in subjects who were receiving PGE_2 in a dosage of 1 mg q.i.d. More recently, Johansson (7) reported that the administration of PGE_2 in a 1 mg dose protected arthritic patients taking indomethacin in a dosage of 50 mg t.i.d. Again, the assessment of the protective effect of the prostaglandin was the measurement of microbleeding. On the basis of endoscopic studies, Karim and colleagues (6) suggested that PGE_2 accelerates healing of gastric ulcers, although this has not been confirmed in large-scale trials.

The mediator that has attracted major interest has been PGE_2, which has been demonstrated in gastric juice. Pace-Asciak (12) showed some time ago that the whole homogenate of rat stomach produced 6-keto-$PGF_{1\alpha}$, a substance later recognized to be the hydrolysis product of PGI_2, or prostacyclin. We have recently shown that the mucosa produces not only PGE_2 and 6-keto-$PGF_{1\alpha}$, but also thromboxane (1).

Figure 1 shows a radiochromatographic scan of the prostaglandins synthesized by bovine gastric mucosal microsomes. The solid line shows that thromboxane B_2 (TXB_2) is a major product of the mucosa. This property appears not to be shared

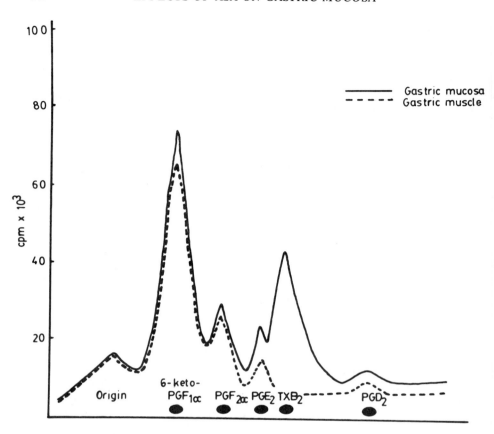

FIG. 1.   Radiochromatogram scan of thin-layer chromatogram of radioactively labeled products following incubation of gastric mucosal and muscle microsomes with ^{14}C-arachidonic acid. From Ali, M., and McDonald, J.W.D (1a), with permission.

by the gastric muscle (dotted line), which produces mainly PGI$_2$. Both tissues form PGI$_2$ and other prostaglandins.

We have also shown that the increase in HC1 secretion that follows pentagastrin stimulation in human volunteers is accompanied by an increase in the output of the prostacyclin hydrolysis product 6-keto-PGF$_{1\alpha}$. We are not yet certain about increases in thromboxane formation under these conditions. Thromboxane B$_2$ is unstable at acid pH. As others have reported, PGE$_2$ is also synthesized under these conditions. The actual cellular site of prostaglandin synthesis in the mucosa is uncertain. If prostaglandins protect against the effects of HC1, one can visualize a physiologic role for increased synthesis following pentagastrin stimulation. In experiments with the bovine abomasum (true stomach, which physiologically resembles the human stomach), we have shown that prostaglandin synthesis from endogenous substrate occurs more rapidly in mucosa from the body of the stomach containing the parietal

TABLE 2. *Radioimmunoassay estimation of 6-keto-PGF₁ synthesized by bovine gastric mucosal and muscle microsomes incubated with arachidonate*

	6-keto-PGF$_1\alpha$ (pmoles/g wet tissue)		
	Endogenous	Saline + AA	Indomethacin + AA
Gastric muscle	17.00 ± 2.90	689.10 ± 91.90	27.00 ± 9.40
Gastric mucosa			
Pylorus	[a]24.30 ± 1.90	659.40 ± 113.50	53.20 ± 20.80
Body	[b]127.00 ± 17.20	1158.50 ± 327.00	127.00 ± 16.20
Cardia	71.60 ± 1.35	1162.10 ± 300.00	97.20 ± 18.90

Results shown represent the mean of 4 or 5 independent experiments (± S.E.M.).
[a]Significantly different from body ($p < 0.01$) and cardia ($p < 0.001$) by Student's t-test.
[b]Significantly different from cardia ($p < 0.05$) by Student's t-test.
From Ali, M., and McDonald, J.W.D. (1a), with permission.

cell than in mucosa from the pyloric or cardiac regions (Table 2) (1a). In the latter areas, the addition of arachidonic acid as substrate greatly enhances prostaglandin synthesis. These studies suggest that parietal cells are the source of the prostaglandin and thromboxane synthesis that follows pentagastrin stimulation. This would be anticipated if the synthesis of these compounds has a physiologic role. The effect of pentagastrin stimulation may be to make substrate available to the cyclo-oxygenase of parietal cells.

Prostaglandins have been shown to exert a number of effects on gastric mucosa, any of which could reasonably account for the protective effect. Prostaglandin E$_2$ inhibits gastric acid secretion (14), but the dosages of PGE$_2$ required to protect the mucosa are lower than those required to block acid secretion. Prostaglandins alter blood flow because of their effects on vascular tone, and it was postulated that the protective action was caused by control of mucosal blood flow (9). However, animal experiments have now shown that other prostaglandins that exert opposite effects on blood flow may be equally protective of the mucosa (15), an observation that appears to rule out control of blood flow as the principal mechanism. Prostaglandins have a direct protective effect on mucosa. Robert has shown that topical application of prostaglandins to mucosa *in vitro* offers protection against a wide variety of agents, including hydrochloric acid, bile salts, and absolute alcohol (11,16). The mechanism of this cytoprotective effect is unknown. Although prostaglandins stimulate secretion of gastric mucus, this effect requires so long an interval that it could not confer an immediate protective effect (15). Prostaglandins may participate in some way in the maintenance of tight junctions between mucosal cells.

CONCLUSION

The principal side effect of acetylsalicylic acid treatment is damage to the gastric mucosa. It appears that this effect, which requires the presence of acid, can be avoided or reduced by neutralizing or preventing acid secretion. The topical effect of acetylsalicylic acid is probably the important one, and it may be possible to avoid damage by the use of enteric-coated acetylsalicylic acid. There is evidence that the damaging effect is due to inhibition of synthesis of a protective prostaglandin and that oral administration of prostaglandins may protect against acetylsalicylic acid effects.

REFERENCES

1. Ali, M., Zamecnik, J., Cerskus, A. L., Stoessl, A. S., Barnett, W. H., and McDonald, J. W. (1977): Synthesis of thromboxane B_2 and prostaglandins by bovine gastric mucosal microsomes. *Prostaglandins*, 14:819–827.

1a. Ali, M., and McDonald, J. W. (1980): Synthesis of thromboxane B_2 and 6-keto prostaglandin $F_{1\alpha}$ by bovine gastric mucosal and muscle microsomes. *Prostaglandins*, 20:245–254.

2. Bowen, B. K., Krause, W. J., and Ivey, K. J. (1977): Effect of sodium bicarbonate on aspirin-induced damage and potential difference changes in human gastric mucosa. *Br. Med. J.*, 2:1052–1055.

3. Brodie, D. A., and Chase, B. J. (1967): Role of gastric acid in aspirin-induced gastric irritation in the rat. *Gastroenterology*, 53:604–610.

4. Cohen, M. M., and Pollett, J. M. (1976): Prostaglandin E_2 prevents aspirin and indomethacin damage to human gastric mucosa. *Surg. Forum*, 27:400–401.

5. Davenport, H. W. (1964): Gastric mucosal injury by fatty and acetylsalicylic acid. *Gastroenterology*, 46:245–253.

6. Fung, W. P., Karim, S. M. M., and Tye, C. Y. (1974): Effect of 15(R)-15-methyl prostaglandin E_2 methyl ester on healing of gastric ulcers. Controlled endoscopic study. *Lancet*, 2:10–12.

7. Johansson, C., Kollberg, B., Nordemar, R., Samuelson, K., and Bergström, S. (1980): Protective effect of prostaglandin E_2 in the gastrointestinal tract during indomethacin treatment of rheumatic diseases. *Gastroenterology*, 78:479–483.

8. Kauffman, G. L., and Grossman, M. I. (1978): Prostaglandin and cimetidine inhibit antral ulcers produced by parenteral salicylates (abstract). *Gastroenterology*, 74:1049.

9. Konturek, S. J., Bowman, J., Lancaster, C., Hancher, A. J., and Robert, A. (1979): Cytoprotection of the canine gastric mucosa by prostacyclin: possible mediation by increased mucosal blood flow. *Gastroenterology*, 76:1173.

10. Levy, M. (1974): Aspirin use in patients with major upper gastrointestinal bleeding and peptic-ulcer disease. *N. Engl. J. Med.*, 290:1158–1162.

11. MacKercher, P. A., Ivey, K. J., Baskin, W. N., and Krause, W. J. (1977): Protective effect of Cimetidine on aspirin-induced gastric mucosal damage. *Ann. Intern. Med.*, 87:676–679.

12. Pace-Asciak, C., and Wolfe, L. S. (1971): A novel prostaglandin derivative formed from arachidonic acid by rat stomach homogenates. *Biochemistry*, 10:3657–3664.

13. Rainsford, K. D. (1977): Gastrointestinal and other side effects from the use of aspirin and related drugs; biochemical studies on the mechanisms of gastrotoxicity. *Agents Actions*, (Suppl.) 1:59–70.

14. Robert, A. (1975): Antisecretory, antiulcer, cytoprotective, and diarrheogenic properties of prostaglandins. In: *Advances in Prostaglandin and Thromboxane Research*, Vol. 1, edited by B. Samuelsson and R. Paoletti, pp. 507-521. Raven Press, New York.

15. Robert, A. (1979): Cytoprotection by prostaglandins. *Gastroenterology*, 77:761–767.

16. Robert, A., Nezamis, J. E., Lancaster, C., and Hanchar, A. J. (1979): Cutoprotection by prostaglandins in rats. Prevention of gastric necrosis produced by alcohol, HCl, NaOH, Hypertonic HaCl, and thermal injury. *Gastroenterology*, 77:433–443.

17. Robert, A. R., Schultz, J. R., Nezamis, J. E., and Lancaster, C. (1976): Gastric antisecretory and antiulcer properties of PHE_2, 15-methyl PGE_2, and 16,16-dimethyl PGE_2. Intravenous oral and intrajejunal administration. *Gastroenterology*, 70:359–370.

18. Robert, A., Stowe, D. F., and Nezamis, J. E. (1971): Prevention of duodenal ulcers by administration of prostaglandin E_2 (PGE_2). *Scand. J. Gastroenterol.*, 6:303–305.

19. Silvoso, G. R., Ivey, K. J., Butt, J. H., Lockard, O. O., Holt, S. D., Sisk, C., Brishin, W. N., MacKercher, P. A., and Hewett, J. (1979): Incidence of gastric lesions in patients with rheumatic disease on chronic aspirin therapy. *Ann. Intern. Med.*, 91:517–520.

20. Whittle, B. J. R., Boughton-Smith, N. K., Moncada, S., and Vane, J. R. (1978): Actions of prostacyclin (PGI_2) and its product, 6-oxo-$PGF_{1\alpha}$ on the rat gastric mucosa *in vivo* and *in vitro*. *Prostaglandins*, 15:955–967.

Acetylsalicylic Acid: New Uses for an Old Drug,
edited by H. J. M. Barnett, J. Hirsh, and
J. F. Mustard. Raven Press, New York © 1982.

Controversial Aspects of the Use of Acetylsalicylic Acid as an Antithrombotic Agent

John G. Kelton

Department of Pathology and Medicine, McMaster University Medical Centre, Hamilton, Ontario, Canada L8N 3Z5

Although for many years it was believed that the blood vessel wall was a passive participant in thrombosis, recent evidence refutes this hypothesis. Cells within the vessel walls synthesize prostaglandin I_2 (PGI_2), or prostacyclin, a potent vasodilator and inhibitor of platelet aggregation. This prostaglandin has the opposite actions to the platelet prostaglandin derivative thromboxane A_2 (TXA_2), which is a vasoconstrictor and platelet aggregator. Acetylsalicylic acid inhibits the prostaglandin pathway. Since PGI_2 is synthesized from the same prostaglandin precursors as platelet TXA_2, it is theoretically possible that the use of acetylsalicylic acid to inhibit platelet TXA_2 could in fact augment thrombosis by inhibiting vessel wall PGI_2. *In vitro* evidence suggests that the endothelial prostaglandin pathway is inhibited by the same acetylsalicylic acid concentration that inhibits the platelet prostaglandin pathway. Direct animal experiments and indirect human evidence suggest that a much higher concentration of acetylsalicylic acid *in vivo* is required to initiate or augment thrombosis through inhibition of vessel wall PGI_2.

Another important difference exists between the vessel wall and platelet prostaglandin pathways. Since platelets lack nuclei, they cannot regenerate new enzymes following inactivation by acetylsalicylic acid. In contrast, endothelial cells can rapidly regenerate inactivated prostaglandin enzymes. Further studies are needed to determine the ideal dosage of acetylsalicylic acid to inactive platelet cyclo-oxygenase yet have little or no effect on vessel wall PGI_2.

Prostaglandin I_2 (PGI_2), a recently described prostaglandin, is synthesized by cells of the vessel wall. Whereas the biochemistry of PGI_2 and its mode of action are understood, its precise physiological role remains uncertain. In this chapter we will briefly review one controversial aspect of PGI_2, its inhibition by acetylsalicylic acid, and present evidence illustrating how animal models of thrombosis may provide better understanding of the role of PGI_2. This summary will also include recent animal thrombotic studies that may prove useful in explaining why the antithrombotic benefit of antiplatelet agents is often restricted to males.

THE EFFECTS OF ACETYLSALICYLIC ACID UPON PROSTAGLANDIN I_2

Prostaglandin I_2: Discovery and Characterization

Platelets do not adhere to undamaged endothelial cells. Possible reasons include:

a. electrostatic repulsion caused by the negatively charged surfaces of the platelet and endothelial cell,

b. production of adenosinediphosphatase (ADP-ase) by the endothelial cells (26,27), and

c. production of prostaglandin I_2 (PGI$_2$) (48).

PGI$_2$ (its stable hydrolysis product, 6-keto PGF$_{1\alpha}$) was initially described in 1971 by Pace-Asciak and Wolfe (52), but these investigators did not characterize its biological properties (52). Five years later, Kulkarni et al. (41) described its vasoactive properties, and subsequently, Moncada and co-workers (48) described the generation of prostaglandin I_2 from prostaglandin precursors and the biological properties of PGI$_2$. PGI$_2$ is the most potent naturally occurring inhibitor of platelet aggregation known, and is also a strong vasodilator (11,35). These properties directly oppose the action of the platelet prostaglandin-like material, thromboxane A$_2$ (21).

Prostaglandin I_2 has the "I" designation because it was the next prostaglandin after prostaglandin H to be characterized. The subscript "2" indicates that it is derived from fatty acids with two unsaturated bonds (32). It has a half-life at 37°C, pH 7.4 of 2–5 min, and at 22°C its activity is gone in 20 min. It is stable in an alkaline medium, particularly when the pH is greater than 8.4 (11,31,35,48). Depending upon the type of tissue tested, PGI$_2$ produces either contraction or relaxation. For example, PGI$_2$ relaxes rabbit mesenteric and celiac arteries and constricts rabbit stomach strip, chick rectum, and guinea pig trachea and ilium (48). These effects can be used to test for its presence (46).

Assays for PGI$_2$

Part of the confusion surrounding PGI$_2$ relates to the multitude of assays that have been devised to measure it. Each of these assays has inherent associated difficulties, and their sensitivities may vary considerably.

Direct chemical assays

At present, there are no direct chemical assays for PGI$_2$. Theoretically, it should be possible to develop thin-layer radiochromatography or radioimmunoassays for immunogenically similar PGI$_2$ analogs (9,17,60). However, the pH instability of PGI$_2$ makes the collection and processing of samples using these assays very difficult.

Direct biological assays

A number of biological assays measure PGI$_2$ activity. Investigators using these assays to quantitate PGI$_2$ must confirm that the substance they are measuring is in fact PGI_2 through such techniques as pH lability, effects on isolated tissues, or measurement of the stable end products of PGI_2. PGI_2 mediates its biological effects through elevation of cyclic AMP (22,62). Therefore, as might be expected, direct measurement of cyclic AMP is likely to prove the most sensitive assay for PGI_2 activity. Recently, such an assay was described and was reported to be sensitive to concentrations of PGI_2 as low as 100 fM (43). Many clinicians measure PGI_2 by assessing its effects on platelet aggregation. Concentrations of PGI_2 as low as 5 to 10nM can be quantitated by measuring the inhibition of ADP or arachidonic acid aggregation (15). Measuring inhibition of serotonin release can achieve a several-fold increase in sensitivity, to a 10pM concentration(67). PGI_2 also causes relaxation of certain tissues at concentrations as low as 10pM (23). However, although these tissue perfusion assays can be used to demonstrate the presence of PGI_2, they are difficult to modify into quantitative assays.

Indirect assays

The breakdown products for PGI_2 can be measured on thin-layer radiochromatography (45), but these systems are insensitive and difficult to quantitate. *In vitro*, most PGI_2 is hydrolyzed to the stable end-product 6-keto-$PGF_{1\alpha}$. A radioimmunoassay has been developed that is sensitive to levels of 6-keto-$PGF_{1\alpha}$ as low as 10pM (56), but recent investigations raise concern about it. Although, *in vitro*, most PGI_2 changes to 6-keto-$PGF_{1\alpha}$, *in vivo* perfusion studies have demonstrated that a significant quantity of PGI_2 is initially oxidized and subsequently hydrolyzed to 6, 15-diketo-$PGF_{1\alpha}$ among other products (57,61,68). Therefore, clinicians using 6-keto-$PGF_{1\alpha}$ radioimmunoassays as an index of PGI_2 activity should demonstrate significant cross-reactivity of their antisera to 6, 15-diketo-$PGF_{1\alpha}$.

The Effects of PGI_2 on Platelet Function

Platelet adhesion

The effects of PGI_2 on platelet adhesion have been assessed in a variety of models. Using a nonflowing system, Czervionke et al. (14) measured the adhesion of chromium(^{51}Cr)-labeled platelets to endothelial cell monolayers.

Adhesion was inhibited by 10nM concentrations of exogenous PGI_2. Similar results were reported in 1980 by Fry et al., who noted that PGI_2 concentrations greater than 25nM maximally inhibited thrombin-induced adhesion of ^{51}Cr-labeled platelets to venous endothelial cells (18). These investigators also reported that it took a much higher concentration of PGI_2 to inhibit the adhesion of platelets to fibroblasts.

Weiss and Turitto (66) assessed the ability of PGI_2 to inhibit adhesion in a flowing system. At high rates of shear (2,600/sec), a 56% reduction in adhesion occurred at 10nM concentrations of exogenous PGI_2. Lower rates of shear (800/sec) required significantly greater concentrations of PGI_2 to inhibit adhesion. At very high rates of shear (2,600/sec), much lower concentrations of PGI_2 could inhibit adhesion.

Higgs et al. (28) reported similar results, and also noted an inverse relationship between the rate of shear and the concentration of exogenous PGI_2 required to inhibit platelet adhesion. Weiss and Turitto (66) also reported that, unlike the weak inhibitory effect of PGI_2 upon platelet adhesion, PGI_2 was a potent inhibitor of platelet thrombus formation.

These observations suggest that high concentrations of PGI_2 are required to inhibit adhesion to endothelial cells (following thrombin stimulation), and only very high concentrations inhibit adhesion to the subendothelial cell layers. Such concentrations are unlikely to be reached in the body (13). In contrast, once the platelet monolayer has formed, PGI_2 can readily limit the size of the subsequent platelet thrombus.

Platelet aggregation

Platelets have a specific receptor for PGI_2 (47,58,59). The binding of PGI_2 to platelets results in stimulation of adenyl cyclase, which causes the production of cyclic AMP from ATP. The cAMP, in turn, causes sequestration of ionized calcium within the platelet cytoplasm and, as a result, most platelet functions are inhibited by PGI_2. PGI_2 inhibits shape change, pseudopod extension, and primary and secondary wave aggregation. The amount of PGI_2 required to inhibit aggregation is related to the strength of the stimulus. Thus, 5 to 10pM concentrations of PGI_2 totally inhibit an ADP-induced aggregation, whereas much higher concentrations are required to inhibit thrombin-induced aggregation (15). This effect of PGI_2 on platelet aggregation occurs *in vitro* as well as *in vivo*. The infusion of 1 µg/min into rabbits reduces by 50% the mortality following the infusion of arachidonic acid (5). Similarly, platelet thrombi are inhibited by low concentrations of PGI_2 in a variety of animal models (28,66).

Inhibition of PGI₂ Production by Acetylsalicylic Acid

If PGI_2 is physiologically important in limiting thrombus size *in vivo*, the administration of drugs that inhibit its production could conceivably cause or augment thrombosis. The same prostaglandin precursors that in the platelet form thromboxane A_2 and thus cause platelet aggregation in the vessel wall also form prostaglandin I_2 (Fig. 1). Therefore, it is possible that inhibiting the platelet prostaglandins through the administration of acetylsalicylic acid could also inhibit PGI_2 formation and cause thrombosis or augment it.

An early hypothesis ("prostaglandin steal hypothesis") suggested that the platelets were the source of substrate for vessel-wall PGI_2 production (53). The adherence of platelets to the subendothelial layer results in the release of thromboxanes and prostaglandin endoperoxides. According to this hypothesis, thromboxane A_2 causes further platelet aggregation, and the endoperoxides enter adjacent endothelial cells where they are transformed into PGI_2, which is then released and blocks further aggregation. Although the hypothesis is physiologically attractive, it suggests that the administration of acetylsalicylic acid, which results in inhibition of the platelet prostaglandin pathway, could also block production of vessel-wall PGI_2 because it

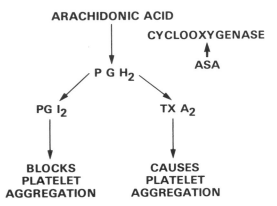

FIG. 1. Diagram of the prostaglandin pathway in platelets and the vessel wall. (TXA$_2$ is produced in platelets, whereas PGI$_2$ is produced in the vessel wall.)

would also block the release of platelet endoperoxides. There is abundant evidence that this theory is incorrect. Both thrombocytopenic and nonthrombocytopenic animals have similar production of vessel wall PGI$_2$ (64). Furthermore, as Needleman and colleagues (49) have reported, the infusion of arachidonic acid but not prostaglandin endoperoxides into an isolated rabbit heart preparation results in the production of PGI$_2$. It is possible that the polar endoperoxides are unable to pass into the endothelial and subendothelial cells. The same investigators have also reported that unless platelet thromboxane synthetase is inhibited, very little platelet endoperoxide is released from the platelets (50). In summary, inhibition of platelet cyclo-oxygenase does not *indirectly* inhibit vessel wall PGI$_2$ production.

Perhaps a more important question is whether *direct* inhibition of vessel wall cyclo-oxygenase can inhibit PGI$_2$. As noted in Fig. 1, vessel-wall cyclo-oxygenase synthesizes the endoperoxides that ultimately form PGI$_2$. Therefore, direct inhibition of the cyclo-oxygenase by acetylsalicylic acid results in decreased production of PGI$_2$.

Two factors may influence the inhibition of PGI$_2$ by acetylsalicylic acid. The first is the sensitivity of vessel-wall cyclo-oxygenase to inhibition by acetylsalicylic acid, and the second relates to the ability of acetylsalicylic acid to diffuse from the circulation into the endothelial and subendothelial layers without being hydrolyzed. Investigations on the effect of acetylsalicylic acid on the vessel-wall PGI$_2$ production will now be summarized.

In isolated enzyme preparations

In 1978, Burch et al. (10), using the techniques they had used earlier to define the dosage of acetylsalicylic acid that inhibits platelet cyclo-oxygenase, studied the inhibition of PGI$_2$ production by acetylsalicylic acid. They reported that inhibition of vessel wall cyclo-oxygenase by acetylsalicylic acid required a concentration some 60 to 250 times higher than was required to inhibit platelet cyclo-oxygenase.

In tissue cultures

In 1977, Baenziger et al. (3) reported that both fibroblasts and smooth muscle cells were capable of synthesizing PGI_2 (quantitated by the inhibition of ^{14}C-serotonin platelet release). They reported that inhibition of PGI_2 production by these tissues was less than one-tenth as sensitive to acetylsalicylic acid as was inhibition of platelet prostaglandin production. In 1979, Czervionke et al. (14) assayed endothelial PGI_2 production using an assay for 6-keto-$PGF_{1\alpha}$. They reported that vessel-wall PGI_2 production was much less sensitive to acetylsalicylic acid than was platelet prostaglandin production. In contrast, Jaffe and co-workers (29) measured PGI_2 production from cultured endothelial cells, using inhibition of platelet serotonin release as an index of PGI_2 activity. They reported that endothelial cell cyclo-oxygenase was as sensitive to inhibition of acetylsalicylic acid as was platelet cyclo-oxygenase.

In vessel wall segments

The inhibition of PGI_2 by acetylsalicylic acid has been assessed *ex vivo*. After infusion of acetylsalicylic acid, vessel wall segments are removed and PGI_2 production is quantitated. These techniques have a number of potential technical difficulties; for example, the basal level of PGI_2 production by vessel wall preparations is highly variable. One potential cause is local thrombin generation during isolation of the segments (8).

In 1978, Basista et al. (4) reported that five times the concentration of acetylsalicylic acid was required to inhibit vessel wall PGI_2 production as was required to inhibit platelet prostaglandin production. In their study, PGI_2 activity was assessed by measuring the inhibition of ADP-induced platelet aggregation.

In 1979, Villa and coworkers (65) investigated the sensitivity of rat platelets and arterial and venous tissue to inhibition by acetylsalicylic acid. PGI_2-like activity was assessed by measuring inhibition of ADP-induced human platelet aggregation. These investigators noted that arterial tissues were seven times less sensitive to the effects of acetylsalicylic acid than were platelets; however, they reported that venous tissue was equally sensitive to the action of acetylsalicylic acid.

With in vitro *models of thrombosis*

In 1978, Kelton et al. (37) related the effects of pretreatment with varying doses of acetylsalicylic acid to the size of thrombi in damaged rabbit jugular vein. In this model, the animals were treated with the test agent and 30 min later the jugular veins were damaged in a standard fashion. The volume of thrombus that developed over the next 6 hr was quantitated by measuring accretion of iodine-125 rabbit fibrinogen. Doses of acetylsalicylic acid as low as 3 mg/kg inhibited platelet-prostaglandin production in this model; however, augmentation of thrombosis did not occur until massive doses of acetylsalicylic acid were used (200 mg/kg). Doses of sodium salicylate that produced equivalent metabolic aberration did not increase thrombus size (Fig. 2). Thrombus was also augmented when tranylcypromine (a PGI$_2$-synthetase inhibitor) was instilled into the vein segments.

Of·interest was the observation that there was no thrombogenic activity if an interval of 2½ hr was interposed between the administration of acetylsalicylic acid and the injury to the jugular veins. This suggested to us that vessel wall PGI$_2$ was rapidly regenerated, presumably through the synthesis of new cyclo-oxygenase enzyme. This hypothesis has been confirmed by other groups using more direct measurements of PGI$_2$ recovery.

Other investigators, using *in vivo* models of thrombosis, have also demonstrated that a much higher dose of acetylsalicylic acid is required to cause or augment thrombosis than to inhibit platelet prostaglandin production (1,16,40,69). These observations suggest that in animals there is a wide differential between the inhibition of platelet-prostaglandin production and the inhibition of vessel-wall PGI$_2$ as assessed by augmentation of thrombosis. However, as with many aspects of PGI$_2$, this area remains controversial. Recently, Buchanan et al. (7) suggested that relatively low concentrations of acetylsalicylic acid result in both inhibition of PGI$_2$ production and increased platelet accumulation onto damaged arterial segments in rabbits.

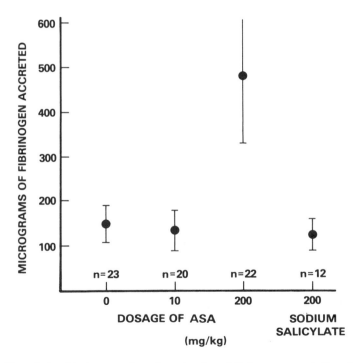

FIG. 2. The relationship between thrombus size (μg of fibrinogen accreted) and dosage of acetylsalicylic acid. In this model of damage-induced venous thrombosis, the rabbits were pretreated with the drug 30 min before the injury. [From Kelton, J. G., et al. (37) with permission.]

In people

One study in which the effect of acetylsalicylic acid on PGI_2 activity in people was measured has been reported. In 1979, Masotti and co-workers (46) measured PGI_2 (stimulated by arm ischemia) by assessing its effect on isolated tissue strips. They determined the dosage of acetylsalicylic acid that inhibited 50% of platelet aggregatory activity (ID_{50}) and the dosage that inhibited 50% of PGI_2 production. Platelet-prostaglandin production was only slightly more sensitive than vessel-wall PGI_2 production to the inhibitory effects of acetylsalicylic acid (ID_{50} of 3.2 to 3.5 mg/kg for platelets and ID_{50} of 4.9 mg/kg for PGI_2). This report is of interest since it suggests that the dosages of acetylsalicylic acid successfully used in most human clinical trials would inhibit PGI_2 production.

Nonetheless, at present there is no evidence that acetylsalicylic acid is thrombotic in humans. This conclusion is based upon a number of observations.

Effects of acetylsalicylic acid on bleeding time. The bleeding time is a simple measure of platelet–vessel wall interaction. The administration of acetylsalicylic acid prolongs the bleeding time through inhibition of platelet function. The cyclo-oxygenase pathway in human platelets is inhibited at doses of acetylsalicylic acid as low as 120 mg, and this dose prolongs the bleeding time and in some situations is antithrombotic. Theoretically, if enough acetylsalicylic acid was given to inhibit vessel wall PGI_2 production, the bleeding time would not be prolonged but would remain normal or potentially shortened. This occurrence has been demonstrated in animals, using either locally administered acetylsalicylic acid or corticosteroids to inhibit PGI_2 (6,7).

In 1978, two groups of investigators suggested that the bleeding time in humans who received high doses of acetylsalicylic acid (2 to 3 g) paradoxically was shortened (51,54). These investigators suggested that in humans this dose of acetylsalicylic acid represented the threshold level for the inhibition of PGI_2. In contrast, a number of other investigators have been unable to demonstrate any shortening of the bleeding time with increasing doses of acetylsalicylic acid as high as 3.9 g (19, 20, 24, 44, 63).

Thrombogenic effects of high-dose acetylsalicylic acid. No studies have been done in which patients were randomized to receive varying doses of acetylsalicylic acid and both the inhibition of PGI_2 and the potential thrombogenicity were assessed. In several studies, however, patients received high doses of acetylsalicylic acid for other reasons, and the occurrence of thrombosis was measured. In 1980, McKenna et al. (44) studied patients who were undergoing orthopedic surgery and were randomized to receive two differerent daily dosages of acetylsalicylic acid. One group received 975 mg/day, while the other received 3.9 g/day. Instead of showing an increased thrombotic tendency, the high-dosage acetylsalicylic acid group demonstrated a significantly lower incidence of venous thrombosis. Although it is possible that the antithrombotic effect of this dosage of acetylsalicylic acid was related to other effects, nonetheless there clearly was no increased thrombogenicity. Patients with rheumatoid arthritis often receive large dosages of acetylsalicylic acid

(3 to 5 g/day) for long periods. In a prospective study of 473 patients with rheumatoid arthritis, Linos et al (42) found no increase in the incidence of cardiovascular or cerebrovascular events when these patients were compared to an age-matched control group. Rather, the men in this study had a 30 to 50% reduction in vascular events.

SEX-RELATED DIFFERENCE IN THE ANTITHROMBOTIC EFFECT

A number of human studies have assessed the effectiveness of acetylsalicylic acid or other antiplatelet agents in preventing arterial thromboembolic disease, venous thrombosis, and thrombosis of arteriovenous shunts. Some of these studies, but not all, have suggested that the major benefit occurs in males (12, 25, 34).

We prospectively studied the potential interaction between acetylsalicylic acid treatment and sex in a randomized study of male and female rabbits, using the previously described model of injury-induced venous thrombosis (38). The results are illustrated in Fig. 3. There was a significant reduction of thrombus size only in the male animals treated with low-dose (10 mg/kg) acetylsalicylic acid. No sex-related differences were observed in the size of thrombus formation in the controls—male and female animals treated with saline. To assess inhibition of the platelet-

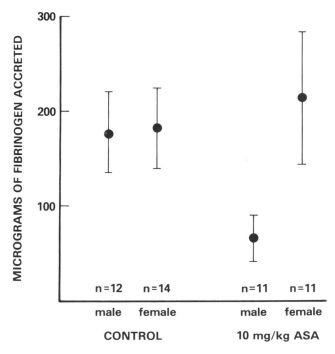

FIG. 3. The relationship between thrombus size (μg of fibrinogen accreted) and the sex of the rabbits. [From Kelton, J. G., et al. (38) with permission.]

prostaglandin pathway, malondialdehyde was measured following stimulation with n-ethylmaleimide. Acetylsalicylic acid treatment produced a significant reduction in MDA production in both sexes, but we detected no sex difference (in MDA production) either before or after acetylsalicylic acid treatment.

These results suggested that male and female rabbits, and, potentially, human platelets, reacted differently after the inhibition of the prostaglandin pathway by acetylsalicylic acid. Further studies were performed to assess the aggregability of human male and female platelets. It has been recognized that platelets from male animals are more sensitive to low levels of aggregating agents than are platelets from female animals (33). It has also been recently reported that the opposite occurs in man; human female platelets are more sensitive to threshold levels of aggregating agents than age-matched human male platelets (30,55). This is surprising, since it is well recognized that human males are at greater risk from thrombosis than are human females. One possible explanation for this observation is that differences in the hematocrit could produce differences in the concentration of ionized calcium, since it is standard practice to collect whole blood into a fixed ratio of citrate anticoagulant without modifying the amount according to the patient's hematocrit. To investigate this possibility, we performed platelet aggregation studies before and after correction of the amount of anticoagulant according to the hematocrit. When platelet aggregation studies were performed in a standard fashion, we noted a significant increase in reactivity of female platelets over male platelets. However, this difference was no longer present after correction for the size of the citrate distribution compartment (39).

Thus, we have concluded that the reported human sex differences in platelet reactivity are an artefact caused by differences in the size of the citrate distribution compartment. We are currently assessing any possible sex-related difference in platelet aggregation *in vitro* before and after the administration of acetylsalicylic acid.

In a further series of experiments, we have demonstrated that hemostatic plug formation is significantly larger in male animals treated with acetylsalicylic acid than in female animals or in sodium salicylate treated animals (36). Although further experimentation is required, these observations suggest that the sex-related differences in the antithrombotic effects of acetylsalicylic acid are related to quantitative differences in the interaction of acetylsalicylic acid-treated platelets and vessel wall.

CONCLUSION

The dosage of acetylsalicylic acid required to inhibit PGI_2 production remains uncertain. However, both *in vitro* and *in vivo* observations suggest that, unlike platelet cyclo-oxygenase—which is inactivated by acetylsalicylic acid for the life-span of that platelet—vessel wall cyclo-oxygenase is rapidly regenerated (within hours) (2). Furthermore, most *in vivo* animal experiments suggest that a much higher dose of acetylsalicylic acid is required to initiate or augment thrombosis than to inhibit platelet prostaglandins. Finally, although the human studies are limited both in design and number of subjects, there is no evidence that high-dose acetylsalicylic acid can cause thrombosis in man.

It is possible that, just as other pathways independent of the prostaglandins lead to platelet aggregation, the vessel wall also has a variety of mechanisms by which to limit thrombosis, and it is only under certain circumstances that inhibition of PGI_2 causes thrombosis in man.

ACKNOWLEDGMENT

Parts of this work were supported by grants from the Canadian and Ontario Heart Foundations.

REFERENCES

1. Amezcua, J. L., Parsons, M., and Moncada, S. (1978): Unstable metabolites of arachidonic acid aspirin and the formation of the haemostatic plug. *Thromb. Res.*, 13:477–488.
2. Baenziger, N. L., Becherer, P. R., and Majerus, P. W. (1979): Characterization of prostacyclin synthesis in cultured human arterial smooth muscle cells, venous endothelial cells and skin fibroblasts. *Cell*, 16:967–974.
3. Baenziger, N. L., Dillender, M. J., and Majerus, P. W. (1977): Cultured human skin fibroblasts and arterial cells produce a labile platelet-inhibitory prostaglandin. *Biochem. Biophys. Res. Commun.*, 78 (1).
4. Basista, M., Dobranowski, J., and Gryglewski, R. J. (1978): Prostacyclin and thromboxane generating systems in rabbit pretreated with aspirin. *Pharmacol. Res. Commun.*, 10:759–763
5. Bayer, B. L., Blass, K. E., and Forster, W. (1979): Anti-aggregatory effect of prostacyclin (PGI_2) in vivo. *Br. J. Pharmacol.*, 66:10–12.
6. Blajchman, M. A., Senyi, A. F., Hirsh, J., Surya, Y., Buchanan, M., and Mustard, J. F. (1979): Shortening of the bleeding time in rabbits by hydrocortisone caused by inhibition of prostacyclin generation by the vessel wall. *J. Clin. Invest.*, 63:1026–1035.
7. Buchanan, M. R., Blajchman, M. A., Dejana, E., Mustard, J. F., Senyi, A. F., and Hirsh, J. (1979): Shortening of the bleeding time in thrombocytopenic rabbits after exposure of jugular vein to high aspirin concentration. *Prostaglandins Med.*, 3:333–342.
8. Buchanan, M. R., Dejana, E., Cazenave, J.-P., Mustard, J. F., and Hirsh, J. (1979): Uncontrolled PGI_2 production by whole vessel wall segments due to thrombin generation *in vivo* and its prevention by heparin. *Thromb. Res.*, 16:551–555.
9. Bunting, S., Moncada, S., Reed, P., Salmon, J. A., and Vane, J. R. (1978): An antiserum to 5,6-dihydro prostacyclin (PGI_1) which also binds prostacyclin. *Prostaglandins*, 15:565–573.
10. Burch, J. W., Baenziger, N. L., Stanford, N., and Majerus, P. W. (1978): Sensitivity of fatty acid cyclooxygenase from human aorta to acetylation by aspirin. *Proc. Natl. Acad. Sci. U.S.A.*, 75:5181–5184.
11. Burch, J. W., and Majerus, P. W. (1979): The role of prostaglandins in platelet function. *Semin. Hematol.*, 16:196–207.
12. Canadian Cooperative Study Group (1979): A randomized trial of aspirin and sulfinpyrazone in threatened stroke. *N. Engl. J. Med.*, 299:53–59.
13. Cazenave, J.-P., Dejana, E., Kinlough-Rathbone, R. L., Richardson, M., Packham, M. A., and Mustard, J. F. (1979): Prostaglandins I_2 and E_1 reduce rabbit and human platelet adherence without inhibiting serotonin release from adherent platelets. *Thromb. Res.*, 15:273–279.
14. Czervionke, R. L., Smith, J. B., Fry, G. L., Hoak, J. C., and Haycraft, D. L. (1979): Inhibition of prostacyclin by treatment of endothelium with aspirin. *J. Clin. Invest.*, 63:1089–1092.
15. Di Minno, G., Silver, M. J., and de Gaetano, G. (1979): Prostaglandins as inhibitors of human platelet aggregation. *Br. J. Haematol.*, 43:637–647.
16. Ellis, E. F., Jones, P. S., Wright, K. F., and Ellis, C. K. (1979): A low dose of oral aspirin inhibits rabbit platelet aggretation but not arterial prostaglandin I_2 synthesis (abstract). Presented at the Fourth International Prostaglandin Conference, Washington, D.C., May 27–31.
17. Fitzpatrick, F. A., and Gorman, R. R. (1978): An antiserum against 9-deoxy-6, 9-epoxy-$PGF_{1\alpha}$ recognizes and binds PGI_2 (prostacyclin). *Prostaglandins*, 15:725–735.

18. Fry, G. L., Czervionke, R. L., Hoak, J. C., Smith, J. B., and Haycraft, D. L. (1980): Platelet adherence to cultured vascular cells: influence of prostacyclin (PGI$_2$). *Blood*, 55:271–275.
19. Girolami, A., Cella, G., Zanon, R. D., Coppelloto, M. G., and Randi, M. L. (1979): Aspirin and bleeding-time (letter). *Lancet* 2:205–206.
20. Godal, H. C., Eika, C., Dybdah, J. G., Daae, L., and Larsen,S.: Aspirin and bleeding-time (letter). *Lancet*, 1:1236.
21. Gorman, R. R. (1979): Modulation of human platelet function by prostacyclin and thromboxane A$_2$. *Fed. Proc.*, 38:83–88.
22. Gorman, R. R., Bunting, S., and Miller, O. V. (1977): Modulation of human platelet adenylate cyclase by prostacyclin (PGX). *Prostaglandins*, 13:377–388.
23. Gryglewski, R. J., and Nicolaou, K. C. (1978): A triple test for screening biological activity of prostacyclin analogues. *Experientia*, 34:1336–1337.
24. Harker, L. A., and Slichter, S. J. (1972): The bleeding time as a screening test for evaluation of platelet function. *N. Engl. J. Med.*, 287:155–159.
25. Harris, W. H., Salzman, E. W., Athanasoulis, C. A., Waltman, A. C., and De Sanctis, R. W. (1977): Aspirin prophylaxis of venous thromboembolism after total hip replacement. *N. Engl. J. Med.*, 297:1246–1249.
26. Heyns, A. du P., Badenhorst, C. J., and Retief, F. P. (1979): A stable non-prostaglandin inhibitor of platelet aggregation in human aorta intima extracts. *S. Afr. Med. J.*, 55:908–910.
27. Heynes, A. du P., van den Berg, D. J., Potgieter, G. M., and Retief, F. P. (1974): The inhibition of platelet aggregation by an aorta intima extract. *Thromb. Diath. Haemorrh.*, 32:417–431.
28. Higgs, E. A., Moncada, A., and Vane, J. R. (1978): Effect of prostacyclin (PGI$_2$) on platelet adhesion to rabbit arterial subendothelium. *Prostaglandins*, 16:17–22.
29. Jaffe, E. A., and Weksler, B. B. (1979): Recovery of endothelial cell prostacyclin production after inhibition by low doses of aspirin. *J. Clin. Invest.*, 63:532–534.
30. Johnson, M., Ramey, W., and Ramwell, P. W. (1975): Sex and age difference in human platelet aggregation. *Nature*, 253:355–357.
31. Johnson, R. A., Lincoln, F. H., Nidy, E. G., Schneider, W. P., Thompson, J. L., and Axen, U. (1978): Synthesis and characterization of prostacyclin, 6-ketoprostaglandin F$_{1\alpha}$, prostaglandin I$_1$, and prostaglandin I$_3$. *J. Am. Chem. Soc.*, 100:7690–7705.
32. Johnson, R. A., Morton, D. R., Kinner, J. H., Whittaker, N., Bunting, S., Salmon, J., Moncada, S., and Vane, J. R. (1976): The chemical structure of prostaglandin X (prostacyclin). *Prostaglandins*, 12:915–928.
33. Johnston, M., and Ramwell, P. W. (1974): Androgen mediated sex difference in platelet aggregation (abstract). *Physiologist*, 17:256A.
34. Kaegi, A., Pineo, G. F., Shimizu, A., Trivedi, H., Hirsh, J., and Gent, M. (1975): The role of sulfinpyrazone in the prevention of arteriovenous shunt thrombosis. *Circulation*, 52:497–499.
35. Kelton, J. G., and Blajchman, M. A. (1980): Prostaglandin I$_2$ (prostacyclin). *Can. Med. Assoc. J.*, 122:175–179.
36. Kelton, J. G., Carter, C. J., and Hirsh, J. (1980): Sex-related differences in the effects of aspirin on hemostatic plug formation in vivo (abstract). *Clin. Res.*, 28:315A.
37. Kelton, J. G., Hirsh, J., Carter, C. J., and Buchanan, M. R. (1978): Thrombogenic effect of high-dose aspirin in rabbits. Relationship to inhibition of vessel wall synthesis of prostaglandin I$_2$-like activity. *J. Clin. Invest.*, 62:892–895.
38. Kelton, J. G., Hirsh, J., Carter, C. J., and Buchanan, M. R. (1978): Sex differences in the antithrombotic effects of aspirin. *Blood*, 52:1073–1076.
39. Kelton, J. G., Powers, P., Julian, J., Boland, V., Carter, C. J., Gent, M., and Hirsh, J. (1980): Sex related differences in platelet aggregation: influence of the hematocrit. *Blood*, 56:38–41.
40. Korbut, R., and Moncada, S. (1978): Prostacyclin (PGI$_2$) and thromboxane A$_2$ interaction in vivo. Regulation by aspirin and relationship with anti-thrombotic therapy. *Thromb. Res.*, 13:489–500.
41. Kulkarni, P. S., Roberts, R., and Needleman, P. (1976): Paradoxical endogenous synthesis of a coronary dilating substance from arachidonate. *Prostaglandins*, 12:337–353.
42. Linos, A., Worthington, J. W., O'Fallon, W., Fuster, V., Whisnant, J. P., and Kurland, L. T. (1978): Effect of aspirin on prevention of coronary and cerebrovascular disease in patients with rheumatoid arthritis. A long-term follow-up study. *Mayo Clin. Proc.*, 53:581–586.
43. McClenaghan, M., and Haslam, R. J. (1980): A sensitive assay for prostacyclin (PGI$_2$) applicable to fresh rabbit blood (abstract). *Fed. Proc.*, 39:323A.
44. McKenna, R., Galante, J., Bachmann, F., Wallace, D. L., Kaushal, S. P., and Meredith, P. (1980): Prevention of venous thromboembolism after total knee replacement by high-dose aspirin or intermittent calf and thigh compression. *Br. Med. J.*, 228:514–517.

45. Marcus, A. J., Weksler, B. B., and Jaffe, E. A. (1978): Enzymatic conversion of prostaglandin endoperoxide H_2 and arachidonic acid to prostacyclin by cultured human endothelial cells. *J. Biol. Chem.*, 253:7138–7141.
46. Masotti, G., Galanti, G., Poggesi, L., Abbate, R., Neri, S. O., and Neri, G. G. (1979): Differential inhibition of prostacyclin production and platelet aggregation by aspirin. *Lancet*, 2:1213–1216.
47. Miller, O. V., and Gorman, R. R. (1979): Evidence for distinct prostaglandin I_2 and D_2 receptors in human platelets. *J. Pharmacol. Exp. Ther.*, 210:134–140.
48. Moncada, S., Gryglewski, R., Bunting, S., and Vane, J. R. (1976): An enzyme isolated from arteries transforms prostaglandin endoperoxides to an unstable substance that inhibits platelet aggregation. *Nature*, 263:663–665.
49. Needleman, P., Bronson, S. D., Wyche, A., Sivakoff, M., and Nicolaou, K. C. (1978): Cardiac and renal prostaglandin I_2. Biosynthesis and biological effects in isolated perfused rabbit tissue. *J. Clin. Invest.*, 61:839–849.
50. Needleman, P., Wyche, A., and Raz, A. (1979): Platelet and blood vessel arachidonate metabolism and interactions. *J. Clin. Invest.*, 63:345–349.
51. O'Grady, J., and Moncada, S. (1978): A paradoxical effect on bleeding time (letter). *Lancet*, 2:780.
52. Pace-Asciak, C., and Wolfe, L. S. (1971): A novel prostaglandin derivative formed from arachidonic acid by rat stomach homogenates. *Biochemistry*, 10:3657–3664.
53. Editorial (1976): P.G.X.: A natural antithrombotic substance. *Lancet*, 2:1005.
54. Rajah, S., Penny, A., and Kester, R. (1978): Aspirin and bleeding time (letter). *Lancet*, 2:1104.
55. Roper, P., Drewinko, B., Hasler, D., Johnston, D., Hester, J., and Freireich, E. J. (1979): Effects of time, platelet concentration, and sex on the human platelet aggregation response. *Am. J. Clin. Pathol.*, 71:263–268.
56. Salmon, J. A. (1978): A radioimmunoassay for 6-keto-prostaglandin $F_{1\alpha}$. *Prostaglandins*, 15:383–397.
57. Salmon, J. A., Mullane, K. M., Dusting, G. J., Moncada, S., and Vane, J. R. (1979): Elimination of prostacyclin (PGI$_2$) and 6-oxo-PGF$_{1\alpha}$ in anaesthetized dogs. *J. Pharm. Pharmacol.*, 31:529–532.
58. Schafer, A. I., Cooper, B., O'Hara, D., and Hardin, R. I. (1979): Identification of platelet receptors for prostaglandin I_2 and D_2. *J. Biol. Chem.*, 254:2914–2917.
59. Siegl, A. M., Smith, J. B., Silver, M. J., Nicolaou, K. C., and Ahern, D. (1979): Selective binding site for (^{3}H) prostacyclin on platelets. *J. Clin. Invest.*, 63:215–220.
60. Smith, J. B., Ogletree, M. A., and Lefer, A. M. (1978): Antibodies which antagonise the effects of prostacyclin. *Nature*, 274:64–65.
61. Sun, F. F., McGuire, J. C., and Taylor, B. M. (1978): Metabolism of prostacyclin (PGI$_2$). *Prostaglandins*, 15:724–735.
62. Tateson, J. E., Moncada, S., and Vane, J. R. (1977): Effects of prostacyclin (PGX) on cyclic AMP concentrations in human platelets. *Prostaglandins*, 13:389–397.
63. Treacher, D., Warlow, C., and McPherson, K. (1978): Aspirin and bleeding-time (letter). *Lancet*, 2:1378.
64. Villa, S., Callioni, A., and de Gaetano, G. (1977): Normal prostacyclin-like activity in vascular tissues from thrombocytopenic rats. *Thromb. Res.*, 11:701–704.
65. Villa, S., Livio, M., and de Gaetano, G. (1979): The inhibitory effect of aspirin on platelet and vascular prostaglandins in rats cannot be completely dissociated. *Br. J. Haematol.*, 42:425–431.
66. Weiss, H. J., and Turitto, V. T. (1979): Prostacyclin (prostaglandin I_2, PGI$_2$) inhibits platelet adhesion and thrombus formation on subendothelium. *Blood*, 33:244–250.
67. Weksler, B. B., Ley, C. W., and Jaffe, E. A. (1978): Stimulation of endothelial cell prostacyclin production by thrombin trypsin and the ionophore A 23187. *J. Clin. Invest.*, 62:923-930.
68. Wong, P. Y.-K., Sun, F. F., and McGiff, J. C. (1978): Metabolism of prostacyclin in blood vessels. *J. Biol. Chem.*, 253:5555–5557.
69. Zimmerman, R., Thiessen, M., Mörl, H., and Weckesser, G. (1979): The paradoxical thrombogenic effect of aspirin in experimental thrombosis. *Thromb. Res.*, 16:843–846.

Acetylsalicylic Acid: New Uses for an Old Drug,
edited by H. J. M. Barnett, J. Hirsh, and
J. F. Mustard. Raven Press, New York © 1982.

Action of Prostaglandin Synthetase Inhibitors on the Ductus Arteriosus: Experimental and Clinical Aspects

*Flavio Coceani and Peter M. Olley

Research Institute and Division of Cardiology, The Hospital for Sick Children, Toronto, Ontario, Canada M5B 1X8

Research in the past few years has proved that a prostaglandin, possibly PGE_2, is responsible for keeping the ductus arteriosus patent in the fetus. This prostaglandin-mediated relaxing mechanism develops at an early age, reaches maximal activity at about 0.7 gestation, and abates thereafter. Conceivably, the loss in prostaglandin activity towards term represents a priming factor for postnatal closure of the vessel. These findings provided the means for pharmacologic manipulation of the ductus in the newborn. Whereas PGE_2, or its structurally related PGE_1, is used for keeping the ductus patent in newborns with certain congenital heart malformations, inhibitors of prostaglandin synthesis are used for closing a persistent ductus in the prematurely born infant. Knowledge of prostaglandin involvement in the ductus arteriosus, and possibly in other fetal functions, has drawn attention to the potential dangers in using acetylsalicylic acid or acetylsalicylic acid-like drugs during pregnancy.

During the past few years, evidence has accrued to prove that prostaglandins and allied compounds are important to fetal homeostasis and adjustments of the fetus at birth. Advances in this area, as in most areas of prostaglandin research, have occurred largely through the use of anti-inflammatory drugs, such as acetylsalicylic acid.

Among the fetal and neonatal functions in which prostaglandins are now implicated, regulation of muscle tone in the ductus arteriosus has a special place for both conceptual and practical reasons. The demonstration that prenatal patency of the ductus is an active process determined by a prostaglandin has led to a reappraisal of the role of this vessel in fetal hemodynamics under both normal and pathological conditions. This knowledge, while providing an effective means for the pharmacologic manipulation of the ductus in the newborn, has drawn attention to the potential dangers to the fetus when the mother is given acetylsalicylic acid or acetylsalicylic

---

*Mailing address: Dr. Flavio Coceani, Research Institute, The Hospital for Sick Children, 555 University Avenue, Toronto, Ontario, Canada M5B 1X8.

acid-like drugs. Moreover, the finding that prostaglandins are well tolerated by the newborn has established a precedent in pediatric therapeutics that is likely to be exploited in several disease states. Indeed, the usefulness of prostaglandins, specifically PGI_2, in managing pulmonary hypertensive disorders of the neonate is currently being evaluated in many centers.

In this chapter, we will review the experimental evidence implicating a prostaglandin in the control of ductal tone, the accent being on the data obtained with inhibitors of prostaglandin synthesis. Clinical experience with the inhibitors in managing persistent patency of the ductus will also be examined. Finally, we will analyze the possible adverse effects of the inhibitors on the fetus.

DUCTUS ARTERIOSUS PATENCY

Biochemical and pharmacological data implicate a prostaglandin, specifically PGE_2, in prenatal patency of the ductus arteriosus (Table 1). Among these data, evidence obtained with inhibitors of prostaglandin synthesis is most compelling. As shown by our work in fetal lambs (Table 2), inhibitors of diverse structure constrict the ductus both *in vitro* (21–23) and *in vivo* (21,72). Their action, though variable in magnitude, may equal that of oxygen. Similar results have been obtained by other investigators studying the same species (14,15,47,54) as well as the rat and the rabbit (85,86). Nonsteroidal anti-inflammatory drugs have been used most often, and their effectiveness as ductus constrictors correlates well with their relative potency in interfering with the cyclo-oxygenase reaction. Whether *in vitro* or *in vivo*, active concentrations of the inhibitors are below the threshold for known unspecific effects. In fact, threshold doses for ductus constriction *in utero* are lower than those required for the anti-inflammatory effect in the adult. Moreover, pharmacologically induced contraction of ductal muscle is promptly and fully reversed by treatment with PGE_1 or PGE_2 (22,30,47,54). Collectively, these data prove that ductal muscle is exquisitely sensitive to the relaxant effect of a prostaglandin and that any fall in the level of the active compound results in sustained contraction.

TABLE 1. *Evidence for the involvement of PGE_2 in prenatal patency of the ductus arteriosus*

1. Ductal tissue from both mature and immature fetuses contains an active enzyme system for synthesizing PGI_2 and its stable byproduct 6-keto-$PGE_{1\alpha}$ and PGE_2, and $PGF_{2\alpha}$ (13,30,73,79,90). Whereas PGI_2 is the major product in specimens of the whole vessel, PGE_2 is thought to be relatively more abundant in the muscle layer (see 20).

2. PGE_2 is a potent ductal relaxant, its action greatly exceeding that of PGI_2 at all gestation ages examined (15–17,19,22,30).

3. Inhibitors of prostaglandin synthesis constrict the fetal ductus *in vitro* (14,15,22,23) and *in vivo* (30,47,54,72,85,86).

4. Reduced glutathione, a compound promoting PGE_2 synthesis (28), relaxes the isolated fetal ductus (21) and its action is nearly completely abolished by pretreatment with indomethacin (*unpublished data*).

TABLE 2. *Constrictor action of inhibitors of prostaglandin synthesis on the lamb ductus arteriosus*

Condition	Control	ETA[a]	Indomethacin		Ibuprofen	
			2.8×10^{-5}M	10 mg/kg/day	4.8×10^{-4}M	20 mg/kg/day
In vitro[b]	3.3 ± 0.5 (9)	4.1 ± 0.3 (7)	9.7 ± 0.4 (4)		6.0 ± 0.5 (6)	
In vivo[c]	27 ± 7 (5)			3.8 ± 1.6 (6)		5.8 ± 2.9 (3)

[a]ETA: 5,8,11,14-eicosatetraynoic acid
[b]Experiments were performed on circular strips of ductus arteriosus from term fetuses. Values (g, grams of tension developed in vitro) indicate the mean (± SEM) tension developed over the applied tension for the number of experiments given in parentheses.
[c]Drugs were given orally to pregnant ewes near term for 3 consecutive days. Values (mm²) indicate the mean (± SEM) lumen area of the vessel at the site of maximal narrowing.

Experiments with acetylsalicylic acid-like drugs also indicate that this prostaglandin-mediated relaxing mechanism develops at an early age (14,23). In fact, the response of the ductus to such drugs is maximal at 0.6 to 0.7 gestation, implying that this mechanism is more active in the premature. However, it must be pointed out that developmental changes, though well documented *in vitro* (14,23), could not be confirmed *in vivo* (81). Reduced bioavailability of the drugs in the developing fetus may explain this apparent inconsistency (81). An additional relevant point is that age-related differences in the sensitivity of the isolated ductus to cyclo-oxygenase inhibitors are most obvious under conditions mimicking neonatal rather than fetal oxygenation. Indeed, an important aspect of the action of the inhibitors is their ability to enhance the response of the immature ductal muscle to oxygen. The latter finding provides the rationale for their use in the prematurely born infant with persistent ductus.

The importance of local versus blood-borne prostaglandins in maintaining ductus patency remains unclear. The occurrence of active prostaglandin-synthesizing enzymes in the ductus and the feasibility of manipulating ductal tone *in vitro* by pharmacological means (Table 1) underline the importance of intramural prostaglandins. However, the demonstration of higher levels of prostaglandins, including possibly PGE_2, in the fetal than in the neonatal circulation (10,33,64,65) implies a role for blood-borne compounds. Consistent with the latter possibility is the finding that the indomethacin-induced constriction of the ductus *in vivo* correlates well with the expected fall in circulating levels of prostaglandins (33). It is quite possible that the PGE_2 acting on ductal muscle is formed both within the vessel wall and outside it.

DUCTUS ARTERIOSUS CLOSURE

Experiments with acetylsalicylic acid and acetylsalicylic acid-like drugs, although crucial for proving the importance of prostaglandins to ductus patency, have also provided some clues to the possible function of these compounds in postnatal closure of the vessel. Early in this research, it was thought that prostaglandins might have a direct role in ductus closure by mediating the constrictor effect of oxygen on ductal muscle (17,89). Consistent with that view was the notion that prostaglandin synthesis requires molecular oxygen (71,82) and the demonstration that contractile effects of prostaglandins on smooth muscle from various sources, including vessels, are uniquely dependent on the presence of oxygen (11,24,29,76,88). $PGE_{2\alpha}$, a constrictor agent occurring in ductal tissue, was considered for such a role (89). However, the finding that inhibitors of prostaglandin synthesis do not either modify or enhance the constrictor response of the mature fetal ductus to oxygen made this idea untenable (see 21).

An alternative possibility, suggested by our *in vitro* work with the inhibitors (22), is that prostaglandins, specifically PGE_2, contribute indirectly to ductus closure by becoming less effective postnatally. If confirmed, our proposal would indicate that the loss in prostaglandin activity during the last third of gestation (see above) is a priming factor for the closure. In this context, it must also be noted that blood levels of prostaglandins fall rapidly after birth (10,65) and, therefore, the neonatal ductus is likely to be relieved of the relaxing influence of both intramural and extramural PGE_2.

CLINICAL EXPERIENCE IN THE NEWBORN

Persistent patency of the ductus arteriosus (PDA) often complicates the clinical course of prematurely born infants. This condition, which may or may not be associated with the respiratory distress syndrome, results from an inadequate response of the immature ductal muscle to oxygen. Until recently, the reduced effectiveness of oxygen was sought in either the immaturity of a hypothetical "oxygen sensor" in muscle cells or the inadequacy of the contractile mechanism (61,69). However, the studies reviewed earlier indicate that the ductus-relaxing action of PGE_2 is an important if not the most important factor in the genesis of PDA. By contrast, PDA beyond the neonatal period probably reflects some structural anomaly of the vessel wall (37) and is unresponsive to pharmacologic manipulation (51,58,60).

Although the rationale for using inhibitors of prostaglandin synthesis in preterm infants with PDA is well founded, the reported success rates vary. Table 3 summarizes the present experience with indomethacin, the most commonly used inhibitor; the incidence of positive responses, i.e. the number of patients with permanent

TABLE 3. *Effiacy of indomethacin in closing a patent ductus arteriosus in premature infants*

| Reference | Patients | | | Route of administration | No. of patients with permanent closure |
	No.	Gestation age (weeks)	Postnatal age (days)		
Friedman et al. (32)	114	29.9 ± 2.7	1–6	p.o.; p.r.; i.v.	92 (81%)
Heymann (45)	60	24–35	ns	p.o.	33 (55%)
Alpert et al. (2)	49	29.1 ± 3	21.2 ± 8.2	p.o.; p.r.	22 (45%)
Halliday et al. (41)	36	27.9 ± 1.9	4–66	p.o.; p.r.	24 (67%)
McCarthy et al. (59)	18	31.1 ± 3	17.1 ± 12	p.o.	7 (39%)
Neal et al. (67)	11	29.8 ± 2.1	16 ± 10	p.o.; p.r.	2 (18%)
Bhat et al. (8)	9	32.2 ± 2.5	12.3 ± 4.4	p.o.	6 (66%)
Vert et al. (94)	7	29.5 ± 1.8	14.4 ± 5.3	p.o.; p.r.	4 (57%)
	11	29 ± 1.5	9.5 ± 2.2	i.v.	9 (82%)
Yeh et al. (98)	27	31.3 ± 2.5	10.8 ± 11.4	i.v.	24 (88%)

All patients received indomethacin at the conventional dose of 0.1–0.3 mg/kg, except for 6 patients in the series of Friedman et al. (32) and all patients in the series of Neal et al. (67), who were given 2.5–5 mg/kg and 0.3–1.1 mg/kg, respectively. Figures are means ± SD; ns = nonspecified; p.o. = per os; p.r. = per rectum.

[a]Success rate was 73% and 33% in patients with postnatal age between 4–14 days and over 14 days, respectively.

[b]Responsive patients had a gestation age of 29.2 ± 1.9 weeks and a postnatal age of 7.7 ± 4.3 days.

[c]It is not specified whether closure of the PDA was permanent in all patients.

closure of the PDA, ranged from a low of 18% to a high of 88%. However, many infants who were considered to be nonresponders by the above criterion, showed clinical or echocardiographic signs of transient constriction of their PDA. Theoretically, there are several explanations for this inconsistency, which relate to the following factors:

a. Structural anomalies of the ductus,

b. varying responses to indomethacin by different kinds of muscle cells in the ductus,

c. variable absorption of orally/rectally administered indomethacin,

d. inadequate inhibition of prostaglandin synthesis and/or "escape" from such inhibition despite contained treatment,

e. changes in ductal reactivity prior to indomethacin therapy,

f. developmental changes in the activity of the prostaglandin-mediated ductus-relaxing mechanism,

g. enhanced formation of relaxant products of the lipoxygenase pathways following blockade of the cyclo-oxygenase pathway by indomethacin, and

h. variable effectiveness of the α-adrenoceptor-mediated contractile mechanism, a presumptive target for indomethacin action.

Several of these factors are probably unimportant. Structural anomalies, consisting of either true defects or gross immaturity of the vessel (38), can account only for a small fraction of the failures. Negative results in infants with exceedingly low birth weight (26,32,49) perhaps fall into this category. The presence of morphologically and functionally distinct muscle layers, though documented in the umbilical artery (80), has not been reported in the ductus. In fact, we have found that bundles of ductal muscle respond as the whole vessel to spasmogens (oxygen, indomethacin) and prostaglandins (*unpublished data*). Contrary to the proposal of McCarthy et al. (59), it is also improbable that the contractile effect of indomethacin is mediated by α-adrenoceptors and hence conditioned by the function of intrinsic nerves. The lamb ductus, which seems to be a good model for the human ductus, lacks an effective adrenergic mechanism and responds forcefully to indomethacin even during α-adrenoceptor blockade (*unpublished data*).

Gestation differences among patients may be important because of their possible influence on the pharmacokinetics of indomethacin and the activity of the prostaglandin-relaxing mechanism. According to Vert et al. (94), premature infants, unlike adults (4), show route-specific variations in the bioavailability of indomethacin and are, therefore, more likely to respond to intravenous therapy. The data presented in Table 3 support this conclusion. Germane to the findings of Vert et al. (94) is our observation in three premature infants that ibuprofen (10–18 mg/kg/day in 3 or 4 doses) is poorly absorbed following either oral or rectal administration (18). No information is available on the pharmacokinetics and efficacy of oral acetylsalicylic acid, except for three infants treated by Heymann et al. (48), only one of whom responded promptly to the drug. It must be stressed, however, that indomethacin has been prepared chiefly as a suspension in aqueous medium for oral and rectal use (8,32,41,45,59,67), which raises questions about the actual dose received by the infants.

Whatever the route of administration, in some patients indomethacin may not attain concentrations that adequately inhibit prostaglandin synthesis in the ductus and other tissues. Premature infants with PDA have higher blood levels of prostaglandins than normal preterm infants or adults (35,56,57) and might therefore be less susceptible to indomethacin. It is significant that we found similar peak concentrations of the drug in the plasma of responders and nonresponders (2).

Animal studies indicate that the prostaglandin mechanism responsible for ductus patency undergoes developmental changes in activity and, consequently, the gestational age of the infant at birth may condition the response to indomethacin. McCarthy et al. (59) reported a higher incidence of positive responses in infants with a postconceptional age (i.e., gestational plus postnatal age) of 33 weeks or younger. However, we could not confirm the importance of the gestational age in our series (2). Moreover, closer scrutiny of the data of McCarthy et al. (59) points to postnatal age as being a more significant factor than gestational age. A similar conclusion is borne out by the study of Halliday et al. (41) and, indirectly, by that of Friedman et al. (32) (Table 3).

Postnatal age could influence the outcome of this therapy in several ways. Ductal reactivity may change during the period preceding indomethacin administration as a result of continued exposure to normal or near-normal oxygen tension, which in itself is ineffective in closing the PDA. Infants may also receive drugs with potential dilator action on the ductus. Two such drugs are furosemide, a diuretic that inhibits prostaglandin catabolism (42) and possibly promotes prostaglandin synthesis (96), and theophylline, a central respiratory stimulant inhibiting phosphodiesterase. Any effect of theophylline on the ductus is likely to be persistent; the half-life of this drug in the neonate is prolonged and it may be transformed into the biologically active caffeine (6).

Finally, indomethacin may fail to close the PDA permanently because, although it inhibits PGE_2 synthesis, it might also promote the synthesis of a vasodilator via the lipoxygenase pathways. Biochemical studies (79) and our studies *in vitro* (23) do indeed suggest the presence of such a product in the ductus.

In conclusion, our analysis indicates that indomethacin is likely to be successful in closing a PDA in premature infants if given intravenously at an early postnatal age. The optimal dosage schedule needs to be defined for each infant on the basis of measurements of indomethacin and PGE_2 in the circulation. However, if the existence of vasoactive products of the lipoxygenase pathways in the ductus is confirmed, a drug interfering with all transformations of arachidonic acid would be a better therapeutic agent than indomethacin or other nonsteroidal anti-inflammatory drugs.

Although indomethacin is a promising new tool for managing infants with PDA, some authors have urged caution (66,84). Potential complications of indomethacin therapy include renal insufficiency (31), platelet dysfunction with the possibility of bleeding (34), reduced formation of pulmonary surfactant (9), and necrotizing enterocolitis (31). However, a review of the clinical experience to date indicates that with the exception of a transient oliguria, side effects are uncommon and do not exceed in frequency or severity those occurring in untreated patients (see 32).

EFFECTS OF ACETYLSALICYLIC ACID AND ACETYLSALICYLIC ACID-LIKE DRUGS ON THE FETUS

The importance of prostaglandins to fetal cardiovascular homeostasis and to fetal functions in general (see 46) raises concern about the use of acetylsalicylic acid and acetylsalicylic acid-like drugs during pregnancy. The fetus may be exposed to such drugs at any stage of gestation and under a variety of circumstances, ranging from therapeutic indications (e.g., rheumatoid arthritis, premature labor) to habitual analgesic consumption or even attempted suicide. In fact, the use of these drugs, whether intermittent or continued, is so widespread that acetylsalicylic acid alone is estimated to affect 25% to 70% of the total pregnancies (see 63).

The potential adverse effects of the inhibitors on the fetus, as gathered from studies in animals, are listed in Table 4. However, the actual incidence of complications is low and variable; moreover, some of these side effects are seemingly absent in humans. Whereas platelet dysfunction is well documented (34), teratogenic effects have been detected only in animals (77,78,87,92). Several investigators have reported a higher incidence of stillbirths in animals treated with acetylsalicylic acid or acetylsalicylic acid-like drugs (1,3,12,43,70,75,77,78,95), however, findings in humans are conflicting (25,83,92). Furthermore, neuronal necrosis has been described in fetal rats only after exposure to certain doses of indomethacin (3). It remains to be determined whether this toxic effect occurs in humans.

Acetylsalicylic acid and acetylsalicylic acid-like drugs are likely to constrict the ductus arteriosus in the human fetus as they do in animals; yet of the very few cases of intrauterine closure of this vessel that have been reported (7,53), some may not even be related to drug treatment. This finding implies either that the human ductus is less sensitive to these drugs or, more likely, that a moderate degree of ductus constriction is well tolerated by the fetus. Indeed, certain animal data indicate that only a severe and prolonged constriction of this vessel interferes with placental blood flow and myocardial performance (see 70).

TABLE 4. *Potential complications of fetal exposure to inhibitors of prostaglandin synthesis*

Fetal death or malformation

Impairment in lung and kidney maturation

Vascular effects (ductus arteriosus, pulmonary circulation)

Neuronal degeneration

Reduction in platelet aggregability

Pulmonary hypertension is a more troublesome complication, and it has been linked to the use of inhibitors of prostaglandin synthesis for preventing premature labor (27,40,53,62,97). Again, the incidence of this complication is quite variable; some authors (50,68) could not detect a single case in a relatively large series of infants. When present, pulmonary hypertension probably reflects an action of these drugs on both the ductus arteriosus and the pulmonary vasculature (53,55). The hypertensive state may persist in the newborn, since, according to animal data, pulmonary vessels fail to undergo the normal postnatal dilation (52) and can, instead, exhibit an exaggerated constrictor response to hypoxia (93).

The reason for the variable incidence of side effects is unclear. Whereas certain factors, such as the dose of inhibitor and the length of treatment, are obviously crucial, the importance of other features either is not known or has not been adequately investigated. For example, it has been known for some time that acetylsalicylic acid and acetylsalicylic acid-like drugs can cross the placenta (3,36,43,44,74,91); however, no information is available on the actual clearance of these drugs, apart from recent data on acetylsalicylic acid (5). Moreover, even this single report on acetylsalicylic acid (5) fails to define how much of the compound is converted to salicylate before reaching the fetus. An additional question concerns the ability of the fetus to eliminate these drugs and, specifically, the importance of the ductus venosus in allowing drugs to escape exposure to metabolic enzymes in the liver (see 39). Finally, it remains to be ascertained if the fatty acid cyclo-oxygenase derived from various fetal organs is uniformly sensitive to the inhibitors and, furthermore, if the fetus has mechanisms to compensate for impairment or loss of any prostaglandin-mediated function.

Although the incidence of side effects and the determining factors remain uncertain and warrant further evaluation, the data obtained so far stress the need for extreme caution in the use of acetylsalicylic acid and acetylsalicylic acid-like drugs during pregnancy.

CONCLUSION

Research in the past few years has proved that prenatal patency of the ductus arteriosus is an active process determined by a prostaglandin. This novel concept has been established largely through the use of inhibitors of prostaglandin synthesis. Knowledge of prostaglandin function in the ductus, and possibly other vessels, has afforded new therapeutic tools for treatment of the newborn; it has also focused attention on the possible adverse effects of acetylsalicylic acid and allied drugs on the fetus.

ACKNOWLEDGMENTS

This review and studies of the authors were supported by the Ontario Heart Foundation and the Upjohn Company.

REFERENCES

1. Aiken, J. W. (1972): Aspirin and indomethacin prolong parturition in rats. Evidence that prostaglandins contribute to expulsion of the fetus. *Nature*, 240:21–25.
2. Alpert, B. S., Lewins, M. J., Rowland, D. W., Grant, M. J., Olley, P. M., Soldin, S. J., Swyer, P. R., Coceani, F., and Rowe, R. D. (1979): Plasma indomethacin levels in preterm newborn infants with symptomatic patent ductus arteriosus: clinical and echocardiographic assessments of response. *J. Pediatr.*, 95:578–582.
3. Altshuler, G., Krous, H. F., Altmiller, D. H., and Sharpe, G. L. (1979): Premature onset of labor, neonatal patent ductus arteriosus, and prostaglandin synthetase antagonists—A rat model of the human problem. *Am. J. Obstet. Gynecol.*, 135:261–265.
4. Alván, G., Orme,, M., Bertilsson, L., Ekstrand, R., and Palmer, L. (1975): Pharmacokinetics of indomethacin. *Clin. Pharmacol. Ther.*, 18:364–373.
5. Anderson, D. F., Phernetton, T. M., and Rankin, J. H. G. (1980): The placental transfer of acetylsalicylic acid in near-term ewes. *Am. J. Obstet. Gynecol.*, 136:814–818.
6. Aranda, J. V., Louridas, A. T., Vitullo, B. B., Thom, P., Aldridge, A., and Haber, R. (1979): Metabolism of theophylline to caffeine in the human fetal liver. *Science*, 206:1319–1321.
7. Becker, A. E., Becker, M. J., and Wagenvoort, C. A. (1977): Premature contraction of ductus arteriosus: a cause of foetal death. *J. Pathol.*, 121:187–191.
8. Bhat, R., Vidyasagar, D., Vadapalli, M., Walley, C., Fisher, E., Hastreiter, A., and Evans, M. (1979): Disposition of indomethacin in preterm infants. *J. Pediatr.*, 95:313–316.
9. Bustos, R., Ballejo, G., Giussi, G., Rosas, R., and Isa, J. C. (1978): Inhibition of fetal lung maturation by indomethacin in pregnant rabbits. *J. Perinat. Med.*, 6:240–245.
10. Challis, J. R. G., Dilley, S. R., Robinson, J. S., and Thorburn, G. D. (1976): Prostaglandins in the circulation of the fetal lamb. *Prostaglandins*, 11:1041–1052.
11. Chandler, J. T., and Strong, C. G. (1972): The actions of prostaglandin E₁ on isolated rabbit aorta. *Arch. Int. Pharmacodyn. Ther.*, 197:123–131.
12. Chester, R., Dukes, M., Slater, S. R., and Walpole, A. L. (1972): Delay of parturition in the rat by anti-inflammatory agents which inhibit the biosynthesis of prostaglandins. *Nature*, 240:37–38.
13. Clyman, R. I. (1980): Ontogeny of the ductus arteriosus response to prostaglandins and inhibitors of their synthesis. *Seminars in Perinatology*, 4:115–124.
14. Clyman, R. I., Mauray, F., Heymann, M. A., and Rudolph, M. A. (1978): Ductus arteriosus: developmental response to oxygen and indomethacin. *Prostaglandins*, 15:993–998.
15. Clyman, R. I., Mauray, F., Rudolph, A. M., and Heymann, M. A. (1980): Age-dependent sensitivity of the lamb ductus arteriosus to indomethacin and prostaglandins. *J. Pediatr.*, 96:94–98.
16. Coceani, F., Bodach, E., White, E. P., Bishai, I., and Olley, P. M. (1978): Prostaglandin I₂ is less relaxant than prostaglandin E₂ on the lamb ductus arteriosus. *Prostaglandins*, 15:551–556.
17. Coceani, F., and Olley, P. M. (1973): The response of the ductus arteriosus to prostaglandins. *Can. J. Physiol. Pharmacol.*, 51:220–225.
18. Coceani, F., and Olley, P. M. (1978): Prostaglandins and the ductus arteriosus. In: *Clinical Pharmacology and Therapeutics: A Pediatric Perspective*, edited by B. L. Mirkin, pp. 169–184. Year Book Medical Publishers, Chicago.
19. Coceani, F., and Olley, P. M. (1980): Considerations on the role of prostaglandins in the ductus arteriosus. In: *Advances in Prostaglandin and Thromboxane Research, Vol. 7*, edited by B. Samuelsson, P. W. Ramwell, and R. Paoletti, pp. 871–878. Raven Press, New York.
20. Coceani, F., and Olley, P. M. (1980): Role of prostaglandins, prostacyclin and thromboxanes in the control of prenatal patency and postnatal closure of the ductus arterious. *Seminars in Perinatology*, 4:109–113.
21. Coceani, F., Olley, P. M., Bishai, I., Bodach, E., and White, E. P. (1978): Significance of the prostaglandin system to the control of muscle tone of the ductus arteriosus. In: *Prostaglandins and Perinatal Medicine, Advances in Prostaglandin and Thromboxane Research, Vol. 4*, edited by F. Coceani and P. M. Olley, pp. 325–333. Raven Press, New York.
22. Coceani, F., Olley, P. M., and Bodach, E. (1975): Lamb ductus arteriosus: effect of prostaglandin synthesis inhibitors on the muscle tone and the response to prostaglandin E₂. *Prostaglandins*, 9:299–308.
23. Coceani, F., White, E. P., Bodach, E., and Olley, P. M. (1979): Age-dependent changes in the response of the lamb ductus arteriosus to oxygen and ibuprofen. *Can. J. Physiol. Pharmacol.*, 57:825–831.

24. Coceani, F., and Wolfe, L. S. (1966): On the action of prostaglandin E₁ and prostaglandins from brain on the isolated rat stomach. *Can. J. Physiol. Pharmacol.*, 44:933–950.
25. Collins, E., and Turner, G. (1975): Maternal effects of regular salicylate ingestion in pregnancy. *Lancet*, 2:335–338.
26. Cooke, R. W. I., and Pickering, D. (1979): Poor response to oral indomethacin therapy for persistent ductus arteriosus in very low birthweight infants. *Br. Heart J.*, 41:301–303.
27. Csaba, I. F., Sulyok, E., and Ertl, T. (1978): Relationship of maternal treatment with indomethacin to persistence of fetal circulation syndrome. *J. Pediatr.*, 92:484.
28. van Dorp, D. A. (1967): Aspects of the biosynthesis of prostaglandins. *Prog. Biochem. Pharmacol.*, 3:71–82.
29. Eckenfels, A., and Vane, J. R. (1972): Prostaglandins, oxygen tension and smooth muscle tone. *Br. J. Pharmacol.*, 45:451–462.
30. Friedman, W. F. (1978): Studies of responses of the ductus arteriosus in intact animals. In: *The Ductus Arteriosus, Report of the Seventy-Fifth Ross Conference on Pediatric Research*, edited by M. A. Heymann and A. M. Rudolph, pp. 35–43. Ross Laboratories, Columbus, Ohio.
31. Friedman, W. F., and Fitzpatrick, K. M. (1980): Effects of prostaglandins, thromboxanes, and inhibitors of their synthesis on renal and gastrointestinal function in the newborn period. *Seminars in Perinatology*, 4:143–156.
32. Friedman, W. F., Kurlinski, J., Jacob, J., DiSessa, T. G., Gluck, L., Merritt, T. A., and Feldman, B. H. (1980): The inhibition of prostaglandin and prostacyclin synthesis in the clinical management of patent ductus arteriosus. *Seminars in Perinatology*, 4:125–133.
33. Friedman, W. F., Printz, M. P., and Kirkpatrick, S. E. (1978): Blockers of prostaglandin synthesis: a novel therapy in the management of the premature infant with patent ductus arteriosus. In: *Prostaglandins and Perinatal Medicine, Advances in Prostaglandin and Thromboxane Research, Vol. 4*, edited by F. Coceani and P. M. Olley, pp. 373–381. Raven Press, New York.
34. Friedman, Z., and Berman, W. (1980): Hematologic effects of prostaglandins and thromboxanes and inhibitors of their synthesis in the perinatal period. *Seminars in Perinatology*, 4:73–84.
35. Friedman, Z., and Demers, L. M. (1978): Essential fatty acids, prostaglandins and respiratory distress syndrome of the newborn. *Pediatrics*, 61:341–347.
36. Garrettson, L. K., Procknal, J. A., and Levy, G. (1975): Fetal acquisition and neonatal elimination of a large amount of salicylate. *Clin. Pharmacol. Ther.*, 17:98–103.
37. Gittenberger-de Groot, A. C. (1977): Persistent ductus arteriosus: most probably a primary congenital malformation. *Br. Heart J.*, 39:610–618.
38. Gittenberger-de Groot, A. C., von Ertbruggen, I., Moulaert, A. J. M. G., and Harinck, E. (1980): The ductus arteriosus in the preterm infant: histologic and clinical observations. *J. Pediatr.*, 96:88–93.
39. Green, T. P., O'Dea, R. F., and Mirkin, B. L. (1979): Determinants of drug disposition and effect in the fetus. *Ann. Rev. Pharmacol. Toxicol.*, 19:285–322.
40. Grella, P., and Zanor, P. (1978): Premature labor and indomethacin. *Prostaglandins*, 16:1007–1017.
41. Halliday, H. L., Hirata, T., and Brady, J. P. (1979): Indomethacin therapy for large patent ductus arteriosus in the very low birth weight infant: results and complications. *Pediatrics*, 64:154–159.
42. Hansen, H. S. (1976):15-Hydroxyprostaglandin dehydrogenase. A review. *Prostaglandins*, 12:647–679.
43. Harris, W. H. (1980): The effects of repeated doses of indomethacin on fetal rabbit mortality and on the patency of the ductus arteriosus. *Can. J. Physiol. Pharmacol.*, 58:212–216.
44. Harris, W. H., and Van Petten, G. R. (1980): The placental transfer of indomethacin in the rabbit and sheep. *Proc. Can. Fed. Biol. Soc.*, 23:38.
45. Heymann, M. A. (1978): Management of PDA with prostaglandin synthetase inhibitors. In: *The Ductus Arteriosus, Report of the Seventy-Fifth Ross Conference on Pediatric Research*, edited by M. A. Heymann and A. M. Rudolph, pp. 84–86. Ross Laboratories, Columbus, Ohio.
46. Heymann, M. A., editor (1980): Prostaglandin Symposium. *Seminars in Perinatology*, 4:1–156.
47. Heymann, M. A., and Rudolph, A. M. (1976): Effects of acetylsalicylic acid on the ductus arteriosus and circulation in fetal lambs *in utero*. *Circ. Res.*, 38:418–422.
48. Heymann, M. A., Rudolph, A. M., and Silverman, N. H. (1976): Closure of the ductus arteriosus in premature infants by inhibition of prostaglandin synthesis. *N. Engl. J. Med.*, 295:530–533.
49. Ivey, H. H., Kattwinkel, J., Park, T. S., and Krovetz, L. J. (1979): Failure of indomethacin to close persistent ductus arteriosus in infants weighing under 1000 grams. *Br. Heart J.*, 41:304–307.

50. van Kets, H., Thiery, M., Derom, R., van Egmond, H., and Baele, G. (1979): Perinatal hazards of chronic antenatal tocolysis with indomethacin. *Prostaglandins*, 18:893–907.
51. Kostis, J. B. (1977): Patent ductus arteriosus. *N. Engl. J. Med.*, 296:106.
52. Leffler, C. W., Tyler, T. L., and Cassin, S. (1978): Effect of indomethacin on pulmonary vascular response to ventilation of fetal goats. *Am. J. Physiol.*, 234:H346–H351.
53. Levin, D. L., Fixler, D. E., Morriss, F. C., and Tyson, J. (1978): Morphologic analysis of the pulmonary vascular bed in infants exposed in utero to prostaglandin synthesis inhibitors. *J. Pediatr.*, 92:478–483.
54. Levin, D. L. Mills, L. J., Parkey, M., Garriott, J., and Campbell, W. (1979): Constriction of the fetal ductus arteriosus after administration of indomethacin to the pregnant ewe. *J. Pediatr.*, 94:647–650.
55. Levin, D. L., Mills, L. J., and Weinberg, A. G. (1979): Hemodynamic pulmonary vascular, and myocardial abnormalities secondary to pharmacologic constriction of the fetal ductus arteriosus. A possible mechanism for persistent pulmonary hypertension and transient tricuspid insufficiency in the newborn infant. *Circulation*, 60:360–364.
56. Lucas, A., and Mitchell, M. D. (1978): Plasma-prostaglandins in pre-term neonates before and after treatment for patent ductus arteriosus. *Lancet*, 2:130–132.
57. Lucas, A., and Mitchell, M. D. (1978): Prostaglandins in patent ductus arteriosus. *Lancet*, 2:937–938.
58. McCarthy, J., Juris, A., Zies, L., Ferrero, F., Kaiser, G., Garcia, O., Tamer, D., Ferrer, P., and Gelband, H. (1977): Failure of indomethacin to close the ductus arteriosus. *Pediatr. Res.*, 11:395.
59. McCarthy, J. S., Zies, L. G., and Gelband, H. (1978): Age-dependent closure of the patent ductus arteriosus by indomethacin. *Pediatrics*, 62:706–712.
60. McGrath, R. L., Wolfe, R. R., Simmons, M. A., and Nora, J. J. (1977). Patent ductus arteriosus (correspondence). *N. Engl. J. Med.*, 296:106.
61. McMurphy, D. M., Heymann, M. A., Rudolph, A. M., and Melmon, K. L. (1972): Developmental changes in constriction of the ductus arteriosus: responses to oxygen and vasoactive agents in the isolated ductus arteriosus of the fetal lamb. *Pediatr. Res.*, 6:231–238.
62. Manchester, D., Margolis, H. S., and Sheldon, R. E. (1976): Possible association between maternal indomethacin therapy and primary pulmonary hypertension of the newborn. *Am. J. Obstet. Gynecol.*, 126:467–469.
63. Mandelli, M., and Morselli, P. L. (1977): Antipyretic and nonsteroid antiinflammatory drugs. In: *Drug Disposition During Development*, edited by P. L. Morselli, pp. 271–309. Spectrum Publications, New York.
64. Mitchell, M. D., Jamieson, D. R. S., Sellers, S. M., and Turnbull, A. C. (1980): 6-Keto-$PGF_{1\alpha}$: concentrations in human umbilical plasma and production by umbilical vessels. In: *Advances in Prostaglandin and Thromboxane Research, Vol. 7*, edited by B. Samuelsson, P. W. Ramwell, and R. Paoletti, pp. 891–896. Raven Press, New York.
65. Mitchell, M. D., Lucas, A., Etches, P. C., Brunt, J. D., and Turnbull, A. C. (1978): Plasma prostaglandin levels during early neonatal life following term and pre-term delivery. *Prostaglandins*, 16:319–326.
66. Nadas, A. S. (1976): Patent ductus revisited. *N. Engl. J. Med.*, 295:563–565.
67. Neal, W. A., Kyle, J. M., and Mullett, M. D. (1977): Failure of indomethacin therapy to induce closure of patent ductus arteriosus in premature infants with respiratory distress syndrome. *J. Pediatr.*, 91:621–623.
68. Neibyl, J. R., Blake, D. A., White, R. D., Kumor, K. M., Dubin, N. H., Robinson, J. C., and Egner, P. G. (1980): The inhibition of premature labor with indomethacin. *Am. J. Obstet. Gynecol.*, 136:1014–1019.
69. Noel, S., and Cassin, S. (1976): Maturation of contractile response of ductus arteriosus to oxygen and drugs. *Am. J. Physiol.*, 231:240–243.
70. Novy, M. J. (1978): Effects of indomethacin on labor, fetal oxygenation, and fetal development in rhesus monkeys. In: *Prostaglandins and Perinatal Medicine, Advances in Prostaglandins and Thromboxane Research, Vol. 4*, edited by F. Coceani and P. M. Olley, pp. 285–300. Raven Press, New York.
71. Nugteren, D. H., and Dorp, D. A. van (1965): The participation of molecular oxygen in the biosynthesis of prostaglandins. *Biochim. Biophys. Acta*, 98:654–656.

72. Olley, P. M., Bodach, E., Heaton, J., and Coceani, F. (1975): Further evidence implicating E-type prostaglandins in the patency of the lamb ductus arteriosus. *Eur. J. Pharmacol.*, 34:247–250.
73. Pace-Asciak, C. R., and Rangaraj, G. (1978): Prostaglandin biosynthesis and catabolism in the lamb ductus arteriosus, aorta and pulmonary artery. *Biochim. Biophys. Acta*, 529:13–20.
74. Parks, B. R., Jordan, R. L., Rawson, J. E., and Douglas, B. H. (1977): Indomethacin: studies of absorption and placental transfer. *Am. J. Obstet. Gynecol.*, 129:464–465.
75. Parks, B. R., Rawson, J. E., and Douglas, B. H. (1977): In-utero death as a possible consequence of prenatal administration of indomethacin. *Pediatr. Res.*, 11:419.
76. Paton, D. M., and Daniel, E. E. (1967): On the contractile response of the isolated rat uterus to prostaglandin E_1. *Can. J. Physiol. Pharmacol.*, 45:795–804.
77. Persaud, T. V. N. (1974): Inhibitors of prostaglandin synthesis during pregnancy. 2. The effects of indomethacin in pregnant rats. *Anat. Anz.*, 136:354–358.
78. Persaud, T. V. N., and Moore, K. L. (1974): Inhibitors of prostaglandin synthesis during pregnancy. 1. Embriopathic activity of indomethacin in mice. *Anat. Anz.*, 136:349–353.
79. Powell, W. S., and Solomon, S. (1978): Biosynthesis of prostaglandins and thromboxanes in fetal tissues. In: *Prostaglandins and Perinatal Medicine, Advances in Prostaglandin and Thromboxane Research, Vol. 4*, edited by F. Coceani and P. M. Olley, pp. 61–74. Raven Press, New York.
80. Roach, M. R. (1976): The umbilical vessels. In: *Perinatal Medicine*, edited by J. W. Goodwin, J. O. Godden, and G. W. Chance, pp. 134–142. Williams & Wilkins, Baltimore.
81. Rudolph, A. M. (1978): The role of the ductus arteriosus in the fetus and postnatal circulatory changes. In: *The Ductus Arteriosus, Report of the Seventy-fifth Ross Conference on Pediatric Research*, edited by M. A. Heymann and A. M. Rudolph, pp. 55–62. Ross Laboratories, Columbus, Ohio.
82. Samuelsson, B. (1965): On the incorporation of oxygen in the conversion of 8,11,14-eicosatrienoic acid to prostaglandin E_1. *J. Am. Chem. Soc.*, 87:3011–3013.
83. Shapiro, S., Monson, R. R., Kaufman, D. W., Siskind, V., Heinonen, O P., and Slone, D. (1976): Perinatal mortality and birth-weight in relation to aspirin taken during pregnancy. *Lancet*, 1:1375–1376.
86. Sharpe, G. L., and Altshuler, G. (1977): Ductal manipulation—a note of caution. *J. Pediatr.*, 90:335–337.
85. Sharpe, G. L., Larsson, K. S., and Thalme, B. (1975): Studies on the closure of the ductus arteriosus. XII. *In utero* effect of indomethacin and sodium salicylate in rats and rabbits. *Prostaglandins*, 9:585–596.
86. Sharpe, G. L., Thalme, B., and Larsson, K. S. (1974): Studies on the closure of the ductus arteriosus. XI. Ductal closure *in utero* by a prostaglandin synthetase inhibitor. *Prostaglandins*, 8:363–368.
87. Slone, D., Heinonen, O. P., Kaufman, D. W., Siskind, V., Monson, R. R., and Shapiro, S. (1976): Aspirin and congenital malformations. *Lancet*, 1:1373–1375.
88. Splawinski, J. A., Nies, A. S., Sweetman, B., and Oates, J. A. (1973): The effects of arachidonic acid, prostaglandin E_2 and prostaglandin $E_{2\alpha}$ on the longitudinal stomach strip of the rat. *J. Pharmacol. Exp. Ther.*, 187:501–510.
89. Starling, M. B., and Elliott, R. B. (1974): The effects of prostaglandins, prostaglandin inhibitors, and oxygen on the closure of the ductus arteriosus, pulmonary arteries and umbilical vessels. *Prostaglandins*, 8:187–203.
90. Terragno, N. A., McGiff, J. C., Smigel, M., and Terragno, A. (1978): Patterns of prostaglandin production in the bovine fetal and maternal vasculature. *Prostaglandins*, 16:847–856.
91. Traeger, A. van, Nöschel, H., and Zaumseil, J. (1973): Zur Pharmakokinetik von Indomethazin bei Schwangeren, Kreissenden und deren Neugeborenen. *Zentralbl. Gynaekol.*, 95:635–641.
92. Turner, G., and Collins, E. (1975): Fetal effects of regular salicylate ingestion in pregnancy. *Lancet*, 2:338–339.
93. Tyler, T., Wallis, R., Leffler, C., and Cassin, S. (1975): The effects of indomethacin on the pulmonary vascular response to hypoxia in the premature and mature newborn goat. *Proc. Soc. Exper. Biol. Med.*, 150:695–698.
94. Vert, P., Bianchetti, G., Marchal, F., Monin, P., and Morselli, P. L. (1980): Effectiveness and pharmacokinetics of indomethacin in premature newborns with patent ductus arteriosus. *Eur. J. Clin. Pharmacol.*, 18:83–88.
95. Waltman, R., Tricomi, V., Shabanah, E. H., and Arenas, R. (1973): The effect of anti-inflammatory drugs on parturition parameters in the rat. *Prostaglandins*, 4:93–106.

96. Weber, P. G., Scherer, B., and Larsson, C. (1977): Increase of free arachidonic acid by furosemide in man as the cause of prostaglandin and renin release. *Eur. J. Pharmacol.*, 41:329–332.
97. Wilkinson, A. R., Aynsley-Green, A., and Mitchell, M. D. (1979): Persistent pulmonary hypertension and abnormal prostaglandin E levels in preterm infants after maternal treatment with naproxen. *Arch. Dis. Child.*, 54:942–945.
98. Yeh, T. F., Thalji, A., Luken, J., Raral, D., Carr, I., and Pildes, R. S. (1979): Intravenous indocin therapy in premature infants with PDA: a double-blind control study. *Pediatr. Res.*, 13:354.

Acetylsalicylic Acid: New Uses for an Old Drug,
·edited by H.J.M. Barnett, J. Hirsh, and
J.F. Mustard. Raven Press, New York © 1982.

The Role of Prostaglandins and Their Inhibitors in Reproduction

*John E. Patrick and John R. G. Challis

*Departments of Obstetrics, Gynecology, and Physiology, University of Western Ontario,
London, Ontario, Canada N6A 4V2*

Uterine contractility, ovarian function, implantation, and parturition are profoundly influenced by the prostaglandins. Therefore, the effects of acetylsalicylic acid and related compounds, especially as they act on the uterus in the young healthy woman, are especially important. Primary dysmenorrhea is an illness that affects many postpubescent females to some degree and represents one of the largest single causes of work loss in young women. Investigators first recognized that the menstrual blood of women suffering from the disorder had high prostaglandin levels. In addition, symptoms of dysmenorrhea were very similar to those produced by systemic administration of prostaglandins. Current management of primary dysmenorrhea is based on attempts to decrease production of prostaglandins or counteract their effects. Nonsteroidal anti-inflammatory agents inhibit cyclic endoperoxide synthesis and some interfere with prostaglandin effects on the uterine muscle. Mefenamic acid and flufenamic acid are two preparations that are especially useful in this regard. Although acetylsalicylic acid and indomethacin are inhibitors of prostaglandin synthetase and should in theory relieve dysmenorrhea, they have not proved to be as effective.

There is also evidence that prostaglandins play an important role in successful implantation of the developing blastocyst in rodents. In addition, they are involved in the regulation of endometrial vascular permeability. The information from animal studies suggests that caution should be exercised when administering prostaglandin-synthetase inhibitors to women of child-bearing potential.

Exogenous prostaglandins induce early abortion by a secondary rather than a primary effect on corpus luteum function. Prostaglandins have an abortifacient action on pregnancies of greater than six weeks, but this action is more complicated than simple direct stimulation of the myometrium. Prostaglandins act on the uterine vasculature to compromise placental function and reduce placental steroidogenesis, which in turn results in increased uterine sensitivity to factors promoting contractility.

Prostaglandins are a final common pathway in regulation of the onset of parturition. Our work supports the hypothesis that the estrogen present in amniotic fluid or maternal blood may gain access to the fetal membranes. The latter, particularly

---

*Mailing address: Dr. J.E. Patrick, Department of Obstetrics and Gynecology, St. Joseph's Hospital, 268 Grosvenor Street, London, Ontario, Canada N6A 4V2

chorion, possess highly potent steroid sulfatase activities that hydrolyze conjugated estrogen. The free estrogen may then exert a labilizing action on lysosomal membranes—the net effect being the same as that of progesterone withdrawal. More than one factor is involved in that a series of steroid and peptide hormonal changes eventually merge along the common pathway to prostaglandin generation.

There is some evidence that acetylsalicylic acid or indomethacin may cross the placenta and exert direct adverse effects on the fetus. At the present time it seems premature to recommend their use for treating or preventing preterm labor. It would be desirable to develop a compound that does not cross the placental barrier or have significant effects on maternal and fetal circulatory dynamics.

The prostaglandins play a central role in the control of uterine contractility, ovarian function, implantation, and parturition. This review will examine effects of acetylsalicylic acid (ASA) and related compounds in the pregnant and nonpregnant uterus. The underlying objective is to review potential advantages and disadvantages of acetylsalicylic acid as they relate to the uterus in young healthy women.

THE ROLE OF ACETYLSALICYLIC ACID AND RELATED COMPOUNDS IN THE NONPREGNANT UTERUS

Primary dysmenorrhea is common in nulliparous women. Approximately 52% of postpubescent females are affected and 10% are incapacitated for 1 to 3 days each month (42). It has been estimated that 140 million working hours are lost annually in the United States because of this disease. It is the largest single cause of work and school absence in young women. The symptoms, which are worse during the first 1 or 2 days of menstruation and are associated only with ovulatory cycles, include lower abdominal cramps, severe lower backache, diarrhea, nausea and vomiting, headaches, dizziness, tiredness, and nervousness.

The pathophysiology of the disease was suggested first by Pickles (27), who isolated a menstrual stimulant in the menstrual fluid of women with primary dysmenorrhea. Later he determined that the menstrual blood of women with primary dysmenorrhea had a higher PFG/PGE ratio than that of control women without the disease (28). Since Pickles's first observation, a series of studies have suggested that prostaglandins are a primary etiologic agent in the syndrome of primary dysmenorrhea. There is a similarity between these symptoms and the side effects produced by systemic administration of prostaglandins for induction of labor or therapeutic abortion.

At least four mechanisms have been proposed to explain how prostaglandins may produce severe dysmenorrhea:

a. Higher concentrations of prostaglandins may induce prolonged painful uterine contractions by producing uterine ischemia (15).

b. Delay in expulsion of menstrual blood caused by cervical stenosis may allow an increased absorption of prostaglandins and explain the improvement produced by cervical dilatation in 60% of cases (15).

c. Myometrial sensitivity to prostaglandins may be increased in certain individuals who respond with intense contractions (13).

d. Local prostaglandins may sensitize uterine nerve endings (15).

More recently, firmer evidence has implicated prostaglandins in the etiology of this disease. Lundström and Green (23) measured $PGF_{2\alpha}$ and 15-keto, 13, 14-dihydro-$PGF_{2\alpha}$ (PGFM) in plasma and endometrial biopsies taken during menstruation. Plasma PGFM concentrations were increased fivefold in women with primary dysmenorrhea, and on the first day of menstruation $PGF_{2\alpha}$ levels in endometrial biopsies were four times higher in women with primary dysmenorrhea than in control subjects.

Present evidence suggests that the symptoms of the majority of women with primary dysmenorrhea result from a prostaglandin effect. Therefore, current management of the condition is based on attempts to decrease production of prostaglandins or to reduce their effects (29). One regimen consists of administering oral contraceptives. These steroids probably suppress primary dysmenorrhea indirectly through their action in preventing ovulation. In addition, oral contraceptive pills may lead to a reduction in the concentration of prostaglandins in menstrual fluid or to lowered sensitivity of the myometrium to prostaglandins (42). Virtually all patients who suffer from primary dysmenorrhea improve on oral contraceptive pills. However, the syndrome is encountered in many women who have no need of contraception and in others who, because of medical complications, cannot use oral contraceptives.

Recently, investigators have suggested the use of agents that inhibit cyclic endoperoxide synthesis in the management of dysmenorrhea. The agents being tested include acetylsalicylic acid, indomethacin, the fenamate compounds, and sodium naproxen. Both mefenamic acid and flufenamic acid also inhibit prostaglandin receptors in the uterine muscle and therefore serve a dual function (22).

In a double-blind crossover trial, Anderson et al. (2) compared the efficacy of mefenamic acid and flufenamic acid with that of a conventional analgesic, dextropropoxyphene hydrochloride–paracetamol. Both fenamates were significantly more effective than conventional therapy in relieving symptoms of primary dysmenorrhea. The two fenamate compounds were similar in terms of effectiveness. Anderson et al. asked patients to record the severity of nine symptoms—abdominal pain, backache, leg pain, headache, faintness, nausea, vomiting, diarrhea, and constipation. Mefenamic acid was superior to both flufenamic acid and analgesic for seven of the nine symptoms and superior to analgesic for all nine. Flufenamic acid was superior to analgesic for eight of the nine.

In the same issue of *Lancet*, Kapadia and Elder (15) reported a double-blind, crossover trial comparing flufenamic acid and a placebo. These investigators concluded that pain, episodes of vomiting, and episodes of diarrhea were significantly reduced in the flufenamic group.

Acetylsalicylic acid and indomethacin are inhibitors of PG synthetase and should, in theory, relieve dysmenorrhea if given before the onset of menstruation. However, the fenamates seem to be more effective, perhaps because of their dual action, namely inhibition of prostaglandin synthesis and of PG action at the level of prostaglandin receptors. This is especially true when treatment is started after the onset of menstruation, as is often necessary in women with irregular cycles.

Generally, the side effects of prostaglandin synthetase inhibitors have not been a major problem. Indeed, Anderson et al. (1) reported a decrease in menstrual blood loss from 119 ml in a control group to 60 ml in women treated with either mefenamic acid or flufenamic acid. Most side effects are mild and tolerable. Persons treated with indomethacin have complained of severe headache, GI symptoms, and drug rash with doses above 75 mg/day (16,24). Nausea, GI discomfort, vomiting, gas and diarrhea, and a variety of other symptoms have been reported with mefenamic acid, but Anderson et al. (2) and Kapadia and Elder (15) did not observe side effects that could be directly attributed to either mefenamic or flufenamic acid.

In summary, it appears that inhibition of prostaglandins is a valid treatment in many women with primary dysmenorrhea. When treatment is commenced after the onset of menstruation, the drugs of choice appear to be mefenamic acid, flufenamic acid, and naproxen. When patients have predictable menstrual cycles, indomethacin or acetylsalicylic acid may be considered if given at least one day before the onset of menses. In patients requiring contraception, the drugs of choice are the oral contraceptive pills, if there are no contraindications to their use.

IMPLANTATION OF THE DEVELOPING OVUM

There is evidence that prostaglandins play a role in successful implantation of the developing blastocyst in the uterus. It was first reported by Gavin et al. (11) and Saksena et al. (32) that indomethacin prevented implantation in the rat and the mouse, as indicated by an absence of implantation swellings. However, since indomethacin also inhibits decidualization in response to artificial stimuli (4,30,33,39), it was not clear whether indomethacin inhibited initiation of implantation or subsequent decidualization.

Kennedy (17) demonstrated in rats that indomethacin given on day 5 of pregnancy inhibited the increase in endometrial vascular permeability on the evening of that day. This effect was present even when the animals were given enough exogenous steroids to initiate implantation, showing that the inhibition produced by indomethacin was independent of any effect on ovarian steroidogenesis. Evans and Kennedy also demonstrated that indomethacin inhibited initiation of implantation in the hamster.

In a recent review, Kennedy (18) examined the question of which prostaglandin might mediate the change in endometrial vascular permeability necessary for successful implantation. He injected rats with Evans-blue dye, which allows one to visualize potential implantation sites in the endometrium, and found that the concentrations of E series prostaglandins were elevated at these sites. Kennedy and Zamecnik (in 17) also measured increased levels of 6-oxo-$PGF_{1\alpha}$, a stable breakdown product of PGI_2, in the uterine dye sites. Kennedy concluded that the prostaglandins involved in regulation of endometrial vascular permeability originated from the endometrial cells themselves, since artificial stimuli induced an increase in permeability without the presence of a developing blastocyst.

Kennedy and Armstrong (in 17) suggested an analogy to the inflammatory response that might indicate that prostaglandins of the E or I series cause vasodilatation and that histamine may increase vascular permeability at the site of implantation of the developing ovum.

These data are from pregnancy in rodents, and it is important to seek similar data concerning implantation of the blastocyst in primates. Indeed, it could be argued that the primary role of prostaglandins in rodents is in the spacing of pregnancies in the horn of the uterus. It is important to determine if prostaglandin synthetase inhibitors or prostaglandin antagonists can interrupt the early stages of pregnancy in primates. The information from animal studies suggests that if women are practicing unprotected intercourse with a view to becoming pregnant, great caution should be exercised when administering prostaglandin synthetase inhibitors for other conditions.

MENSTRUAL INDUCTION AND ABORTION

It is now well established that prostaglandins $F_{2\alpha}$ and E_2 and their synthetic analogs terminate pregnancy regardless of gestational age. It has been assumed that prostaglandins produce abortion by acting as a primary uterine stimulant. However, recent evidence suggests that termination of early pregnancies may not be caused simply by uterine stimulation.

Menstrual Induction

The corpus luteum must function properly for the first 6 weeks of a human pregnancy, or abortion will result. The corpus luteum supports the developing conceptus with progesterone and estrogen through the first 6 weeks of gestation, after which time the placenta takes over this endocrine role. In human pregnancy, excision of the corpus luteum earlier than the 6th week results in abortion; furthermore, one cause of early abortion in humans is inadequate function of this structure. Therefore, it seems probable that a better understanding of factors controlling corpus luteum function during early pregnancy may lead to new treatments for infertility.

In some species, prostaglandins have a direct luteolytic effect, and this may also be true in humans. In sheep, the life span of the corpus luteum is prolonged after hysterectomy, and it has been suggested that prostaglandins produced in the ipsilateral uterine horn provoke corpus luteum regression in the nonpregnant estrous cycle. In humans, hysterectomy does not prevent corpus luteum regression during the cycle, an observation that has led investigators to examine whether PGs of ovarian origin may be responsible for luteolysis. Challis (5) examined various tissues in the human ovary and found a high concentration of prostaglandins in the corpus albicans. A high concentration in this site may be either the result or the cause of breakdown of the corpus luteum.

To examine this question further, investigators have recently measured intrauterine pressure with a microballoon and simultaneously collected frequent samples of peripheral venous plasma in women given vaginal suppositories containing a synthetic prostaglandin analog (Upjohn #36,384) in a triglyceride base. Concentrations of the analog were measured by radioimmunoassay of 15-methyl PGF. The object of the study was to determine whether the menstrual induction effect of Upjohn #36,384 was primarily luteolytic or was a result of uterine muscular stimulation. This regimen did not terminate all pregnancies, but whether pregnancy was terminated or not, there was a long delay between the onset of treatment and the increase in resting uterine pressure and in cyclic pressure changes in the uterus. Resting uterine pressure always increased before cyclic uterine pressures, and an increase in cyclic uterine pressures was greater when treatment resulted in early abortion (8). It was interesting that maximum cyclic pressures of the uterus increased when concentrations in 15-methyl PG were falling, and this suggested that vaginal prostaglandin therapy did not act exclusively as an oxytocic agent. It was important that as 15-methyl PGF concentrations rose, progesterone and estradiol levels fell in parallel with human chorionic gonadotrophin concentrations and that the levels of these three hormones continued to fall after the decline in 15-methyl PGF values. Human chorionic gonadotrophin is known to be responsible for maintenance of adequate corpus luteum function. These studies suggested that primary action of prostaglandins in menstrual induction was as an antiluteotrophic agent. It was hypothesized that prostaglandins might diminish uterine blood supply to the developing conceptus and thus produce placental anoxia. As a result of anoxia of the placental site, the production of the luteotrophic agent HCG decreased and, in turn, decreased the corpus luteal stimulation necessary to produce progesterone and estradiol to support the developing conceptus. Therefore, it appears that in humans, exogenous prostaglandins induce early abortion by a secondary rather than a primary effect on corpus luteum function.

Abortion

Csapo (7) and others have also postulated that prostaglandins have an abortifacient action in pregnancies of greater than 6 weeks' gestation and that this action is more complicated than direct uterine stimulation. Csapo studied a group of women who were treated with a vaginal suppository containing 3 mg of Upjohn #36,384 to induce a therapeutic abortion and demonstrated a decrease in progesterone and estradiol levels, which preceded maximum uterine contractility and coincided with an increase in 15-methyl prostaglandin F levels. These workers concluded that prostaglandins act primarily on the uterine vasculature to compromise placental function and therefore to reduce placental steroidogenesis. The decrease in placental steroidogenesis resulted in an increased uterine sensitivity that was probably caused by increased endogenous production and release of prostaglandin secondary to the decreased steroidal action on the myometrium.

There is also evidence that pretreatment with indomethacin prolongs the induction interval in women who are given hypertonic saline intra-amniotically to induce therapeutic abortion (41). This provides further evidence that although exogenous prostaglandins may initiate the process, endogenous prostaglandins are important in the actual abortion. Observations concerning the influence of prostaglandins on luteotrophic function and placental steroidogenesis make it apparent that a considerable amount of investigation will be needed to define the role of antiprostaglandin substances and prostaglandin analogs in treating and preventing early abortion.

PARTURITION

Preterm labor and prematurity make a considerable contribution to perinatal mortality. Rush et al. (31), after reviewing all deliveries between 1973 and 1974 in the John Radcliffe Hospital in Oxford, England, discovered that 5.1% of all deliveries were preterm (less than 37 completed weeks of pregnancy). This 5.1% of deliveries accounted for 65% of early neonatal deaths; furthermore, 35% of newborns died as a result of premature labor of unknown cause. These statistics emphasize the need for a better understanding of the natural mechanisms of parturition.

Parturition in Animals

In a series of experiments carried out in fetal sheep in the late 1960s, Liggins and collaborators (20) obtained evidence concerning the role of the fetus in the initiation of parturition. Hypophysectomy or adrenalectomy of the fetal lamb in utero produced a prolongation of pregnancy, whereas the infusion of adrenocorticotrophin (ACTH) or glucocorticoid hormones into the fetal lamb induced preterm delivery. Infusions of these compounds into the mother had no influence on the length of gestation (20). These studies gave rise to the concept that activation of the fetal pituitary–adrenal axis was one of the mechanisms that triggered parturition.

Thorburn and others (37) subsequently demonstrated that the plasma of fetal lambs contains an increased concentration of cortisol during the last 7 to 10 days before parturition. This increase is independent of changes in plasma binding of cortisol and reflects an increase in the rate of cortisol secretion by the fetal adrenal gland. It is now known that the rise in fetal plasma cortisol concentration is only one link in a chain of endocrine events leading up to parturition. The rise in fetal cortisol is followed by a decrease in the concentration of progesterone in maternal plasma, which occurs 2 to 5 days before birth (37). The fall in placental progesterone output is precipitated by the increase in fetal cortisol through induction in the placenta of 17α-hydroxylase activity, which results in metabolism of progesterone in the placenta to 17α, 20α-dihydroxy progesterone, an inactive metabolite (37). Under the influence of fetal cortisol, the increased availability of 17α-hydroxylated C_{21} steroids in the placenta contributes to a steep rise in unconjugated estrogen concentrations in maternal blood during the last 12 to 14 hr before parturition (37). The fall in progesterone and increase in estrogen lead to an increase in prostaglandin production that is first observed as an elevation in the concentration of prostaglandin $F_{2\alpha}$ in the maternal utero-ovarian vein at the time of parturition (10).

The fall in maternal plasma progesterone and rise in unconjugated estrone and estradiol appear to cause the placenta, myometrium, decidua, and fetal membranes to increase prostaglandin production. Therefore, the concentration of prostaglandin

$F_{2\alpha}$ in the utero-ovarian vein increases in parallel with the increase in the estrogen concentrations at normal term, or during an intrafetal infusion of ACTH or dexamethasone and after maternal administration of estrogen (37).

Parturition can be induced in hypophysectomized fetal sheep by infusion of ACTH into the fetus. These animals are delivered without a rise in maternal estrogen concentrations, but placental progesterone decreases and prostaglandin synthesis is elevated (10). It is possible that progesterone withdrawal alone may be a sufficient stimulus to prostaglandin production in these animals.

During the second stage of labor, oxytocin is secreted by the mother, following activation of the Ferguson reflex by pressure of the fetal presenting part on the vagina. Oxytocin not only acts on the myometrium to enhance uterine activity but also stimulates increased prostaglandin $F_{2\alpha}$ secretion from both the myometrium and the maternal placenta, which insures rapid delivery of the fetus once the cervix has dilated. Steroids are also involved in oxytocin release and action; e.g., the amount of oxytocin released in response to vaginal distension is greater in an estrogen-dominated animal than in one treated with progesterone. It is also possible that estrogen increases both the number and affinity of uterine oxytocin receptors, thereby enhancing oxytocin action on the target organ.

Finally, prostaglandins may be considered as part of the final pathway leading to myometrial contractility. It has recently been suggested that prostaglandins may be a stimulus to formation of gap junctions between adjacent myometrial cells. Gap junctions are thought to form pathways of low resistance that facilitate electrical conductivity between adjacent cells (10). Until full term these structures are not seen in uterine muscle in large numbers. Their presence may be important in the development of synchronous uterine contractility. The prostaglandins also interact with the adenylate cyclase system in myometrium and influence the availability of free calcium. Therefore, prostaglandin E_2 and $F_{2\alpha}$ decrease stimulation of cyclic AMP, which results from beta-agonist action on the myometrium and may decrease the ATP-dependent binding of calcium to the intracellular membrane.

Studies of Human Parturition

Regulation of onset of labor in humans is not completely understood, but it seems clear that prostaglandins are a final common pathway to parturition.

In general, it has been believed that anencephaly in the absence of polyhydramnios predisposes to prolongation of gestation. However, in 1973, after studying 147 anencephalic infants delivered in Amsterdam between 1931 and 1972, Swaab and Honnebier (35) found that for the group as a whole the mean length of gestation was 36.6 weeks, which was shorter than for the control population (39.6 weeks). However, a significant number of the anencephalic fetuses presented with polyhydramnios, which is known to predispose to preterm labor. When anencephalic fetuses with polyhydramnios were excluded, the mean length of pregnancy was 39.7 weeks, which was not significantly different from that of the control population. Furthermore, infants in the anencephalic group showed a much wider variation about the mean; 41% of births were premature and 35% were postmature, a distribution similar to that reported following experimental anencephaly in rhesus monkeys (26). These studies of humans and monkeys suggest that, unlike the sheep, human fetuses play a role only in the fine tuning of gestational length.

Much research effort has been expended in determining human cortisol concentrations in various body fluids with respect to parturition, but there is little evidence that cortisol in the primate plays a role analogous to that of cortisol in fetal sheep in the initiation of parturition.

In some species it is well established that progesterone helps to maintain uterine quiescence; this effect is mediated through suppression of the spontaneous generation and propagation of action potentials in the uterus. In primates the role of progesterone is less clear since, in most reports, concentrations of this steroid do not decrease before spontaneous labor. In fact, measurements of progesterone binding in maternal plasma show that free progesterone concentrations rise with the approach of parturition.

Recent work has focused on the suggestion that there may be local regulation of effective progesterone concentrations within the pregnant uterus and particularly at the level of the fetal membranes in humans. Progesterone metabolism by fetal membranes may be substantial by mid-pregnancy, but decreases by two- to sixfold near term, perhaps because the steroid is no longer available for metabolism (25). Recently, a progesterone-binding protein has been described in human chorion and amnion that may influence the availability of progesterone in late pregnancy (25,34). Schwartz et al. (34) propose that although peripheral progesterone measurements give no evidence of progesterone withdrawal, progesterone-binding capacity in fetal membranes increases after 37 weeks and may induce a local progesterone withdrawal. This action could reduce progesterone concentrations in lysosomes in the human fetal membranes and trigger the steps that lead to an increase in prostaglandin production at labor. At present there is little justification for administering large amounts of progesterone to women presenting in preterm labor and little reason to suspect that progesterone withdrawal, with the possible exception of local change due to progesterone binding proteins, is a prerequisite to the onset of human parturition.

It is not yet clear if estrogen is involved in the mechanism of onset of parturition in humans. In general, labor at term is preceded by an increase in concentration of maternal peripheral plasma estradiol during the final 5 to 6 weeks of pregnancy and by a more rapid increase in the concentration of estradiol in amniotic fluid during the final 20 days (14,40). There is no terminal increase in estradiol concentrations in maternal peripheral venous plasma, such as is seen during the last 24 hours of pregnancy in sheep.

In women and rhesus monkeys, estrone sulfate is quantitatively the major estrogen in the amniotic fluid. Its concentration more than doubles during the last 15 to 20 days of pregnancy. Diczfalusy et al. (9) have shown that estrone sulfate can gain access to the fetus and to fetal membranes from the amniotic fluid. In experiments performed before the 20th week of gestation, these investigators injected tritiated estrone sulfate intra-amniotically and recovered most of the radioactivity from the fetal membranes in an unconjugated form.

In patients with placental sulfatase deficiency, estrogen production is low, and these patients often have prolonged gestation and may fail to respond to induction of labor (21). In this condition, the cervix is small, tight, and hard, and does not ripen easily, which suggests that estrogen may be a stimulus to cervical ripening as well as myometrial contractility. In support of the hypothesis that estrogen is involved in the onset of human parturition, it has been demonstrated that in some women at term, large doses can stimulate uterine contractions but not labor.

At the present time, evidence suggests that estrogen may be involved in human parturition and may provide a link between the fetus and its mother. Whether the active estrogen is in maternal plasma or amniotic fluid remains to be determined, and this question will not be answered until the main site of action for estrogen is established. If the major estrogen effect is on prostaglandin production in fetal membranes, its concentration in amniotic fluid, from which it can be taken up and metabolized in fetal membranes, may be important.

Pulsatile release of maternal oxytocin increases with progression of labor, and sensitivity of the uterus to oxytocin rises during late pregnancy—changes that may be caused by the stimulatory effect of circulating estrogens on the concentration of oxytocin receptors in the uterus. Despite its widespread use to initiate or stimulate labor, the role of oxytocin in the initiation of human parturition has been poorly defined. Schwarz et al. (34) have suggested that its role may be to insure involution of the uterus once the products of conception have been delivered.

Three major lines of evidence suggest that prostaglandins contribute to parturition. These are (a) changes in prostaglandin production near term, (b) effects of inhibitors of prostaglandins, and (c) effects of exogenous prostaglandins.

The concentrations of prostaglandin F metabolites rise progressively in urine throughout late pregnancy and in peripheral blood at the time of parturition. During labor, concentrations of PGE and PGF rise in amniotic fluid, and this increase correlates well with progressive dilatation of the cervix. At full dilatation, the concentration of PGF in amniotic fluid exceeds the concentration of PGE.

Retrospective studies of women who had ingested acetylsalicylic acid for long periods during pregnancy showed that they had significantly longer pregnancies and longer labors than matched controls. Furthermore, indomethacin has been used to suppress myometrial activity and prolong pregnancy in rhesus monkeys and to prevent or treat preterm labor in women (38).

There is considerable evidence that the major site of PG production is within the pregnant uterus. The fetal membranes and decidua may be the principal tissues involved. MacDonald et al. (25) suggested that phospholipase A_2 is the major regulatory step and demonstrated that the PG rise in amniotic fluid in women in labor was accompanied by a parallel rise in unesterified arachidonic acid, which was preferentially released over other fatty acids. They also showed that fetal membranes were richly endowed with fatty acid precursors of arachidonic acid production and that the amnion in particular had appreciable phospholipase activity.

When unesterified arachidonic acid, but not oleic acid, was administered intra-amniotically to women requesting therapeutic abortion, uterine activity and abortion ensued. However, intra-amniotic injection of arachidonic acid was ineffective in women who had ingested acetylsalicylic acid. It is important that not all investigators were able to induce abortion with purified arachidonic acid. Finally, Thorburn (36) has proposed that the cyclo-oxygenase system may be of greater importance in parturition than has been recognized to date, but current concepts of prostaglandin metabolism suggest that the major regulatory step is the availability of unesterified arachidonic acid.

Phospholipase A_2 is a lysosomal enzyme, and it has been proposed that factors that regulate lysosomal stability might control the level of tissue phospholipase activity. Although Gustavii (12) initially proposed that decidual lysosomes were particularly susceptible to fracture, recent evidence suggests that arachidonic acid liberation occurs mainly in the fetal membranes, particularly in the amnion. It is possible that steroids regulate the activity of phospholipids through their effects on lysosomal stability.

MacDonald et al. (25) have suggested that the appearance of a high-affinity binding protein for progesterone in the fetal membranes induces a local progesterone withdrawal. If progesterone is normally involved in maintaining lysosomal stability, its withdrawal could result in increased phospholipase A_2 activity. These investigators and Gustavii have drawn an analogy between endocrine interactions at parturition and those at the end of the menstrual cycle.

Our own work supports an alternative hypothesis. We propose that estrogen, present in amniotic fluid either as a sulfoconjugate or as free steroid, gains access to fetal membranes. It is known that fetal membranes, particularly chorion, possess highly potent steroid sulfatase activities and could hydrolyse the conjugated estrogen present in amniotic fluid (6). The free estrogen then might exert a direct labilizing effect on lysosomal membranes and influence their function through synthesis of new protein according to classical receptor theory. The net result would be the same as progesterone withdrawal. Phospholipase A_2 activity would be increased and prostaglandin synthesis initiated. Because prostaglandin itself can directly influence lysosomal fragility, this would provide a positive feedback mechanism.

It is likely that in normal women, more than one of the above-mentioned factors are involved in the stimulus to prostaglandin production. The influence of the fetus may be in proportion to its participation in estrogen synthesis, although still unelucidated factors controlling production of the progesterone-binding protein may also have a fetal component.

Therefore, evidence is accumulating that a series of steroid and peptide hormonal changes eventually merge along the final common pathway to prostaglandin generation. It is likely that any one or all of the steroids mentioned can influence prostaglandin production. The sheep fetus plays a prominent role in the onset of parturition through its production of cortisol, which influences both progesterone and estrogen production. The human fetus, through its secretion of C_{19} steroids, has some influence on estrogen production, but apparently little direct influence on progesterone. Human fetuses seem to have a reduced influence on the control of parturition, unless one considers the amnion and chorion as fetal structures. Hence it seems probable that the timing of human parturition is still very much influenced by the products of conception.

SAFETY OF INHIBITORS OF PROSTAGLANDIN SYNTHESIS DURING PREGNANCY

The final common pathway in parturition is production of prostaglandins and their effects on uterine smooth muscle. Therefore, clinicians have asked investigators whether prostaglandin synthetase inhibitors might be safe for use in the prevention or treatment of preterm labor.

Maternal anemia, gastrointestinal bleeding, and postpartum hemorrhage have been reported to be associated with the use of salicylates during pregnancy, but the major concern regarding these substances is their possible actions on the fetus (19). Prostaglandins may have significant roles in fetal life. It has been suggested that the most important effects of naturally occurring prostaglandins are in the maintenance of the ductus arteriosus and the renal, mesenteric, uteroplacental, and probably the cerebral and coronary arteries in a relaxed or dilated state during fetal life. These effects have been reviewed in detail by Levin (19).

There is little direct evidence that acetylsalicylic acid or indomethacin produces congenital abnormalities in human fetuses. Some studies have indicated that there is an increase in fetal anomalies and in fetal and neonatal deaths when the mothers ingest salicylate (19). Furthermore, a variety of reports have suggested that maternal ingestion of indomethacin or salicylate before birth may induce premature constriction of the ductus arteriosus and pulmonary hypertension in the newborn (19).

Both indomethacin and salicylate cross the placenta in rabbits, sheep and rhesus monkeys. Salicylate ingested before delivery is present in the plasma of newborns, and plasma concentrations of salicylate remain elevated for a longer period than concentrations in maternal plasma (3). In addition, the kinetics of acetylsalicylic acid and indomethacin metabolism vary with age; for example, both drugs are eliminated more slowly in newborns than in adults (3).

Although it is not yet possible to recommend the use of prostaglandin synthetase inhibitors in the treatment or prevention of preterm labor, it may eventually be possible to make use of such inhibitors, particularly if a compound can be developed that does not cross the fetal barrier or have significant effects on maternal or fetal circulatory dynamics.

ACKNOWLEDGMENTS

We wish to thank Drs. Tom Kennedy, Al Yuzpe and Peter Mitchell for their help with this review. Parts of this work were supported by grants-in-aid from the Medical Research Council of Canada, The Richard and Jean Ivey Foundation, and the Physicians' Services Incorporated Foundation.

REFERENCES

1. Anderson, A. B. M., Haynes, P. J., Guillebaud, J., and Turnbull, A. C. (1976): Reduction of menstrual-blood loss by prostaglandin-synthetase inhibitors. *Lancet*, 1:774–776.
2. Anderson, A. B. M., Haynes, P. J., Fraser, I. S., and Turnbull, A. C. (1978): Trial of prostaglandin-synthetase inhibitors in primary dysmenorrhea. *Lancet*, 1:345–348.
3. Berman, W., Friedman, Z., and Vidyasagar, D. (1980): Pharmacokinetics of inhibitors of prostaglandin synthesis in the perinatal period. *Seminars in Perinatology*, 4:67–72.
4. Castracane, V. D., Saksena, S. K., and Slaikl, A. A. (1974). Effect of IUD's, prostaglandins and indomethacin on decidual cell reaction in the rat. *Prostaglandins*, 6:397–404.
5. Challis, J. R. G., Calder, A. A., Dilley, S., Forster, C. S., Hillier, K., Hunter, D. J. S., MacKenzie, I. A., and Thorburn, G. D. (1976): Production of prostaglandin E and F by corpora lutea, corpora albicantes and stroma from the human ovary. *J. Endocrinol.*, 68:401–408.
6. Challis, J. R. G., and Greenblatt, E. (1980): Metabolism of [³H] oestrone sulphate by fetal membranes, placenta and uterine tissues from pregnant rabbits. *J. Reprod. Fertil.*, 58:13–18.
7. Csapo, A. I., and Pulkkinen, M. O. (1979): The mechanism of prostaglandin action on the pregnant human uterus. *Prostaglandins*, 17:283–299.
8. Csapo, A. I., and Pulkkinen, M. O. (1979): The mechanism of prostaglandin action on the early pregnant human uterus. *Prostaglandins*, 18:479–490.
9. Diczfalusy, E., Tillinger, K.-G., Wiqvist, N., Levitz, M., Condon, G. P., and Dancis, J. (1963): Disposition of intra-amniotically administered estriol-16-C¹⁴ and estrone-16-C¹⁴ sulfate by women. *J. Clin. Endocrinol. Metab.*, 23:503–509.
10. Garfield, R. E., Sims, S., and Daniel, E. E. (1977): Gap junctions: their presence and necessity in myometrium during parturition. *Science*, 198:958–960.
11. Gavin, M. A., Dominquez Fernandez-Tejerina, J. C., Montanes De Las Heras, M. F., and Vijil Maeso, E. (1974): Efectos de un inhibitor de la biosintesis de las prostaglandinas (indometacina) sobre la implantacion en la rata. *Reproduccion*, 1:177–183.
12. Gustavii, B., and Brunk, U. (1974): Lability of human decidual cells. *In vivo* effects of hypertonic saline. *Acta Obstet. Gynecol. Scand.*, 53:271–274.
13. Halbert, D. R., Demers, L. M., and Darnell Jones, D. E. (1976): Dysmenorrhea and prostaglandins. *Obstet. Gynecol. Surv.*, 31:77–81.
14. Jolivet, A., and Gautray, J. P. (1978): Liquide amniotique: aspects hormonaux de la maturation foetale et du declenchement du travail. In: *INSERM, Endocrinologie prénatale et parturition*, edited by L. Cedard and C. Sureau, p. 11. INSERM, Paris.
15. Kapadia, L., and Elder, M. G. (1978): Flufenamic acid in treatment of primary spasmodic dysmenorrhea. *Lancet*, 1:348–350.
16. Kauppila, A., and Ylikorkala, O. (1977): Indomethacin and tolfenamic acid in primary dysmenorrhea. *Eur. J. Obstet. Gynecol. Reprod. Biol.*, 7:59–71.
17. Kennedy, T. G. (1977): Evidence for a role for prostaglandins in the initiation of blastocyst implantation in the rat. *Biol. Reprod.*, 16:286–291.
18. Kennedy, T. G. (1980): Prostaglandins and the endometrial vascular permeability changes preceding blastocyst implantation and decidualization. *Prog. Reprod. Biol.*, 1:234–243.
19. Levin, D. L. (1980): Effects of inhibition of prostaglandin synthesis on fetal development oxygenation and the fetal circulation. *Seminars in Perinatology*, 4:35–44.
20. Liggins, G. C. (1969): The foetal role in the initiation of parturition in the ewe. In: *Foetal Autonomy*, edited by G. E. W. Wolstenholme and M. O'Connor, p. 218. Churchill, London.
21. Liggins, G. C., Forster, C. S., Grieves, S. A., and Schwartz, A. L. (1977): Control of parturition in man. *Biol. Reprod.*, 16:39–56.
22. Lindner, H. R., Zor, U., Bauminger, S., Tsafriri, A., Lamprecht, S. A., Koch, Y., Antebi, A., and Schwartz, A. (1974): Use of prostaglandin synthetase inhibitors in analyzing the role of prostaglandins in reproductive physiology. In: *Prostaglandin Synthetase Inhibitors*, edited by H. J. Robinson, and J. R. Vane, pp. 271–287. Raven Press, New York.
23. Lundström, V., and Green, K. (1978): Endogenous levels of prostaglandin F₂ₐ and its main metabolites in plasma and endometrium of normal and dysmenorrheic women. *Am. J. Obstet. Gynecol.*, 130:640–646.
24. Lundström, V., Green, K., and Wiqvist, N. (1976): Prostaglandins, indomethacin and dysmenorrhea. *Prostaglandins*, 11:893–907.
25. MacDonald, P. C., Porter, J. C., Schwarz, G. E., and Johnston, J. M. (1978): Initiation of parturition in the human female. *Seminars in Perinatology*, 2:273–286.

26. Novy, M. J., Walsh, S. W., and Kittinger, G. W. (1977): Experimental fetal anencephaly in the rhesus monkey: effect on gestational length and fetal and maternal plasma steroids. *J. Clin. Endocrinol. Metab.*, 45:1031–1038.
27. Pickles, V. R. (1957): A plain muscle stimulant in the menstruum. *Nature*, 180:1198–1199.
28. Pickles, V. R., Hall, W. J., Best, F. A., and Smith, G. N. (1965): Prostaglandins in endometrium and menstrual fluid from normal and dysmenorrheic subjects. *J. Obstet. Gynaecol. Brit. Comm.*, 72:185–192.
29. *Population Reports (1980):* Series G, Number 8, pp. 96–97. The Johns Hopkins University, Baltimore.
30. Rankin, J. C., Ledford, B. E., Jonsson, H. T., and Baggett, B. (1979): Prostaglandins, indomethacin and the decidual cell reaction in the mouse uterus. *Biol. Reprod.*, 20:399–404.
31. Rush, R. W., Keirse, M. J. N. C., Howat, P., Baum, J. D., Anderson, A. B. M., and Turnbull, A. C. (1976): Contribution of preterm delivery to perinatal mortality. *Br. Med. J.*, 2:965–968.
32. Saksena, S. K., Lau, I. F., and Chang, M. C. (1976): Relationship between oestrogen, prostaglandin $F_{2\alpha}$ and histamine in delayed implantation in the mouse. *Acta Endocrinol. (Copenh.)*, 81: 801–807.
33. Sannes, N., Baulieu, E-E., and Le Goascogne, C. (1976): Prostaglandin(s) as inductive factor of decidualization in the rat uterus. *Mol. Cell Endocr.*, 6:153–158.
34. Schwartz, B. E., Milewich, L., Grant, N. F., Porter, J. C., Johnston, J. M., and MacDonald, P. C. (1977): Progesterone binding and metabolism in human fetal membranes. *Ann. N.Y. Acad. Sci.*, 286:304–310.
35. Swaab, D. F., and Honnebier, W. J. (1973): The influence of removal of the fetal rat brain upon intrauterine growth of the fetus and the placenta and on gestation length. *J. Obstet. Gynaecol. Br. Comm.*, 80:590–597.
36. Thorburn, G. D. (1977): The fetus, pregnancy and parturition. *Ann. Rech. Vet.*, 8:428–437.
37. Thorburn, G. D., Challis, J. R. G., and Robinson, J. S. (1979): Endocrine control of parturition. In: *Biology of the Uterus*, edited by R. M. Wynn, p. 653. Plenum Press, New York.
38. Thorburn, G. D., and Challis, J. R. G. (1979): Endocrine control of parturition. *Physiol. Rev.*, 59:863–918.
39. Tobert, J. A. (1976): A study of the possible role of prostaglandins in decidualization using a nonsurgical method for the instillation of fluids into the rat uterine lumen. *J. Reprod. Fertil.*, 47:391–393.
40. Turnbull, A. C., Anderson, A. B. M., Flint, A. P. F., Jeremy, J. Y., Keirse, M. J. N. C., and Mitchell, M. D. (1977): Human parturition. In: *The Fetus and Birth*, edited by J. Knight and M. O'Connor, p. 427. Elsevier, Amsterdam.
41. Waltman, R., Tricomi, V., and Palav, A. (1973): Aspirin and indomethacin—effect on instillation-abortion time of mid-trimester hypertonic saline induced abortion. *Prostaglandins*, 3:47–58.
42. Ylikorkala, O., and Dawood, M. (1978): New concepts in dysmenorrhea. *Am. J. Obstet. Gynecol.*, 130:833–847.

Acetylsalicylic Acid: New Uses for an Old Drug,
edited by H. J. M. Barnett, J. Hirsh, and
J. F. Mustard. Raven Press, New York © 1982.

Central and Peripheral Mechanisms for the Antialgesic Action of Acetylsalicylic Acid

Tony L. Yaksh

Departments of Neurologic Surgery and Pharmacology, Mayo Clinic, Rochester, Minnesota 55901

This chapter briefly reviews the neural substrates whereby acetylsalicylic acid might exert its antinociceptive actions. The likelihood that acetylsalicylic acid is acting through the inhibition of prostaglandin synthetase strongly argues that prostaglandins or some member of the arachidonic acid cascade plays a role in the transmission of nociceptive stimuli. A variety of evidence reviewed in the chapter suggests that the role of prostaglandins is to facilitate the processing of nociceptive stimuli in the body. The antinociceptive effects of acetylsalicylic acid are therefore explained in terms of its ability to prevent the hypersensitivity accompanying this facilitated transmission of nociceptive information. Evidence suggests that the prostaglandins may exert a direct action on peripheral free nerve endings to facilitate the activation of nociceptive terminals and within the central nervous system, particularly in the spinal cord, to inhibit tonic modulatory systems. In either place, inhibition of prostaglandin synthesis would serve to reduce a facilitated transmission associated with the inflammatory response and reduce the hypersensitivity associated with such chronic stimulation.

Early investigators reported upon the analgesic efficacy of acetylsalicylic acid (23). Although often maligned as being relatively inactive in experimental tests, this drug has been used extensively in clinical practice for over 70 years. Clinical trials support its analgesic effectiveness in certain types of chronic pain, particularly that associated with skeletomuscular disorders such as arthritic inflammation (30,35). Perhaps the principal misunderstanding regarding the use of acetylsalicylic acid in pain is that it deals most efficiently with certain types of pain and that its maximum effect is limited. As we will see below, it is likely that its activity is truncated not because it is ineffective as an active drug but because the system through which nonsteroidal anti-inflammatory agents exert their effects is *facilitative* to the substrate through which pain information travels and is not an essential link between somatic stimulation and the perceptual processes in the central nervous system. To delineate the mechanisms of action of acetylsalicylic acid in particular and nonsteroidal analgesics in general, extensive investigations have been carried out to examine the effects of these drugs in conventional animal models. As shown in Fig. 1, simple animal tests commonly employed as analgesic assays, that is the tail flick (a spinal

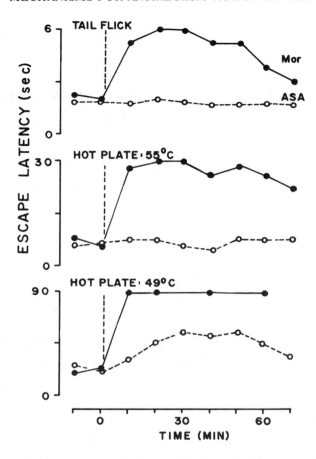

FIG. 1. Time course of the effect of morphine (Mor: ●—●: 10 mg/kg, i.p.) or acetylsalicylic acid (ASA: ○—○: 25 mg/kg, i.p.) on the escape latency on the tail flick test *(top panel)*, the 55°C hot plate *(middle panel)*, or the 49°C hot plate *(bottom panel)*. Each curve represents the mean of 6 to 12 animals. Percent variation was less than 10% of the mean. The drugs were injected at the period indicated by the vertical dashed line.

reflex) and hot plate (55°C) tests, are not altered even by large doses of acetylsalicylic acid. In contrast, morphine, in a dose-dependent fashion, will elevate the pain threshold over a wide range of stimulus strengths. This is not to say that acetylsalicylic acid is necessarily ineffective in response to thermal stimuli; for example, when one employs an extremely sensitive animal test (namely the hot plate test, wherein the stimulus temperature is maintained at 49 or 55°C), systemically administered, nonsteroidal, anti-inflammatory agents can achieve a mild elevation in the response latency.

The tests described above are thought of as simple threshold tests; that is, the animal responds as soon as it receives the appropriate stimulus information. Thermal pain is thought to be communicated by small myelinated or unmyelinated fiber systems (29,44). Upon activation of these systems, the animal performs either a reflex (tail flick) or operant (vocalization, licking of the hind paws) escape response. Thus, the duration of exposure to noxious stimulus is limited by the time required for transmission over the appropriate spinal and brain-stem reflex arcs. As a rule, tests in which the stimulus and resulting neural activation are abbreviated are largely *not* affected by anti-inflammatory agents. This has classically held both in animal and human experimental pain models (2).

In contrast to thermal and electrical threshold tests, the tests that are most sensitive to the effects of the anti-inflammatory "acetylsalicylic acid-like" agents provide clues to the mechanisms underlying the actions of these agents. Two characteristics of these tests are that the stimulus is associated with tissue damage or inflammation and that the stimulus is chemical.

Pressure applied to the rat's paw will produce a stimulus-dependent effort to escape. Figure 2 shows results of experiments using this test, which was devised by Randall and Selitto (40). As is clearly seen, the injection of a small amount of saline into the foot pad has very little effect on the pressure threshold. Also, whereas morphine produces a clear increase in the amount of pressure the animal is willing to accept, acetylsalicylic acid or similar agents are without effect. Again, these results are similar to those observed when one utilizes a simple pain *threshold* measure, whether the stimulus be thermal, electrical or, in this case, mechanical. In contrast, if one induces an inflammatory response by treating an animal with an intraplantar injection of an irritant such as carageenine (13,16,47), brewer's yeast (40), or in this case a dilute solution of formalin, the paw becomes inflamed and warm to the touch, and edema results. In addition, as shown in the bottom part of Fig. 2, the paw becomes *hypersensitive* to the stimulus; that is, a pressure that previously did not evoke an escape response, now evokes such a response, indicating that what earlier was innocuous is now painful. In this preparation, morphine is also able to produce an increase in the antinociceptive threshold. In contrast to the previous experiments in the uninflamed *normal* paw, acetylsalicylic acid shows a clear ability to elevate the pain threshold. Under these circumstances, it is important to note that although the morphine effect is not maximal, a slight increase in dose would completely block the pressure threshold. In contrast, higher doses of acetylsalicylic acid-like compounds do *not* completely block the response to mechanical pressure; these compounds generally reverse only the hyperalgesic component. Here there is a clear analogy to the clinical situation in chronic somatic pain, such as that seen with arthritis or inflammation. Acetylsalicylic acid-like agents have a similar effect on the writhing response evoked by the intraperitoneal injection of an irritant such as phenylbenzoquinone (25) or the incapacitating effects of intra-articular injections of urate crystals (7,11,43,45). It has been suggested that the pain associated with tissue damage originates from the liberation of endogenous factors that may activate sensory endings of small fibers known to transmit nociceptive information. The search for such factors, reviewed elsewhere (8,34), has been extensive. Briefly, bradykinin, serotonin, and histamine are present in damaged

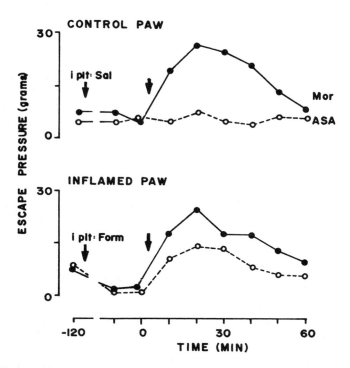

FIG. 2. Pressure (*grams*) required to evoke an escape response versus the time after the systemic injection of morphine (MOR: ●—●: 10 mg/kg, i.p.) or acetylsalicylic acid (ASA: ○—○: 25 mg/kg, i.p.). The top panel indicates the effect of such treatment on thresholds obtained following the intraplantar injection of 50 μl of sterile saline at the time indicated by the first arrow. The bottom panel indicates the effect of such treatment on the escape pressure threshold in an animal in which formalin (10%: 50 μl) was injected into the plantar surface at the time indicated by the first arrow. Each curve represents the mean and standard error of 5 to 12 animals. The error variance was less than 10% of the mean value.

tissue and are capable of activating such fiber systems. Lim (31) has suggested that these agents may interact with perivascular sensory afferents. These agents do not produce their effects by a direct central action, as is shown by the blockade of their nociceptive effects by rhizotomy (19) and the absence of aversive responses after spinal administration (41,51). Bradykinin, for example, induces extreme pain when administered to blister bases in humans (28). In animals, the intra-arterial administration of bradykinin produces clear signs of behavioral aversion, even in the lightly anesthetized animal (20), and evokes discharges in nociceptive neurons in the spinal cord by afferent activation (3,4,42). Figure 3 presents the effects of increasing doses of intra-arterial bradykinin on the pupil diameter of the anesthetized cat (33); increasing doses increase the magnitude and duration of the dilation. If one stimulates (in the same animal) the sciatic nerve at an intensity that is associated with the activation of small fibers and that would evoke escape behavior in an unanesthetized animal, one observes a significant increase in the diameter of the

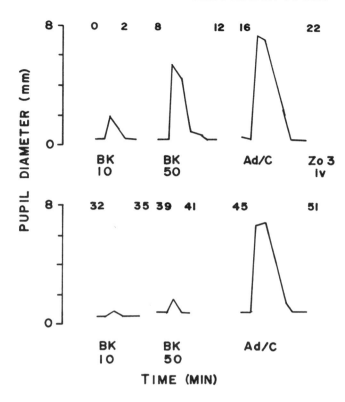

FIG. 3. Effect on pupil diameter in the chloralose-urethanized cat (in millimeters: ordinate) as a function of the intra-arterial injection of bradykinin, 10 μg (BK10) or bradykinin, 50 μg (BK50), or bilateral stimulation of the sciatic nerve at high intensity (Aδ/C). The numbers over each record indicate the real time in minutes; the bottom panel is a continuation of the experiment in the top panel. At 22 minutes after the first bradykinin injection, zomepirac sodium (ZO 3, i.v.) was administered intravenously and the bradykinin and sciatic nerve stimulation sequence repeated in the bottom panel. This figure presents the results observed in a single animal.

pupil. In such a preparation, spinal transections or cold block of the cord block the effects of both bradykinin and electrical stimulation on pupil size. Classical physiology indicates that such responses are mediated by the autonomic reflex arcs activated by painful stimuli. In Fig. 3, the intrathecal administration of zomepirac sodium, an anti-inflammatory agent, significantly reduces the bradykinin-evoked increases in pupil size. In contrast, this agent has little if any effect on the magnitude of the pupil dilatation evoked by the brief electrical stimulus applied to the sciatic nerve. Such results indicate that the pupillary reflex was still functional, and that the intra-arterial bradykinin effect was inhibited at a point peripheral to the axon stimulus, e.g. presumably at the nerve endings. The question of central versus peripheral sites of action for acetylsalicylic acid will be discussed in greater detail below.

The existence of a broad category of compounds that possess acetylsalicylic acid-like analgesic activity has puzzled investigators for a number of years. In the early 1970s, Vane (46) noted that many of these agents had the ability to antagonize the synthesis of prostaglandins by inhibiting the membrane-bound enzyme, cyclo-oxygenase. While it was true that the prostaglandin-synthetase inhibitors also exerted other effects, such as uncoupling oxidative phosphorylation and altering leukocytic migration and protein synthesis, these effects were obtained only at doses considerably higher than those required to inhibit prostaglandin synthetase, and at blood levels higher than those achieved in analgesic therapeutic regimens (14). These results suggested that some mediator derived from the arachidonic acid cascade may play a role in the transduction and/or transmission of nociceptive information.

As noted above, following tissue damage, local sites become hyperalgesic; i.e., previously innocuous stimuli applied to the region have a noxious quality. In addition to being the putative mediator of the inflammatory response, prostaglandins have been found in a variety of inflamed tissues and exudates (1,5,6,17,18,21). For example, the levels of stable prostaglandins in skin following a local burn are elevated to 20 to 40 times that observed in unaffected skin (32). Considerable work

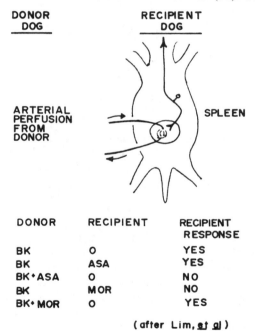

DONOR	RECIPIENT	RECIPIENT RESPONSE
BK	0	YES
BK	ASA	YES
BK·ASA	0	NO
BK	MOR	NO
BK· MOR	0	YES

(after Lim, *et al*)

FIG. 4. An adaptation of the experimental paradigm employed by Lim and his colleagues (32) in demonstrating the peripheral action of acetylsalicylic acid. As described in the text, the spleen of the recipient dog received its arterial perfusion from the donor dog. The listing at the bottom of the figure indicates the injections made into the donor dog's arterial perfusion (donor) and into the recipient's arterial perfusion (recipient). The third column indicates whether the recipient displayed the typical agitation response as a result of the bradykinin injection.

by Ferreira and colleagues (13), however, does not suggest that the prostaglandins are themselves mediators of the pain of inflammation. It has been shown that systemic injection of agents that yield painful sensations (9,10,12) uniquely facilitates the activation of peripheral pain terminals by *sensitizing* the peripheral receptor to mechanical and chemical stimuli. In 1976 Handwerker (22) observed that the discharge of peripheral C-fibers was proportional to the intensity of a locally applied thermal stimulus. The rate of afferent discharge was near zero until skin temperatures began to reach 45 to 50°C. The addition of prostaglandin E_2 (1–3 μg/min) to the fluid perfusing the receptive field produced a dose-dependent increase in the discharge rate of the fibers at every stimulus intensity. The addition of even high doses of prostaglandin E_2 to the skin perfusate had little effect on afferent activity at the lowest stimulus, indicating that the prostaglandins alone were not evoking discharge. The net effect, therefore, of increasing the levels of a member of the arachidonic acid cascade at the peripheral locus is to decrease the stimulus intensity required to evoke a given level of activity in afferent fibers associated with the pain response.

A peripheral locus for the analgesic action of acetylsalicylic acid-like drugs is suggested by the elegant experiments of Lim and colleagues, whose general paradigm is presented schematically in Fig. 4 (32). When studying the pain response of a dog (recipient) whose spleen, though normally innervated, received its blood supply from a second dog (donor), they observed that bradykinin administered into the splenic circulation of the recipient dog evoked signs of agitation. Injection of acetylsalicylic acid-like drugs into the circulation of the recipient had little effect on the response of this dog to the nociceptive stimulus. In contrast, acetylsalicylic acid-like drugs administered into the splenic circulation of the recipient dog blocked the pain response; this suggests that these agents act at perivascular receptors in the spleen of the recipient dog. Since acetylsalicylic acid administered to the recipient dog did not reach its spleen (it was being perfused by the donor dog), the drug's failure to block the bradykinin effect indicated that in this preparation a significant degree of pain relief was not associated with an action on the CNS of the recipient dog. This was in contrast to the effects of opiates whose administration into the recipient circulation blocked the response, suggesting that opiates act not on the perivascular receptors in the spleen activated by the bradykinin given via the donor cross perfusion, but more centrally, presumably in the brain and spinal cord.

Other direct evidence that acetylsalicylic acid-like compounds may act peripherally is suggested by the observation that injections of small amounts of acetylsalicylic acid-like drugs into the inflamed region attenuate the nociceptive response (13).

Thus it appears reasonable to assume that inhibition of the synthesis of some member of the arachidonic acid cascade by the nonsteroidal, anti-inflammatory agents could produce a significant degree of analgesia by the peripheral inhibition of the synthesis of agents that potentiate the response of peripheral nerve fibers to somatic stimuli. It also appears that prostaglandins alone do not mediate the pain response; rather they facilitate the generation of an ongoing message. This explains the limited effectiveness of cyclo-oxygenase inhibitors in controlling pain. They are effective only in those situations where the arachidonic acid cascade has been activated. In animal models, this activation is associated with the presence of tissue damage or the use of a chemical stimulus to activate free nerve endings.

In spite of evidence that inhibitors of prostaglandin synthesis exert their action on a peripheral system, there has been an increasing awareness that they may also exert a central action on neuronal transmission. If the effects of acetylsalicylic acid-like drugs were all peripheral, it is puzzling how such agents, which have comparatively little effect on inflammation, could be active as acetylsalicylic acid-like drugs. Thus, acetaminophen and acetylsalicylic acid are similar in their ability to relieve pain, but the former has little if any peripheral anti-inflammatory effect. Significantly, although having little effect on prostaglandin synthetase in peripheral tissue, these agents are both quite potent in brain enzyme systems (15).

The central action of these drugs can be directly assessed by injecting them into the CNS. During the past four years, we have been studying the existence and role of modulatory systems within the spinal cord. We considered that these acetylsalicylic acid-like agents might exert an effect via a spinal substrate involving prostaglandins.

By insertion of a small catheter down the lumbar space through the cisternal magna, a chronic injection preparation can be obtained (48) and used to determine the effects of altering prostaglandin levels in the spinal cord of the intact and unanesthetized animal. Figure 5 shows the effects of injecting intrathecal acetylsalicylic acid or zomepirac sodium on the writhing response evoked by the intraperitoneal injection of dilute acetic acid. As can be seen, the intrathecal administration of saline had no effect on the time course of the irritant effect. In contrast, intrathecal acetylsalicylic acid (100 μg) or zomepirac sodium (30 μg) attenuated the writhing effect but did not block it. In the bottom graph, which shows the dose-response curve for these two agents, it can be seen that (a) Zomax was 3 to 10 times more potent than acetylsalicylic acid, and (b) maximum inhibition was achieved with the 30 μ dose, suggesting a plateau of effectiveness (higher doses had no greater effect). We know that the effect was not peripheral because 100 μg of drug given intravenously had little influence on the response. These observations concerning a central effect corroborate earlier reports by Ferreira and colleagues (13), who observed that the intraventricular administration of prostaglandin synthesis inhibitors reduced the hyperalgesia associated with the intraplantar injection of an irritant such as carageenine. All these observations taken together suggest that at some point in the neuraxis, increases in the levels of prostaglandins facilitate the processing of the pain message. Figure 6 presents the results of one such series of experiments in which increases in the levels of $PGF_{2\alpha}$ in the spinal cord produced a decrease in the nociceptive threshold to mechanical pressure; i.e., it produced hyperalgesia. Ferreira and colleagues (13) observed that the intraventricular administration of prostaglandins also enhanced the hyperalgesia produced by intraplantar carageenine. In an important finding, they observed that the intraplantar injection of prostaglandins in conjunction with a simultaneous intracerebral injection produced an intense hyperalgesia.

With regard to a central action, it is known that the levels of prostaglandins in the central nervous system normally are low. Therefore, if the central action of prostaglandin-synthesis inhibitors is on a prostaglandin-facilitating mechanism, one

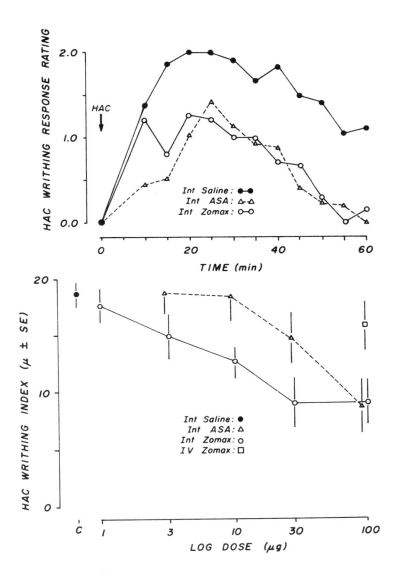

FIG. 5. (*Top*) Effect of the intrathecal administration of saline (●—●), acetylsalicyclic acid (ASA: Δ—Δ: 100 μg) or zomepirac sodium (ZOMAX: ○—○: 30 μg) on the writhing response induced by the intraperitoneal injection of acetic acid (HAC: 1.5 ml, 4% solution). Experiments were carried out double-blind. The intrathecal injections were made 10 min before the administration of the acetic acid. (*Bottom*) Dose-response data for intrathecal saline (●), intrathecal acetyl-salicylic acid (INT ASA: Δ—Δ), intrathecal zomepirac sodium (INT ZOMAX: ○—○) or intravenous zomepirac sodium (IV ZOMAX:□) on the acetic-acid writhing index. The index was calculated as the area under the individual curves presented in the top figure. Each point represents the mean and standard error of 6 to 18 rats.

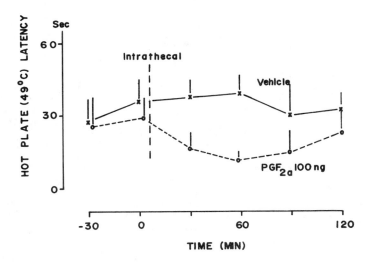

FIG. 6. The response latency on the 49°C hot plate as a function of time after the intrathecal injection of prostaglandins $F_{2\alpha}$(100 ng) or saline vehicle (*vehicle*) at the time zero indicated by the vertical line. Each curve represents the mean and standard error of 5 to 7 animals.

must determine what mechanism underlies the synthesis of prostaglandins. Ramwell and Shaw (37) have demonstrated that somatic stimulation provokes the release of prostaglandin from the sensory cortex of the anesthetized cat. That the release was limited to the contralateral cortex argues that the change was not caused simply by a nonspecific effect such as an elevation in blood pressure or the trauma of the surgical procedure. These investigators also demonstrated that stimulation of the peripheral nerve would generate a stimulus-dependent increase in the levels of the prostaglandins released from frog hemisected spinal cord (38). Recently, we demonstrated the release of prostaglandins $F_{2\alpha}$ from the spinal cord of the intact but anesthetized cat following high-intensity stimulation of the sciatic nerve (S. Romero and T. Yaksh, unpublished observations).

These observations, which show increasing extracellular levels of prostaglandins in cortex and cord associated with prolonged noxious stimulation, in conjunction with experiments in which intrathecal injections of these drugs provoke hyperalgesia, suggest that some component of the peripheral pain message may be facilitated by the activation of a prostaglandin-synthetase-sensitive mechanism.

Though their central role in *facilitating* the pain message is not understood, it is known that prostaglandins can exert a powerful control over the release of a variety of neurotransmitters. Of particular interest is the fact that prostaglandins have been shown to inhibit the release of transmission through sympathetic ganglia (24) and depress the release of norepinephrine from hypothalamic brain slices. Recently, we demonstrated in the spinal cord that peripheral stimuli activate an intrinsic modulatory system that is associated with the activation of *descending* monoamine pathways (49). A variety of experiments have shown that these descending pathways, which

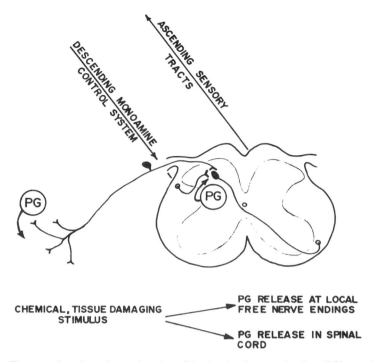

CHEMICAL, TISSUE DAMAGING
STIMULUS

PG RELEASE AT LOCAL
FREE NERVE ENDINGS

PG RELEASE IN SPINAL
CORD

FIG. 7. The tentative sites where elevation of the levels of prostaglandins (PG) may facilitate the transmission of nociceptive stimuli. As indicated in the bottom of the figure, chemical or tissue-damaging stimuli will release PGs at local free nerve endings and release PGs from the spinal cord. Activation of the primary afferent input activates ascending sensory pathways that reflexly activate (at the brainstem level) descending monoamine pathways that exert a modulatory control over dorsal-horn sensory processing. This model is described in the text.

release norepinephrine and serotonin, are capable of exerting a powerful modulatory influence on spinal function (41,51). We believe that these descending pathways are reflexively activated by high-intensity peripheral somatic stimulation (50). This suggests that the hyperalgesia that is produced by intraventricular or intrathecal administration of prostaglandins may be the result of inhibiting the release of this descending modulatory monoamine transmitter. Our demonstration of the release of prostaglandins in the spinal cord following somatic input suggests that this amount of prejunctional inhibition by prostaglandins would to that degree increase the intensity of the pain message. It seems likely that a portion of the systemic and all of the intrathecal effects of prostaglandin-synthesis inhibitors are the result of reducing the concentration of prostaglandins in spinal cord and that the associated increased insensitivity to otherwise innocuous stimuli is the result of a facilitated processing of nociceptive information. It is significant that pharmacological inhibition of norepinephrine terminals by the intrathecal administration of α-adrenergic blocking agents will evoke a hyperalgesia comparable to that produced by the intrathecal injection of PGF_2 described above (36). Other alternatives also exist. Kadlec and colleagues (27) have provided indirect evidence of an interaction between the generation of prostaglandins and changes in endorphin release from guinea-pig ileum.

Figure 7 shows the points at which prostaglandins may act to facilitate the transmission of noxious stimuli. Clearly, prostaglandins are released at peripheral nerve terminals in the presence of a variety of chemical stimuli and of stimuli that produce frank tissue damage and resultant inflammation. The evidence cited above supports the idea that the presence of increased levels of prostaglandins, although not essential for the generation of the pain message, facilitates transmission and augments the sensory response for any intensity of stimulus. Within the central nervous system it has been observed that large quantities of extracellular prostaglandins accumulate in response to peripheral nerve stimulation. Increasing the levels of prostaglandin activity within the neuraxis by intraventricular or intrathecal administration increases the sensitivity of the animal to a noxious stimulus. The mechanisms underlying this central action are not entirely clear, but it appears that these descending monoamine pathways exert both a tonic and reflexly activated control over the rostrad transmission of nociceptive information. The data indicating that prostaglandins may inhibit the release of norepinephrine from such CNS terminals therefore suggest that the magnitude of the ascending sensory message is in part a balance between the release of monoamines and the release of prostaglandins— with the levels of prostaglandins in the cord governing the effectiveness of the monoamine system. In all cases, therefore, the inhibition of prostaglandin synthesis could block pain transmission only to the extent that the prostaglandin system was facilitating the processing of pain information. This suggests (a) why prostaglandin synthesis inhibitors are relatively effective against enduring stimuli such as those associated with inflammation or tissue damage and (b) why the antialgesic effect of acetylsalicylic acid is limited—that is, a ceiling effect is observed in both clinical and animal work (2,39). The effect of acetylsalicylic acid is limited because the system that it inhibits serves only to facilitate pain processing, not to mediate it entirely. In contrast, systems mediated by morphine may inhibit the release of the pain transmitter from the primary afferents (26). Thus, activation of an opiate receptor in the spinal cord can totally block the transmission of noxious stimuli through the spinal synaptic circuitry. This difference in part explains other differences between the properties of analgesia produced by the opiates and by the prostaglandin-synthesis inhibitors. Opiates exert their effects via a receptor system that is subject to the development of tolerance. In contrast, acetylsalicylic acid-like agents act by virtue of their ability to inhibit the *synthesis* of a key facilitative mediator. The inhibition of enzyme function is not subject to such a loss of effectiveness with repeated use. Thus, the effectiveness of acetylsalicylic acid, unlike that of many analgesic drugs, does not decline with repeated usage.

ACKNOWLEDGMENT

I would like to thank Ms. Gail Harty for her technical assistance and Ms. Ann Rockafellow for preparing this manuscript. Some of this work was supported in part by grants from McNeil Laboratories and the Mayo Foundation.

REFERENCES

1. Arthurson, F., Hamberg, M., and Jonsson, C. E. (1973): Prostaglandins in human blister fluid. *Acta Physiol. Scand.*, 87:270–276.
2. Beecher, H. K. (1957): The measurement of pain. *Pharmacol. Rev.*, 9:59–290.
3. Besson, J. M., Conseiller, C., Hamann, K. F., and Maillard, M. C. (1972): Modifications of dorsal horn cell activities in the spinal cord after intra-arterial injection of bradykinin. *J. Physiol. (Lond.)*, 221:189–205.
4. Besson, J. M., Guilbaud, G., and LeBars, D. (1975): Descending inhibitory influences exerted by the brain stem upon the activities of dorsal horn Lamina V cells induced by intra-arterial injection of bradykinin into the limbs. *J. Physiol.*, 248:725–739.
5. Bhattacherjee, P., and Phylactos, A. (1977): Increased prostaglandin synthetase activity in inflamed tissues of the rabbit eye. *Eur. J. Pharmacol.*, 44:75–80.
6. Blackham, A., Farmer, J. B., Radziwonik, H., and Westwick, J. (1974): The role of prostaglandins in rabbit mono-articular arthritis. *Br. J. Pharmacol.*, 51:45–53.
7. Brune, K., Bucher, K., and Walz, D. (1974): The avian microcrystal arthritis. II. Central versus peripheral effects of sodium salicylate, acetaminophen and colchicine. *Agents Action*, 4:27–33.
8. Chahl, L. A. (1979): Pain induced by inflammatory mediators. In: *Mechanisms of Pain and Analgesic Compounds*, edited by R. F. Beers, Jr., and E. G. Bassett, pp. 273–284. Raven Press, New York.
9. Collier, J. G., Karim, S. M. M., Robinson, B., and Somers, K. (1968): Action of prostaglandins A_2, B_1, E_2, $F_{2\alpha}$ on superficial veins of man. *Br. J. Pharmacol.*, 44:374P–375P.
10. Collier, H. O. J., and Schneider, C. (1974): Nociceptive response to prostaglandins and analgesic actions of aspirin and morphine. *Nature*, 236:241–243.
11. Faires, J. S., and McCarty, D. J., Jr. (1962): Acute arthritis in man and dog after intrasynovial injection of sodium urate crystals. *Lancet*, 2:682–685.
12. Ferreira, S. H. (1972): Prostaglandins, aspirin-like drugs and analgesia. *Nature*, 200:240–243.
13. Ferreira, S. H., Lorenzetti, B. B., and Correa, F. M. A. (1978): Central and peripheral antialgesic action of aspirin-like drugs. *Eur. J. Pharmacol.*, 53:39–48.
14. Ferreira, S. H., and Vane, J. R. (1974): New aspects of the mode of action of nonsteroid anti-inflammatory drugs. *Ann. Rev. Pharmacol.*, 14:57–73.
15. Flower, R. J., and Vane, J. R. (1972): Inhibition of prostaglandin synthetase in brain explains the anti-pyretic activity of paracetamol (4-acetamido-phenol). *Nature*, 240:410–411.
16. Garcia Leme, J., Hamamura, L., Leite, M. P., and Rocha e Silva, M. (1973): Pharmacological analysis of the acute inflammatory process induced in the rat's paw by local injection of carageenine and by heating. *Br. J. Pharmacol.*, 48:88–96.
17. Goldyne, M. E., Winkelmann, R. K., and Ryan, R. J. (1973): Prostaglandin activity in human cutaneous inflammation: Detection by radioimmunoassay. *Prostaglandins*, 4:737–748.
18. Greaves, M. W., Sodergaard, J., and McDonald-Gibson, W. (1971): Recovery of prostaglandins in human cutaneous inflammation. *Br. Med. J.*, 2:258–260.
19. Guzman, F., Braun, C., and Lim, R. K. S. (1962): Visceral pain and the pseudo-affective response to intra-arterial injection of bradykinin and other algesic agents. *Arch. Int. Pharmacodyn. Ther.*, 136:352–384.
20. Guzman, F., Braun, C., Lim, R. K. S., and Rodgers, D. W. (1964): Narcotic and non-narcotic analgesics which block visceral pain evoked by intra-arterial injection of bradykinin and other algesic agents. *Arch. Int. Pharmacodyn. Ther.*, 149:571–588.
21. Hamberg, M., and Jonsson, C.-E. (1973): Increased synthesis of prostaglandins in the guinea pig following scalding injury. *Acta Physiol. Scand.*, 87:240–245.
22. Handwerker, H. O. (1976): Influences of algogenic substances and prostaglandins on the discharge of unmyelinated cutaneous nerve fibers identified as nociceptors. *Adv. Pain Res. Ther.*, 1:41–45.
23. Hanzlik, P. J. (1927): *Actions and Uses of the Salicylates and Cinchophen in Medicine*. Williams & Wilkins, Baltimore.

24. Hedqvist, P., Stjarne, L., and Wennmalm, A. (1971): Facilitation of sympathetic neurotransmission in the cat spleen after inhibition of prostaglandin synthesis. *Acta Physiol. Scand.*, 83:430–432.
25. James, G. W. L., and Church, M. K. (1978): Hyperalgesia after treatment of mice with prostaglandins and arachidonic acid and its antagonism by anti-inflammatory–analgesic compounds. *Arzneim. Forsch.*, 28:804–809.
26. Jessell, T. M., and Iversen, L. L. (1977): Opiate analgesics inhibit substance P release from rat trigeminal nucleus. *Nature*, 268:549–551.
27. Kadlec, O., Seferna, I., and Masek, K. (1980): Modulatory role of prostaglandins on cholinergic neurotransmission in the guinea pig. In: *Advances in Prostaglandin and Thromboxane Research, Vol. 8*, edited by B. Samuelsson, P. W. Ramwell, and R. Paoletti, pp. 1255–1257. Raven Press, New York.
28. Keele, C. A., and Armstrong, R. (1964): *Substances Producing Pain and Itch*. Williams & Wilkins, Baltimore.
29. LaMotte, R. H., and Campbell, J. N. (1978): Comparison of responses of warm and nociceptive C-fiber afferents in monkey with human judgments of thermal pain. *J. Neurophysiol.*, 41:509–528.
30. Lasagna, L. (1970): The clinical pharmacology of analgesics and analgesic antagonists. In: *The Pharmacology of Pain, Vol. 9*, edited by R. K. S. Lim, pp. 113–120. Pergamon Press, New York.
31. Lim, R. K. S. (1967): Pain mechanisms. *Anesthesiology*, 28:106–110.
32. Lim, R. K. S., Guzman, F., Rodgers, D. W., Goto, K., Braun, G., Dickerson, G. D., and Engle, R. J. (1964): Site of action of narcotic analgesics determined by blocking bradykinin-evoked visceral pain. *Arch. Int. Pharmacodyn. Ther.*, 152:25–59.
33. Loewy, A. D., Araugo, J. C., and Kerr, F. W. L. (1973): Pupillodilator pathways in the brainstem of the cat: Anatomical and electrophysiological identification of a central autonomic pathway. *Brain Res.*, 60:65–94.
34. Lynn, B. (1977): Cutaneous hyperalgesia. *Br. Med. Bull.*, 33:103–108.
35. Moertel, C. G., Ahmann, D. L., Taylor, W. F., and Schwartau, N. (1974): Relief of pain by oral medications. A controlled evaluation of analgesic compounds. *JAMA*, 29:55–59.
36. Proudfit, H. K., and Yaksh, T. L. (1980): Alterations in nociceptive threshold and morphine-induced analgesia following the selective depletion of spinal cord monoamines. *Proc. Soc. Neurosci.*, 6:433.
37. Ramwell, P. W., and Shaw, J. E. (1966): Spontaneous and evoked release of prostaglandins from cerebral cortex of anesthetized cats. *Am. J. Physiol.*, 211:125–134.
38. Ramwell, P. W., Shaw, J. E., and Jessup, R. (1966): Spontaneous and evoked release of prostaglandins from frog spinal cord. *Am. J. Physiol.*, 211:998–1004.
39. Randall, L. O. (1963): Non-narcotic analgesics. In: *Physiological Pharmacology, Vol. 1. The Nervous System. Part A, Central Nervous System Drugs*, edited by W. S. Root and F. G. Hofmann, Academic Press, New York.
40. Randall, L. O., and Selitto, J. J. (1957): A method for measurement of analgesic activity on inflamed tissue. *Arch. Int. Pharmacodyn. Ther.*, 111:409–419.
41. Reddy, S. V. R., Maderdrut, J. L., and Yaksh, T. L. (1980): Spinal cord pharmacology of adrenergic agonist-mediated antinociception. *J. Pharmacol. Exp. Ther.*, 213:525–533.
42. Satoh, M., Doi, T., Kawasaki, K., Akaide, A., and Takagi, H. (1976): Effect of indomethacin and other anti-inflammatory agents on activation of dorsal horn cells in the spinal cord induced by intra-arterial bradykinin. *Jpn. J. Pharmacol.*, 26:309–314.
43. Smolin, L. N. (1976): The peripheral mechanisms of sensitization of inflamed tissues. In: *Somatosensory and Visceral Receptor Mechanisms: Progress in Brain Research, Vol. 43*, edited by A. Iggo and O. B. Ilyensky, pp. 307–309. Elsevier, Amsterdam.
44. Torebjork, H. E. (1974): Afferent C units responding to mechanical, thermal and chemical stimuli in human non-glaborous skin. *Acta Physiol. Scand.*, 92:374–396.
45. Van Arman, C. G., Carlson, R. P., Risley, G. A., Thomas, R. H., and Nuss, G. W. (1970): Inhibitory effects of indomethacin, aspirin and certain other drugs on inflammations induced in rat and dog by carageenine, sodium and ellagic acid. *J. Pharmacol. Exp. Ther.*, 175:459–472.
46. Vane, J. R. (1971): Inhibition of prostaglandin synthesis as a mechanism of action for aspirin-like drugs. *Nature (New Biol.)*, 291:233–238.
47. Winter, C. A., and Flataker, L. (1965): Reaction threshold to pressure in edematous hindpaws of rats and responses to analgesic drugs. *J. Pharmacol. Exp. Ther.*, 150:165–171.

48. Yaksh, T. L., and Rudy, T. A. (1976): Chronic catheterization of the spinal subarachnoid space. *Physiol. Behav.*, 17:1031–1036.

49. Yaksh, T. L., and Rudy, T. A. (1978): Narcotic analgesics: CNS sites and mechanisms of action as revealed by intracerebral injection techniques. *Pain*, 4:299–359.

50. Yaksh, T. L., and Tyce, G. M. (1980): Resting and K+ evoked release of serotonin and norepinephrine *in vivo* from the rat and cat spinal cord. *Brain Res.*, 192:113–146.

51. Yaksh, T. L., and Wilson, P. R. (1979): Spinal serotonin terminal system mediates antinociception. *J. Pharmacol. Exp. Ther.*, 208:446–453.

Acetylsalicylic Acid: New Uses for an Old Drug,
edited by H. J. M. Barnett, J. Hirsh, and
J. F. Mustard. Raven Press, New York © 1982.

Temperature Regulation, Fever, and Antipyretics

*Keith E. Cooper, W. L. Veale, and N. W. Kasting

*Division of Medical Physiology, the University of Calgary, Calgary,
Alberta, Canada T2N 1N4*

Body temperature is maintained constant by a balance in the rate of heat production and the rate of heat loss. Heat loss involves control of the blood flow through the skin, which is partly dependent upon temperature-sensing mechanisms within the hypothalamus and partly on reflexes generated from temperature sensors in the skin. Sweating, another avenue of heat loss, similarly seems to depend on information arriving at the brain from the skin and from sensing the temperature of the blood reaching the hypothalamus region. Heat retention in the adult is also brought about by skin vasoconstriction. In man both heat loss and heat retention are to a large extent controlled by behavioral means.

A variety of drugs that affect the synthesis or receptor binding of any of the transmitter substances can be expected to have an effect on body temperature. Furthermore, it is likely that other parts of the brain, including the limbic system, are involved in the behavioral aspects of thermoregulation.

Fever is thought to be mediated by the generation of endogenous pyrogens. Endogenous pyrogen or pyrogens appear to act in the brain principally in the preoptic area, but they may also act in other regions of the brain to excite the heat conservation mechanisms and the heat production mechanisms, thereby raising body temperature. Recent evidence suggests that a humoral feedback mechanism in the brain may tend to limit the height of fever. In a wide variety of species, fever has an important survival value. In mammals with blood-borne infections it plays an important role in increasing survival, chiefly in the first 6 hours or so. Therefore, the use of antipyretics may be unwise.

Acetylsalicylic acid is an inhibitor of prostaglandin synthetase. Minute amounts of prostaglandins of the 'E' series produce fever when injected into the same regions in which micro-injections of endogenous pyrogen also produce fever. The levels of prostaglandins in the cerebrospinal fluid have been correlated with the onset of fever and with its suppression by acetylsalicylic acid and other antipyretics. On the other hand, other investigators have been able to suppress prostaglandin release without altering the fever and vice versa. Animals that have suffered total ablation of the parts of the brain that respond to prostaglandin with fever are still able to

---

*Mailing address: Dr. K.E. Cooper, Professor of Medical Physiology, University of Calgary, Calgary, Alberta, Canada T2N 1N4

get fever from intravenous pyrogens. Also, injection into the cerebrospinal fluid of substances that block the receptor sites for the 'E' series prostaglandins does not prevent fever from intravenous pyrogen; and other substances that block protein synthesis but have no effect on prostaglandin production appear to be good antipyretics when injected into the cerebrospinal fluid. Thus the modes of action of a number of different antipyretics seem to vary, and various types of actions have been postulated for the antipyretics, including acetylsalicylic acid.

This brief review deals with the action of antipyretics, in particular salicylate, on body temperature in health and during fever.

The human body can be considered as a core consisting of the intracranial, intrathoracic, and intra-abdominal contents, the temperature of which is regulated with remarkable precision close to 37°C, and a shell made up of the skin, subcutaneous tissues, muscles, and limbs. In extremes of thermal environment, the shell temperature can fluctuate widely in the process of defending the core temperature. Five physiologically controlled processes act to retain or dissipate heat from the shell during short-term perturbations of body or environmental temperature. These are:

a. behavioral, e.g., varying the amount of clothing or altering the shelter temperature (this is probably the most significant mechanism used by man);

b. vasomotor, e.g., control of the blood flow in the skin;

c. sweating, the mechanism that allows evaporation of water secreted on to the skin surface (its efficiency is greatly increased by acclimatization to heat);

d. respiratory heat loss (panting), a mechanism used by man only in extreme heat conditions but of great importance in many animals;

e. shivering, or metabolic heat production from random muscle contraction. Changes in basal metabolism caused by increased thyroid hormone production or by alterations in fat metabolism represent long-term adaptations to cold exposure, and not rapid immediate responses to thermal changes.

In determining the type and extent of these effector responses, the brain uses afferent information derived from many sources. Behavioral thermoregulation depends on assessment of the environmental conditions by many senses. Temperature is sensed by neural transducers in the skin and many other body sites, but particularly in the central nervous system. Thermosensitive neurones have been detected in the preoptic and anterior hypothalamic areas (PO/AH), in the septal region, the midbrain, the brainstem, and the spinal cord. The highest density of such thermosensitive units is in the PO/AH. The widespread existence of such thermosensitive structures is not surprising if one considers that thermoregulatory processes have been retained in the central nervous system during evolution, with the more precise mechanisms "layered" at higher and higher levels (26). The afferent information is integrated and translated into effector action principally within the preoptic and hypothalamic areas of the brain, with participation of the septal areas and much of the midbrain, spinal cord, and the higher brain areas.

The brain circuitry, the complex connections of which have not yet been unravelled, is assisted by a number of synaptic transmitter substances. It is clear that both norepinephrine (NE) and 5-hydroxytryptamine (5-HT) are transmitter agents in hypothalamic thermoregulatory synapses. In the primates and many other mammals, it is likely that 5-HT is involved in pathways that drive effector mechanisms leading to a rise in body temperature (13,24). Similarly, in these species, NE tends to be used in synapses, the activation of which leads to a fall in body temperature. However, in other species, the role of these monoamines may be reversed (5). In addition, evidence from many experiments suggests models of synaptic connections in which the neurons driving the effector mechanisms for heat production and retention "branch" to inhibit the mechanisms for heat loss and *vice versa* (3). It is also clear that thermoregulatory circuits may employ a number of other neuro-transmitters, such as dopamine (7), acetylcholine (21) and histamine (21). The action of monoamines in thermoregulation has some importance in relation to the clinical use of monoamine-oxidase inhibitors, since there is evidence that these drugs can potentiate fever.

A further concept, as yet not fully understood, is that a balance between the concentrations of Ca^{++} and Na^+ in the posterior hypothalamus may determine the body temperature "set point" (25). In microperfusion studies, the thermoregulatory response to altering the Ca^{++} and Na^+ concentrations in fluid perfusing brain tissue are specific to the posterior hypothalamus. Although the full significance of this observation is not yet clear, it could be of major importance in helping us understand the activity of the "final common pathways" of the thermoregulatory effectors and of the action of drugs on them.

There has been controversy as to whether prostaglandins contribute to the mediation of normal thermoregulatory responses. The consensus is that, in most species, prostaglandins are not part of the normal thermoregulatory process (10). Thus the occasionally reported hypothermic action of some antipyretic agents in nonfebrile animals is related to an action unassociated with prostaglandin synthesis.

An understanding of the antipyretic action of salicylate and other antipyretics requires an appreciation of the current concept of the mechanism of fever—namely, pathological elevation of body temperature by mechanisms initially outside the normal thermoregulatory processes that drive the thermoregulatory effector systems to conserve and produce heat. There is evidence that endotoxins interact with such cells as blood leucocytes (1), reticuloendothelial cells, and perhaps other cell types, causing them to release a pyrogenic substance known as "endogenous pyrogen." Endogenous pyrogen is a peptide of molecular weight of 15,000 daltons, which may occur in the circulation as a trimer of 45,000 dalton molecular weight (11). There is increasing evidence that the main blood-cell type releasing endogenous pyrogen is the monocyte. Certainly, the evidence favors the release of endogenous pyrogen as essential to the fever in infection, cell damage, and allergy.

Endogenous pyrogen (EP) reaches the cerebral circulation and is alleged to enter the brain (although there is still little evidence for this) to cause fever. The mechanism by which EP causes fever is the subject of controversy; it is commonly stated that EP causes the release of prostaglandins of the "E" series (PGE) and that PGE acts on hypothalamic neurones to drive the heat conservation and production pathways (22,23). The main evidence for PGE involvement in fever is as follows:

a. Microinjection or tissue perfusion of PGE into the PO/AH or the cerebral ventricles in minute quantities causes fever, and the loci of injection in which PGE induces fever correspond precisely with the sites of action of injected EP. All species respond similarly to such PGE microinjection, if they respond at all (14,29,34).

b. The concentration of PGE in cerebrospinal fluid, derived from lateral ventricle to cisterna magna perfusion, rises and falls as the body temperature increases and decreases in fever (12).

c. Drugs that inhibit the synthesis of PGE are antipyretic (15,30).

d. Brain tissue is capable of synthesizing PGE.

e. Exogenous and endogenous pyrogens cause fever when microinjected into the PO/AH, but do so only after a significant latent period. Similarly injected PGE induces fever with little or no latent period.

Although this evidence seems strongly to suggest a major role for PGE in the genesis of fever and to implicate PGE-synthesis inhibition in the action of antipyretic drugs, there is growing evidence that the PGE pathway is not the only essential mechanism of fever. The evidence against the sole role of PGE as a final mediator in fever is as follows:

a. Ablation of the PO/AH in the rabbit is such that intra-ventricular injection of PGR, or injection of PGE into the lesion site, does not prevent fever due to intravenous pyrogen. However, the character of the fever is different (33).

b. The action of PGE on thermosensitive PO/AH neurones does not consistently mimic that of EP.

c. Intraventricular PGE antagonists, which block PGE fever, do not prevent EP fevers (9). But arachidonic acid injected into the cerebral ventricles causes fever that is blocked by indomethacin but not by prostaglandin antagonists, suggesting that endoperoxides or thromboxanes may be more important than prostaglandins (20).

d. Salicylate, a poor antipyretic in the rabbit, can be intravenously infused in a dose that prevents the rise in PGE concentration in CSF but does not prevent the fever.

e. Intravenously injected, cyclohexamide, a protein-synthesis inhibitor, attenuates fever due to intraventricular EP (8,28). It does not alter the fever caused by intraventricular arachidonic acid (8).

Thus, it appears that although PGE might be involved in the genesis of fever, there are other fever mechanisms that do not depend on its synthesis and action, and one of these may involve PG precursors or thromboxanes.

For centuries, the role of fever in the body's defense against infection has been in question. In recent years, Kluger and his colleagues (18) have adduced powerful evidence that fever has a protective effect and a survival value. Vertebrates that principally use behavioral thermoregulation, such as some lizards, fish, and indeed some Crustacea, respond to infection by raising their body temperatures. This they do by spending more time in the sun or by seeking warmer water. If this rise in temperature is prevented, the mortality associated with infection is much higher. Other evidence suggests that survival in the rabbit is enhanced by fever during a blood-borne infection, and that suppression of fever by systemic or hypothalamic administration of salicylate during the first 6 hours of infection increases the mortality rate (32). The way in which fever protects the infected organism is not fully understood. One mechanism may be related to the reduction in plasma iron that accompanies early fever, thereby reducing the supply of a necessary bacterial metabolite (19). Also, the inflammatory response may be enhanced by fever (2), but many facets of its survival value remain to be elucidated.

Antipyretic drugs have been known for many centuries (17), but their modes of action, in the main, still elude our understanding. Some steroids, such as cortisol, may be antipyretic, and there is some evidence that these substances can inhibit the synthesis of EP. The chemical structures of other antipyretic substances, including salicylic acid and its derivatives—especially acetylsalicylic acid, acetanilid, acetaminophen, phenacetin, antipyrine, aminopyrine and indomethacin—are shown in Fig. 1. In antipyretic doses, these drugs have little effect on normal body temperature, but in higher doses, the more lipid-soluble compounds, such as aminopyrine, can lower the temperature in nonfebrile animals. It is likely that indomethacin and salicylate do not inhibit EP formation or limit its passage into the brain. Salicylate acts at the same loci in the hypothalamus to reduce fever as prostaglandin acts to cause fever (31), and it may also have actions elsewhere. If we accept the hypothesis that one element in the production of fever is the release of PGE or its precursors

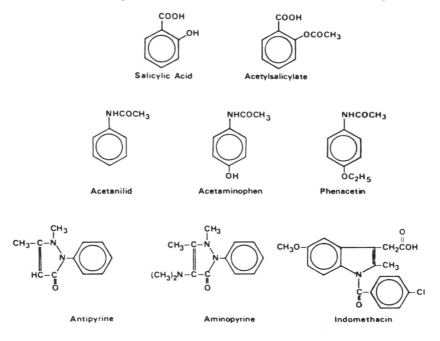

FIG. 1. Some antipyretic substances.

into the PO/AH, then the inhibition of PGE synthesis may be one mode of action of salicylate. It is also possible that antipyretics directly compete with EP for receptor sites on PO/AH thermoregulatory neurones (4). There is, however, some neurophysiological evidence that this may not be the case (27). Whether the antipyretics could affect the postulated Ca^{++}/Na^{+} set-point mechanism in the posterior hypothalamus is an interesting speculation. Certainly, there is some evidence from ion fluxes that this ratio may alter during the rising and falling phases of body temperature in fever.

In large overdoses, salicylate may cause fever, but this is a consequence of the uncoupling of oxidative phosphorylation in most tissues. This action is quite distinct from its normal therapeutic action in fever.

A new and most interesting concept is that the brain produces its own endogenous antipyretic, at a rate determined by the height of the fever, and possibly as a feedback mechanism to limit fever to its useful protective level. There is evidence that, in the sheep, this endogenous antipyretic is arginine vasopressin (AVP) and that it acts in the septal region (6,16). The evidence for this includes the following observations:

a. Tissue perfusates from the septal region contain AVP, and its concentration dramatically rises in fever.

b. AVP perfused through the septal area in very small amounts suppresses fever.

c. AVP perfused through the septal area does not reduce normal body temperature.

d. AVP-containing neurons project from the supraoptic, suprachiasmatic, and paraventricular nuclei to the septal region.

e. Perfusion of the septal region with either AVP antibody or AVP analogs— which are not antipyretic—greatly enhances fever.

f. Some antipyretics also suppress fever when perfused through the septal area. In addition, there is evidence that naturally occurring AVP suppresses fever from a day or two before to a few hours after the term of pregnancy, an observation that is of obvious significance but is little understood. There is also some evidence that AVP present in the ventricular CSF can provoke seizures similar to those seen in febrile convulsions in children. Thus, in elucidation of the mechanism of therapeutic antipyresis, the possible role of endogenous peptide antipyretics may be considered.

The protective value of fever should lead us to reappraise the use of antipyretics. Clearly, in excessively high fevers they may be of benefit, and they may be important in protecting against the teratogenic effect of fever in early pregnancy. Possibly, they are important in reducing the risk of febrile convulsions in children. Otherwise, the increased comfort induced by a few milligrams of acetylsalicylic acid has to be weighed against the possible therapeutic value of the fever. It is clear that we are only at the beginning of our understanding of fever and antipyretic drug action.

REFERENCES

1. Beeson, P. B. (1948): Temperature elevating effect of a substance obtained from polymorphon-uclear leucocytes. *J. Clin. Invest.*, 27:525–531.

2. Bernheim, H. A., Bodel, P. T., Askenase, P. W., and Atkins, E. (1978): Effects of fever on host defense mechanisms after infection in the lizard *Dipsosaurus dorsalis*. *Br. J. Exp. Pathol.*, 59:76–84.
3. Bligh, J. (1973): *Temperature Regulation in Mammals and Other Vertebrates*. North-Holland, Amsterdam.
4. Clark, W. G., and Cumby, H. R. (1975): The antipyretic effect of indomethacin. *J. Physiol. (Lond.)*, 248:625–638.
5. Cooper, K. E., Cranston, W. I., and Honour, A. J. (1965): Effects of intraventricular and intrahypothalamic injection of noradrenaline and 5-HT on body temperature in conscious rabbits. *J. Physiol. (Lond.)*, 181:852–864.
6. Cooper, K. E., Kasting, N. W., Lederis, K., and Veale, W. L. (1979): Evidence supporting a role for endogenous vasopressin in natural suppression of fever in the sheep. *J. Physiol. (Lond.)*, 295:33–45.
7. Cox, B., and Potkonjak, D. (1967): The effect of ambient temperature on the actions of tremorine on body temperature and on the concentration of noradrenaline, dopamine, 5-hydroxytryptamine and acetylcholine in rat brain. *Br. J. Pharmacol. Chemother.*, 31:356–364.
8. Cranston, W. I., Dawson, N. J., Hellon, R. F., and Townsend, Y. (1978): Contrasting actions of cyclohexamide on fever caused by arachidonic acid and by pyrogen. *J. Physiol. (Lond.)*, 285:35P.
9. Cranston, W. I., Duff, G. W., Hellon, R. F., and Mitchell, D. (1976): Effect of a prostaglandin antagonist on the pyrexia caused by PGE_2 and leucocyte pyrogen in rabbits. *J. Physiol. (Lond.)*, 256:120P.
10. Cranston, W. I., Hellon, R. F., and Mitchell, D. (1975): Is brain prostaglandin synthesis involved in responses to cold? *J. Physiol. (Lond.)*, 249:425–434.
11. Dinarello, C. A., and Wolff, S. M. (1977): Partial purification of human leucocytic pyrogen. *Inflammation*, 2:179–189.
12. Feldberg, W., and Gupta, K. P. (1973): Pyrogen fever and prostaglandin activity in cerebrospinal fluid. *J. Physiol. (Lond.)*, 228:41–53.
13. Feldberg, W., and Myers, R. D. (1963): A new concept of temperature regulation by amines in the hypothalamus. *Nature*, 200:1325.
14. Feldberg, W., and Saxena, P. N. (1971): Further studies on prostaglandin E_1 fever in cats. *J. Physiol. (Lond.)*, 219:739–745.
15. Flower, R. J., and Vane, J. R. (1972): Inhibition of prostaglandin synthetase in brain explains the antipyretic activity of paracetamol (4-acetamidophenol). *Nature*, 240:410–411.
16. Kasting, N. W., Veale, W. L., and Cooper, K. E. (1978): Evidence for a centrally active endogenous antipyretic near parturition. In: *Current Studies of Hypothalamic Function. Part II, Metabolism and Behaviour*, edited by K. Lederis and W. L. Veale, pp. 63–71. Karger, Basel.
17. Kasting, N. W., Veale, W. L., and Cooper, K. E. (1980): Fever and its role in disease: rationale for antipyretics. In: *Pyretics and Antipyretics*, edited by A. S. Milton (*in press*). Springer Verlag, Berlin.
18. Kluger, M. J. (1979): *Fever, Its Biology, Evolution and Function*. Princeton University Press, Princeton, N. J.
19. Kluger, M. J., and Rothenburg, B. A. (1979): Fever and reduced iron: their interaction as a host defense response to bacterial infection. *Science*, 203:374–376.
20. Laburn, H., Mitchell, D., and Rosendorff, C. (1977): Effects of prostaglandin antagonism on sodium arachidonate fever in rabbits. *J. Physiol. (Lond.)*, 267:559–570.
21. Lomax, P., and Green, M. D. (1974): Histamine and temperature regulation. In: *Proceedings, 2nd Symposium on Temperature Regulation and Drug Action*, pp. 82–94. Karger, Basel.
22. Milton, A. S., and Wendlandt, S. (1970): A possible role for prostaglandin E_1 as a modulator for temperature regulation in the central nervous system of the cat. *J. Physiol. (Lond.)*, 207:76–77.
23. Milton, A. S., and Wendlandt, S. (1971): Effects on body temperature of prostaglandins of the A, E, and F series on injection into the third ventricle of unanaesthetized rats and rabbits. *J. Physiol. (Lond.)*, 218:325–336.
24. Myers, R. D. (1966): Release of chemical factors from the diencephalic region of the unanaesthetized monkey during changes in body temperature. *J. Physiol. (Lond.)*, 188:50–51.
25. Myers, R. D., and Veale, W. L. (1971): The role of sodium and calcium ions in the hypothalamus in the control of body temperature of the unanaesthetized cat. *J. Physiol. (Lond.)*, 212:411–430.
26. Satinoff, E. (1974): Neural integration of thermoregulatory responses. In: *Limbic and Autonomic Nervous System: Advances in Research*, edited by Leo V. Dicara, pp. 41–83. Plenum Press, New York.

27. Schoener, E. P., and Wang, S. C. (1975): Leucocytic pyrogen and sodium acetylsalicylate on hypothalamic neurons in the cat. *Am. J. Physiol.*, 224:185–190.
28. Siegert, R., Phillip-Dormston, W. K., Radsak, K., and Menzel, H. (1975): Inhibition of Newcastle disease virus-induced fever in rabbits by cyclohexamide. *Arch. Virol.*, 48:367–373.
29. Stitt, J. T. (1973): Prostaglandin E$_1$ fever induced in rabbits. *J. Physiol. (Lond.)*, 232:163–179.
30. Vane, J. R. (1971): Inhibition of prostaglandin synthesis as a mechanism of action of aspirin-like drugs. *Nature*, 231:232–235.
31. Vaughn, L. K., Veale, W. L., and Cooper, K. E. (1979): Sensitivity of hypothalamic sites to salicylate and prostaglandin. *Can. J. Physiol. Pharmacol.*, 57:118–123.
32. Vaughn, L. K., Veale, W. L., and Cooper, K. E. (1980): Fever and survival in a mammal: effects of central pyresis. In: *Thermoregulatory Mechanisms and Their Therapeutic Implications*, pp. 115–120. Karger, Basel.
33. Veale, W. L., and Cooper, K. E. (1975): Comparison of sites of action of prostaglandin and leucocyte pyrogen in brain. In: *Temperature Regulation and Drug Action*, pp. 218–226. Karger, Basel.
34. Veale, W. L., and Whishaw, I. Q. (1976): Body temperature responses at different ambient temperatures following injections of prostaglandin E$_1$ and noradrenaline into the brain. *Pharmacol. Biochem. Behav.*, 4:143–150.

Acetylsalicylic Acid: New Uses for an Old Drug,
edited by H. J. M. Barnett, J. Hirsh, and
J. F. Mustard. Raven Press, New York © 1982.

DISCUSSION

W. R. Soller: Dr. Patrick stated that fenamate acids inhibit prostaglandin receptors as well as their synthesis and that acetylsalicylic acid inhibits PG synthesis but presumably not the receptors. Apparently acetylsalicylic acid must be given one day before the onset of dysmenorrhea, yet fenamates may be given on the day of onset. Does this suggest that the stable PGs, possibly stored in the uterus, and not the unstable endoperoxides with short half-lives are responsible for the manifestations of primary dysmenorrhea?

J. E. Patrick: This is a major controversy in dysmenorrhea. Although it is true that the fenamates probably have a dual role, that is, the blocking of receptors as well as synthesis, clinical studies suggest that acetylsalicylic acid and indomethacin may be useful in the management of this disorder but indicate that pretreatment is essential to success. These agents don't seem to work if given after onset of the cycle. I have no information on the issue of storage.

J. Hirsh: Concerning the dose of acetylsalicylic acid and related gastric mucosal lesions, is there a dose below which one does not see such lesions?

J. W. D. McDonald: Some publications purport to show erosions with lower doses, and others suggest a dose-response relationship for microscopic bleeding. Most of the studies have been done in patients with rheumatoid arthritis and followed by endoscopy. The patients are almost always on substantial doses of acetylsalicylic acid, such as 2400 mg/day.

Frank Rosenberg: Dr. McDonald, the U. S. Atomic Energy Commission recently sponsored the search for a "universal antidote" to radiation. As part of this program, they did a study of acetylsalicylic acid in cancer patients who received large doses of radiation to the abdominal area. They found that acetylsalicylic acid prevented diarrhea, nausea, and vomiting of the radiation-sickness syndrome. Do you have any further information?

McDonald: I was not aware of that report. This may be analogous to the experience in patients with inflammatory bowel disease, in whom some of the inflammation seems to be caused by prostaglandins and is inhibited by the salicylate released from salazopyrine. I suspect that, with radiation, the lesions are primarily in the intestine rather than in the stomach.

Rosenberg: In the Silvoso study, do you recall how long after the last ingestion endoscopy was done? Literature reports suggest that in the study of potential gastric irritants, the incidence of erythema and surface erosions depends in part on the interval between drug administration and endoscopy. Second, in your gastric irritation model, have you seen a difference in potency between indomethacin, naproxen, and the salicylates?

McDonald: I believe that the morning dose of acetylsalicylic acid was given before endoscopy, as part of a chronic experiment in patients who had taken acetylsalicylic acid for 3 months. Mucosal effects, which can be identified microscopically by biopsy, and the erythema are said to disappear within 1 to 2 hours of ingestion. Clinically, erythema and erosions are seen to disappear within a couple of days of cessation of acetylsalicylic acid. Obviously, an ulcer takes longer to heal.

P. Needleman: Could Dr. Coceani tell us what happens to make the normal ductus close at birth? What is there about a high oxygen surge that closes the normal ductus?

F. Coceani: I don't really know. However, I can speculate on the basis of certain facts. First, the guinea pig's ductus is peculiar in being utterly unresponsive to all inhibitors of prostaglandin synthesis. In other words, its patency apparently does not depend on prostaglandins, yet it constricts forcefully in response to oxygen. Second, the relaxant response of the lamb ductus to exogenous prostaglandin is much greater, at least *in vitro*, with low as opposed to high oxygen tensions. This partial blockade of the response to exogenous prostaglandin can be reversed by pretreatment with inhibitors of prostaglandin synthesis. Based on this, we can speculate that the prostaglandin and oxygen-sensitive mechanisms work independently. Oxygen acts directly on muscle, and then, beyond this, withdrawal of the prostaglandin effect is a complementary mechanism inducing closure. However, the role of the autonomic nervous system must also be considered.

Recently, we analyzed the response to autonomic agents in the guinea pig as compared with the lamb ductus, because of this difference in the prostaglandin mechanism. The guinea pig has an active adrenergic nervous system that includes both contractile alpha and relaxant beta activities. The lamb seems to have an inconsistent alpha mechanism and a very weak beta mechanism. In the guinea pig, effectiveness of the alpha mechanism increases with the increase in oxygen tension. It is therefore tempting to speculate that in the guinea pig, the beta-adrenergic mechanism compensates, at least in part, for the lack of the prostaglandin mechanism but that activation of alpha adrenoceptors contributes to postnatal closure of the vessel.

Needleman: Is there any analogy with closure of the umbilical artery and its surge of oxygen content?

Coceani: The umbilical artery differs from the ductus arteriosus in being able to synthesize thromboxane A_2 and in responding to this compound with a forceful contraction.

Needleman: It's pretty hard to find thromboxane in the umbilical artery — you see mostly prostaglandin E and prostacyclin.

Coceani: But you don't find it at all in the ductus arteriosus.

Needleman: It has been reported that imidazole blocks the ulcerogenic effects of acetylsalicylic acid on the gastrointestinal tract. How does that fit with the finding that the gastric mucosa makes thromboxane? Is it possible that if the metabolism were shunted away from thromboxane, the ulcerogenic effects of acetylsalicylic acid-like drugs might be prevented?

McDonald: I was not aware of this observation. I am pleased that someone has confirmed that mucosa does make thromboxane in addition to 6-keto-$PGF_{1\alpha}$. Would you like to enlarge on your hypothesis?

Needleman: Mucosa throughout the gastrointestinal tract makes thromboxane, not just the gastric portion. This interesting set of cells has the capacity to make PGE, PGI, and thromboxane, and it may be that whatever orchestrates these pathways controls the local reactions. I would like to draw out Dr. Kelton, because his data, using high doses of acetylsalicylic acid, suggest that the principal problem relates to arachidonic acid metabolism and thromboxane formation. Do you believe the prostacyclins are not very important?

Kelton: I don't know — this could turn out to be true. Just as we fixed our attention on the prostaglandin pathway in platelets while ignoring other pathways, we may now find that the vessel wall has other ways to limit thrombosis, one of which is PGI_2. It is possible that under extraordinary circumstances thrombosis can be augmented or caused by inhibition of PGI_2.

Rosenberg: Some people say that the acetylsalicylic acid trial failed because the acetylsalicylic acid was too high and inhibited prostacyclin formation, but recent data have shown that this is not a reasonable explanation.

May I point out to Drs. Needleman and Kelton that at a dose of 200 mg/kg in the rabbit, other effects must be considered, like disturbed acid-base balance, which may influence thrombogenesis.

Kelton: That is correct. We used a sodium salicylate control, which caused equal metabolic aberration, and observed no change in thrombus size. In addition, we instilled tranylcypromine in the veins and observed an increase in thrombus size (2). We suggest that this effect is related to PGI_2 inhibition.

H. J. M. Barnett: Dr. Kelton showed various methods by which the differential inhibition of thromboxane and PGI₂ can be demonstrated. In all of these methods, was there any sex difference? Was there any difference between male and female in arachidonic content of body tissues?

Kelton: We have divided all of our data by sex of the animal, and there is no difference in augmentation of thrombosis. With respect to inhibition of thrombosis and platelet accumulation in damaged vessels, there is an augmentation inhibition in the female animals but this is significantly greater in the male animals. We have studied differential inhibition of the prostaglandin pathway by measuring not only MDA but also the prostaglandin breakdown product, thromboxane B₂. Once again, we can see no difference. It is unlikely that the sex effect is related to differences in the metabolism of acetylsalicylic acid. We believe that there is something different about the way male and female platelets react with damaged vessel walls following inhibition with acetylsalicylic acid (1).

Unidentified: In the early 1950s, Keats and Lasagna indicated that the benzomorphan series of drugs were strongly analgesic in man, acting centrally, yet when used in the rat-tail flick and other standard analgesic tests, they showed no effect whatsoever. Could you comment on the differences you saw between acetylsalicylic acid and morphine in the rat-tail flick test, when other strongly acting central analgesics are negative?

Yaksh: I would note first that the benzomorphans are *not* strongly analgesic in man; they are extremely weak in comparison to morphine. We have demonstrated that the benzomorphans do not exert a direct effect on the spinal cord. Pentazocine, for example, does not block the tail flick when given intrathecally. On the other hand, if you modify the tail flick or the hot-plate test to make it into a weak test with a long reaction latency, the benzomorphans can be shown to possess a mild threshold-elevating property. It has also been shown that the partial agonists—and that is in fact what they are—have analgesic efficacy on measures like the writhing test. This difference between partial agonists and the full agonists such as morphine is probably caused in part by the type of receptors with which they interact. In recent years, opiate-binding studies have suggested the existence of multiple populations of opiate receptors. In addition, more recent work has indicated that receptor populations may differ within the brain and even between the dorsal and ventral horns of the spinal cord. Therefore, it is quite likely that these drugs may act on different receptors. I would also like to point out that Martin et al. have demonstrated the antinociceptive effect of the benzomorphans on the spinalized dog reflexes. These drugs act on the spinal cord, but not in a way comparable to that of the opiates. With regard to acetylsalicylic acid or other inflammatory agents—they *do not* block the tail flick under any conditions.

Rosenberg: Lin and co-workers have shown that the benzomorphan analgesics do act centrally. Also, as the temperature of the hot plate is lowered too far, one begins to pick up the anti-anxiety, muscle-relaxant, and tranquilizing agents as false positives.

McDonald: Earlier, Dr. Rosenberg asked about the relative potency of nonsteroidal drugs as inhibitors of mucosal prostaglandin synthesis. Acetylsalicylic acid is intermediate in potency, if you look at almost any tissue in the body. Indomethacin is the most potent, with acetylsalicylic acid approximately equipotent to phenylbutazone.

REFERENCES

1. Kelton, J. G., Carter, C. J., and Hirsh, J. (1980): Sex-related differences in the effects of aspirin on hemostatic plug formation in vivo (abstract). *Clin. Res.*, 28:315A.
2. Kelton, J. G., Hirsh, J., Carter, C. J., and Buchanan, M. R. (1978): Thrombogenic effect of vessel wall synthesis of prostaglandin I₂-like activity. *J. Clin. Invest.*, 62:892–895.

Acetylsalicylic Acid: New Uses for an Old Drug,
edited by H. J. M. Barnett, J. Hirsh, and
J. F. Mustard. Raven Press, New York © 1982.

Coronary Prostacyclin Synthesis and Models for Its Modulation by Interaction with Platelets

John Turk and *Philip Needleman

Departments of Pharmacology and Medicine, Jewish Hospital and Washington University Medical School, St. Louis, Missouri 63110

In isolated perfused rabbit hearts, an endogenous prostaglandin-like substance fulfills the criteria of mediating the changes in coronary resistance produced by certain vasoactive substances. The primary arachidonate metabolite produced both in isolated perfused hearts and in isolated coronary arteries is prostacyclin (PGI_2). In addition, the major site of cardiac prostacyclin synthesis appears to be in the coronary vasculature itself. Using the isolated perfused mesenteric vascular bed, one can readily demonstrate that the smooth muscle cells synthesize prostaglandins even in the absence of endothelial cells. Blood vessels readily synthesize prostaglandins from intrinsic arachidonate. However, when platelets adhere to damaged vessels, an exchange of prostaglandin precursor may take place. Our evidence suggests that platelets can contribute endoperoxide precursor to blood vessel for prostacyclin synthesis only when the platelet thromboxane synthetase is inhibited. Platelet lipoxygenase products readily inactivate vascular prostacyclin synthetase in cell-free systems but do not appear to be released from intact platelets.

Early studies in this laboratory on resistance changes in the coronary vessels of isolated perfused rabbit hearts indicated that the vasodilation induced by hypoxia was not accompanied by prostaglandin biosynthesis (22), whereas the vasodilation produced by exogenous bradykinin was associated with a dose-dependent release of a material that behaved like prostaglandin E_2 (PGE_2) when assayed on a battery of superfused test organs (21,23). This latter observation was of interest in view of the possible involvement of the kallikrein-kinin system in the response to human occlusive coronary artery disease (29). In addition, the PGE_2-like material seemed to mediate the effects of bradykinin on the coronary vasculature, since peptide-induced vasodilation and production of the prostaglandin-like substance were prevented by indomethacin (21,23). Subsequent studies involving selective radiolabeling of

---

*Mailing address: Dr. P. Needleman, Department Head, Washington University School of Medicine, St. Louis, Missouri 63110.

coronary vascular or myocardial lipid pools with ^{14}C-fatty acids demonstrated that bradykinin selectively induced the release of vascular arachidonic acid and this release was efficiently coupled to prostaglandin biosynthesis. Hypoxia induced release of fatty acids from myocardial lipid pools as well, but this was accompanied by little prostaglandin synthesis (10,11,34). The coronary vasculature thus appears to be the major site of cardiac prostaglandin production.

Although the prostaglandin-like substance released from coronary vessels by bradykinin resembled PGE_2 on bioassay and in some chromatographic systems, perfusion of isolated rabbit hearts with exogenous PGE_2 itself did not produce vasodilation. Perfusion with the prostaglandin precursor arachidonic acid produced vasodilation, suggesting the possibility that the coronary vessels were converting arachidonic acid to a novel metabolite with vasodilator activity (14). The coronary venous effluent from hearts perfused with either bradykinin or arachidonate was subsequently shown to contain an arachidonate metabolite that differed from PGE_2 both chemically and chromatographically (12). This substance is now known to be 6-keto-prostaglandin $F_{1\alpha}$ (6KF), an arachidonate metabolite first identified in the homogenates of rat stomach (27). 6KF is chemically stable but biologically inert and arises from the rapid isomerization of the biologically active species 6(9)-oxy-11,15-dihydroxyprosta-5β-dienoic acid (prostacyclin) (13,27). Prostacyclin appears to be the major arachidonate metabolite produced by coronary vessels (34).

Before the chemical structure of prostacyclin was established, Vane and co-workers (1,4) had established that its precursor was the prostaglandin endoperoxide PGH_2 (6) and that prostacyclin was a potent inhibitor of platelet aggregation (1,4). In contrast, the principal product of PGH_2 in blood platelets is thromboxane A_2 (8). This labile material is a potent vasoconstrictor and induces platelet aggregation before its isomerization to the biologically inert product, thromboxane B_2 (8).

Since prostacyclin appears to be synthesized in all vascular sources so far examined, it has been proposed that continuous vascular synthesis of prostacyclin occurs as a homeostatic mechanism to prevent platelet adhesion and aggregation on normal vascular endothelium (1,4,18). Vascular injury would lead to a local decrease in prostacyclin production and promote platelet accumulation at the site of the injury for hemostasis and vascular repair (18). In addition, the low levels of cyclo-oxygenase activity observed in some vessel preparations (1,4) led to the speculation that blood platelets, which contain a highly active cyclo-oxygenase (1,4,18), may contribute part of the endoperoxide PGH_2 used for vascular prostacyclin synthesis.

Observations from this laboratory bring several aspects of this model into question. First, isolated perfused rabbit mesenteric vessels readily generate prostacyclin either from exogenous arachidonate in the perfusate or from endogenous arachidonate provided by bradykinin stimulation (30). This suggests the presence of an active vascular cyclo-oxygenase. Second, denuding the vessels of endothelial cells by perfusion with hypotonic fluid did not affect the ability of the vessels to generate prostacyclin from either exogenous or endogenous arachidonate (30). This prostacyclin synthesis presumably occurred in the intact vascular smooth muscle cells, and hence it appears that endothelial injury has little effect on local prostacyclin production.

Finally, exogenous PGH_2 in the perfusate to mesenteric vascular preparations with intact endothelium was not converted to prostacyclin (30), suggesting that the labile and polar endoperoxide could not gain access to vascular prostacyclin synthetase from the extracellular space. However, some conversion of exogenous PGH_2 to prostacyclin was observed after hypotonic vascular injury (30). In addition, it is possible that platelets must be present before PGH_2 can be transferred to vascular cells.

To examine this possibility, the membrane lipids of washed human platelets were pre-labeled with ^{14}C-arachidonic acid (26). Treatment of such preparations with thrombin results in liberation of membrane-derived ^{14}C-arachidonic acid, which is converted to ^{14}C-PGH_2 by the platelet cyclo-oxygenase. The ^{14}C-PGH_2 is then converted to ^{14}C-thromboxane B_2 (TxB_2) by thromboxane synthetase (26). The question of whether any ^{14}C-PGH_2 escapes the platelet or is transferred to vascular tissue by the platelet was addressed by including bovine aortic microsomes or aortic rings in the incubation mixture. If transfer of the radiolabeled endoperoxide to these sources of vascular prostacyclin synthetase occurs, generation of the prostacyclin isomerization product [14]C-6KF should be observed. However, co-incubation of bovine aortic rings or microsomes and platelets prelabeled with ^{14}C-arachidonic acid, and stimulation with thrombin resulted in the generation only of ^{14}C-TxB_2 without demonstrable [14]C-6KF (26). This does not support the transfer of ^{14}C-PGH_2 from the platelet to vascular prostacyclin synthetase. When the thromboxane synthetase inhibitor imidazole (20,25) was included in the incubation mixture, however, thrombin stimulation did result in the generation of [14]C-6KF (26). This demonstrated that inhibition of the metabolism of the labile endoperoxide ^{14}C-PGH_2 within the platelet allowed the species to escape the platelet for utilization by vascular prostacyclin synthetase (Fig. 1A).

This observation raised the question of whether inhibition of the metabolism of other arachidonate metabolites in the platelet might permit their escape from the platelet. Of particular interest in this regard is the platelet-lipoxygenase product 12-hydroperoxy-5,8,10,14-eicosatetraenoic acid (12-HPETE) (7). Shortly after the discovery of prostacyclin synthetase, Vane and co-workers (17) had demonstrated that the enzyme was inactivated by 15-hydroperoxy-arachidonic acid. It has subsequently been shown that the enzyme is inactivated by a number of hydroperoxy-fatty acids (31) including 12-HPETE (5). The inactivation appears to result from the generation of a highly reactive oxidant, possibly the hydroxyl radical, from organic hydroperoxides (5,37).

The physiologic significance of the platelet lipoxygenase pathway remains uncertain but the possibility exists that vascular prostacyclin synthesis may be modulated by the platelet lipoxygenase product 12-HPETE. Siegel and co-workers (32,33) have recently suggested that high concentrations of indomethacin promote accumulation of 12-HPETE to 12-hydroxy-5,8,10,14-eicosatetraenoic acid (12-HETE). It is conceivable that 12-HPETE might escape from the platelet under these conditions, in a situation analogous to that for PGH_2 and imidazole, described above.

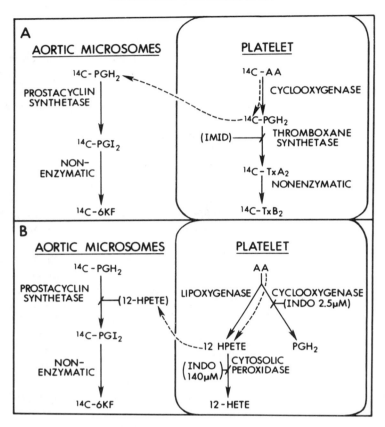

FIG. 1. Schema of platelet–aortic microsome systems. **A.** Washed human platelets were prelabeled with ^{14}C-arachidonic acid (AA) and incubated with bovine aortic microsomes. Thrombin treatment released membrane-bound ^{14}C-AA, which was converted to ^{14}C-PGH$_2$ by platelet cyclo-oxygenase. In the absence of imidazole (IMID), ^{14}C-thromboxane B$_2$ (TxB$_2$) was formed from ^{14}C-PGH$_2$; no escape of ^{14}C-PGH$_2$ from the platelet occurred; and no ^{14}C-6-keto-prostaglandin F$_{1\alpha}$ (6KF) was formed. In the presence of IMID, thromboxane synthetase was inhibited and ^{14}C-PGH$_2$ escaped from the platelet (dotted lines) and was converted to ^{14}C-6KF by prostacyclin synthetase in the aortic microsomes (26). **B.** Washed human platelets were incubated with bovine aortic microsomes. Exogenous arachidonic acid (AA) is the substrate for both lipoxygenase and cyclo-oxygenase. Cyclo-oxygenase inhibition with 2.5 μM indomethacin (INDO) diverts AA through the lipoxygenase. Inhibition of a cytosolic peroxidase by 140 μM INDO may result in accumulation of 12-HPETE (32,33). If 12-HPETE escapes the platelet (dotted lines), inactivation of prostacyclin synthetase should result and be reflected by failure to convert exogenous ^{14}C-PGH$_2$ to ^{14}C-6KF (36).

To determine whether 12-HPETE generated *in situ* would inactivate vascular prostacyclin synthetase and whether 12-HPETE generated in the intact platelet could escape the platelet when its degradation was inhibited by high concentrations of indomethacin, the following experimental strategy was employed: a) A lipoxygenase source (washed human platelets) (16) or the supernatant of lysed platelets (centrifuged at 100,000 g) (33) was treated with 2.5 μM or 140 μM indomethacin. (The lower dose inhibited cyclo-oxygenase but not 12-HPETE peroxidase. The higher dose inhibited both activities) (32,33). b) Bovine aortic microsomes (26) were added as a source of prostacyclin synthetase. c) Arachidonic acid was added as a lipogenase substrate. (Indomethacin diverted arachidonate through the lipoxygenase to 12-HPETE and prevented the generation of unlabelled PGH_2.) d) The prostacyclin synthetase substrate ^{14}C-PGH_2 (2,24) was added. e) Prostacyclin synthetase activity was reflected by the generation of ^{14}C-6KF from exogenous ^{14}C-PGH_2 in this system. Production of 12-HPETE and its liberation from the platelet would be expected to inactivate prostacyclin synthetase (Fig. 1B).

Excellent conversion of ^{14}C-PGH_2 to ^{14}C-6KF was observed in this system in the absence of lipoxygenase substrate. The addition of arachidonic acid resulted in inactivation of prostacyclin synthetase as reflected in failure to convert ^{14}C-PGH_2 to ^{14}C-6KF. Mediation of this inactivation by a platelet lipoxygenase product was demonstrated by the lack of inactivation observed when either a) the lipoxygenase inhibitor (7) eicosatetraynoic acid (ETYA) was included in the incubation or b) a platelet lipoxygenase source was not included (36). When the supernatant of lysed platelets was employed as the lipoxygenase source, only 0.5 μM arachidonic acid was required to produce half-maximal inactivation of prostacyclin synthetase. When intact platelets were employed as the lipoxygenase source, 35 μM and 80 μM arachidonic acid were required to produce half-maximal and complete inactivation of prostacyclin synthetase, respectively. High concentrations of indomethacin did not influence the dose of arachidonic acid required to inactivate prostacyclin synthetase with either lipoxygenase source (36).

Suspensions of washed platelets were found to aggregate fully on exposure to 2 to 8 μM arachidonic acid, and on exposure to 80 μM arachidonic acid the suspensions exhibited a slow diminution in optical density without formation of visible aggregates (Fig. 2A). The probability that this optical behavior reflected platelet lysis was supported by the demonstration of an arachidonic acid concentration-dependent release of lactate dehydrogenase (LDH) activity from platelet suspensions exposed to concentrations of arachidonic acid exceeding 20 μM (Fig. 2B). It therefore appears that the prostacyclin synthetase inactivation observed in the whole platelet-aortic microsomal system depends on platelet lysis with release of 12-HPETE or lipoxygenase and not on release of 12-HPETE from the intact platelet.

One possibility for the failure of high-dose indomethacin to potentiate prostacyclin inhibition in this system is that inhibition of the 12-HPETE peroxidase may retard the generation of an oxidant from 12-HPETE. Recent evidence suggests that intact organic hydroperoxides do not directly inhibit prostacyclin synthetase and that the inhibition is mediated by an oxidant generated from the hydroperoxides by peroxidase action (5). The influence of high concentrations of indomethacin on the time course of prostacyclin synthetase inactivation was therefore examined by varying the time of exposure of the aortic microsomes to the 12-HPETE generating system. With washed platelets (lipoxygenase source) and aortic microsomes (prostacyclin synthetase source), the incubation period after the addition of 80 μM arachidonic acid (lipoxygenase substrate) and before the addition of ^{14}C-PGH_2 (prostacyclin synthetase substrate)

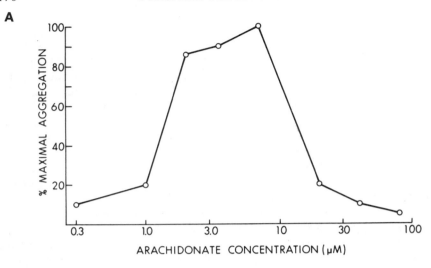

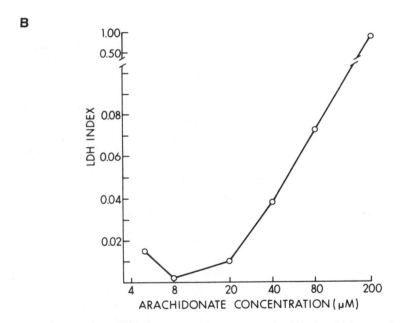

FIG. 2A. Platelet aggregation induced by exogenous arachidonic acid. Suspensions of washed human platelets (16) were stirred at 37° C in a Payton dual channel aggregometer and the optical density of the suspensions recorded by continuous graphic display. Various doses of arachidonic acid were introduced as solution in 0.9% NaCl (pH 8.5). The percent maximal aggregation was calculated as 100 times the ratio of the change in optical density 5 min after the introduction of a given dose of arachidonic acid over the change in optical density 5 min after the introduction of 7 μM arachidonic acid. **FIG. 2B.** Arachidonic acid concentration dependence of lactate dehydrogenase release from platelets. Suspensions of washed platelets were treated with 2.5 μM indomethacin and then incubated with arachidonic acid (4 to 200 μM) for 5 min at 37°C. The platelets were removed from suspension by sedimentation for 30 sec in a microfuge.

was varied from 0 to 5 min. The degree of prostacyclin synthetase inactivation increased with the duration of this pre-incubation period, with half-maximal inactivation occurring at about 2 min. The presence of high concentrations of indomethacin did not influence the time course of inactivation (Fig. 3A). Using the supernatant of lysed platelets as a lipoxygenase source in this system, 80 μM arachidonic acid produced complete inactivation at the earliest time tested (30 sec) and at all subsequent times (not shown). When 4 μM arachidonic acid was used in the platelet lysate system, the degree of prostacyclin synthetase inactivation could again be shown to vary with the length of the incubation period after addition of arachidonic acid and before addition of ^{14}C-PGH$_2$. Half-maximal inactivation occurred at about 30 sec, and the time course of inactivation was not influenced by high-dose indomethacin with this lipoxygenase source either (Fig. 3B). The absence of an indomethacin effect may reflect the presence of an indomethacin-insensitive peroxidase in the aortic microsomes, such as that associated with other microsomal sources of prostacyclin synthetase (5).

The low dose of arachidonic acid and the short time period required to inactivate prostacyclin synthetase in the platelet lysate-aortic microsomal system suggest that modulation of prostacyclin synthesis by lipoxygenase products could occur in cells containing both lipoxygenase and prostacyclin synthetase activities. Vascular tissue has recently been shown to produce lipoxygenase products (3). In addition, although it does not appear that 12-HPETE is released from platelets, it is still possible that lipoxygenase products are transferred from platelets to vascular tissue during the platelet adhesion process. Such transfer could be one mechanism by which platelets modulate the response to vascular injury. In selected animal models the proliferative lesions developing after experimental vascular injury may be prevented by thrombocytopenia (19) and dipyridamole (9), although acetylsalicylic acid may afford little protection (Needleman, P., Sivakoff, M., and Hsueh, W., *unpublished results*). If platelet cyclic AMP were elevated by dipyridamole (28), inhibition of phospholipase activity should result (16) and reduce substrate availability for lipoxygenase.

In summary, coronary prostacyclin synthesis appears to be the major form of cardiac prostaglandin synthesis and appears to mediate the coronary resistance changes induced by the vasoactive peptide bradykinin. Two models for the modulation of vascular prostacyclin synthesis by blood platelets have been examined: a) Transfer of prostaglandin H$_2$ from the platelet to vascular prostacyclin synthetase does not occur unless platelet thromboxane synthesis is inhibited by imidazole; b) vascular prostacyclin synthesis is readily inactivated by platelet lipoxygenase products in cell-free systems, but 12-HPETE does not appear to be released from the intact platelet.

FIG. 2B *(contd).* The supernatant was assayed for lactate dehydrogenase (LDH) activity (15). This value was designated LDH (experimental). The LDH in control supernatants derived from platelet suspensions not exposed to arachidonic acid was designated LDH (control). The total LDH activity of platelet suspensions was estimated from the activity present in detergent (0.1% Triton) solubilized suspensions and was designed LDH (total). The LDH index was calculated as [LDH (experimental) − LDH (control)] divided by LDH (total).

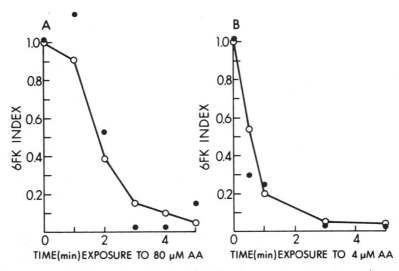

FIG. 3. Time dependence of inactivation of aortic microsomal prostacyclin synthetase with platelet lipoxygenase sources and arachidonic acid. In **A** the lipoxygenase source was washed human platelets (0.5 cc) (16), and in **B** it was the 100,000 g supernatant (0.5 cc) of platelets lysed by freeze-thawing (33). The lipoxygenase sources were treated with 2.5 μM indomethacin (*open circles*) or 140 μM indomethacin (*closed circles*). Bovine aortic microsomes (50 μl, 200 μg protein) (26) were then added as a source of prostacyclin synthetase. The lipoxygenase substrate arachidonic acid was then added at a final concentration of 80 μM **(A)** and 4 μM **(B)**. The prostacyclin synthetase substrate ^{14}C-PGH$_2$ (75,000 cpm) (2,24) was added 0 to 5 min after addition of arachidonic acid and incubated for 5 min. All incubations were performed with continuous stirring at 37° C in a Payton dual channel aggregometer. At the end of the incubation period, reactions were terminated by the addition of 50 μl or 2N formic acid. The mixtures were then extracted twice with ethyl acetate (1 cc). The extracts were concentrated and subjected to thin layer chromatography in solvent system A9 (13). Thin layer radiochromatograms were generated, peak assignment performed, and radioactive products quantitated as described previously (26,35). For each incubation the cpm from the ^{14}C-6KF peak was divided by the sum of cpm for the peaks for PGE$_2$ and HHT. This ratio was divided by the corresponding ratio from an otherwise identical incubation mixture without lipoxygenase substrate. The resulting number was designated the 6KF index and was taken as an estimate of prostacyclin synthetase activity. cpm = counts/min.

REFERENCES

1. Bunting, S., Gryglewski, R., Moncada, S., and Vane, J. R. (1976): Arterial walls generate from prostaglandin endoperoxides a substance (prostaglandin X) which relaxes strips of mesenteric and celiac arteries and inhibits platelet aggregation. *Prostaglandins*, 12:897–913.
2. Gorman, R., Sun, F., Miller, O., and Johnson, R. (1977): Prostaglandins H$_1$ and H$_2$. Convenient biochemical synthesis and isolation. Further biological and spectroscopic characterization. *Prostaglandins*, 13:1043–1056.
3. Greenwald, J. E., Branchine, J. R., and Wong, L. K. (1979): The production of the arachidonate metabolite HETE in vascular tissue. *Nature*, 281:588–589.
4. Gryglewski, R. J., Bunting, S., Moncada, S., Flower, R. J., and Vane, J. R. (1976): Arterial walls are protected against deposition of platelet thrombi (prostaglandin X) which they make from prostaglandin endoperoxides. *Prostaglandins*, 12:685–711.
5. Ham, E. A., Egan, R. N., Soderman, D. D., Gale, P. N., and Kuehl, F. A. (1979): Peroxidase dependent deactivation of prostacyclin synthetase. *J. Biol. Chem.*, 254:2191–2194.

6. Hamberg, M., and Samuelsson, B. (1973): Detection and isolation of an endoperoxide intermediate in prostaglandin biosynthesis. *Proc. Natl. Acad. Sci. U. S. A.*, 70:899–903.

7. Hamberg, M., and Samuelsson, B. (1974): Prostaglandin endoperoxides. Novel transformation of arachidonic acid in human platelets. *Proc. Natl. Acad. Sci. U. S. A.*, 71:3400–3404.

8. Hamberg, M., Svenson, J., and Samuelsson, B. (1975): Thromboxanes: a new group of biologically active compounds derived from prostaglandin endoperoxides. *Proc. Natl. Acad. Sci. U. S. A.*, 72:2994–2998.

9. Harker, L. A., Ross, R., Slichter, S. J., and Scott, R. J. (1976): Homocysteine-induced arteriosclerosis. The role of endothelial cell injury and platelet response in its genesis. *J. Clin. Invest.*, 58:731–741.

10. Hsueh, W., Isakson, P. C., and Needleman, P. (1977): Hormone selective lipase activation in the isolated rabbit heart. *Prostaglandins*, 13:1073–1091.

11. Hsueh, W., and Needleman, P. (1978): Sites of lipase activation and prostaglandin synthesis in isolated, perfused rabbit hearts and hydronephrotic kidneys. *Prostaglandins*, 16:661–681.

12. Isakson, P. C., Raz, A., Denny, S., Pure, E., and Needleman, P. (1977): A novel prostaglandin is the major product of arachidonic acid metabolism in rabbit heart. *Proc. Natl. Acad. Sci. U. S. A.*, 74:101–105.

13. Johnson, R., Morton, D. R., Kinnis, J. H., Gorman, R., McGuire, J., and Sun, F. (1976): The chemical structure of prostaglandin X (prostacyclin). *Prostaglandins*, 12:915–928.

14. Kulkarni, P. S., Roberts, R., and Needleman, P. (1976): Paradoxical endogenous synthesis of coronary dilating substance from arachidonate. *Prostaglandins*, 12:337–353.

15. Lowry, O. H., and Passonneau, J. V. (1972): *A Flexible System of Enzymatic Analysis.* Academic Press, New York.

16. Minkes, M., Stanford, N., Chi, M., Roth, G., Raz, A., Needleman, P., and Majerus, P. W. (1977): Cyclic adenosine 3'-5' monophosphate inhibits the availability of arachidonate to prostaglandin synthetase in human platelet suspensions. *J. Clin. Invest.*, 59:449–454.

17. Moncada, S., Gryglewski, R. J., Bunting, S., and Vane, J. R. (1976): A lipid hydroperoxide inhibits the enzyme in blood vessel microsomes that generates from prostaglandin endoperoxides the substance (prostaglandin X) which prevents platelet aggregation. *Prostaglandins*, 12:715–737.

18. Moncada, S., and Vane, J. R. (1975): Arachidonic acid metabolites and the interactions between platelets and blood vessel walls. *N. Engl. J. Med.*, 300:1142–1147.

19. Moore, S., Friedman, R. J., Singal, D. P., Gauldre, J., and Blajchman, M. (1976): Inhibition of injury-induced thromboatherosclerotic lesions by antiplatelet serum in rabbits. *Thromb. Diath. Haemorrh.*, 35:70–81.

20. Needleman, P., Bryan, B., Wyche, A., Bronson, S. P., Eakins, K., Ferrendelli, J. A., and Minkes, M. (1977): Thromboxane synthetase inhibitors as pharmacologic tools: Differential biochemical and biological effects on platelet suspensions. *Prostaglandins*, 14:897–907.

21. Needleman, P., Key, S. L., Denny, S. E., Isakson, P., and Marshall, G. R. (1975): Mechanism and modification of bradykinin induced coronary vasodilation. *Proc. Natl. Acad. Sci. U. S. A.*, 72:2060–2063.

22. Needleman, P., Key, S., Isakson, P., and Kulkarni, P. S. (1975): Relationship between oxygen tension, coronary vasodilation and prostaglandin biosynthesis in the isolated rabbit heart. *Prostaglandins*, 9:123–134.

23. Needleman, P., Marshall, G. R., and Sobel, B. (1975): Hormone interactions in the isolated rabbit heart. Synthesis and coronary vasomotor effects of prostaglandins, angiotension and bradykinin. *Circ. Res.*, 37:802–808.

24. Needleman, P., Minkes, M., and Raz, A. (1976): Thromboxanes, selective biosynthesis and distinct biological properties. *Science*, 143:163–165.

25. Needleman, P., Raz, A., Ferrendelli, J. A., and Minkes, M.: Application of imidazole as a selective inhibitor of thromboxane synthetase in human platelets. *Proc. Natl. Acad. Sci. U. S. A.*, 74:1716–1720.

26. Needleman, P., Wyche, A., and Raz, A. (1979): Platelet and blood vessel arachidonate metabolism and actions. *J. Clin. Invest.*, 63:345–349.

27. Pace-Asciak, C., and Wolff, L. S. (1971): A novel prostaglandin derivative formed from arachidonic acid by rat stomach homogenates. *Biochemistry*, 10:3657–3669.

28. Pidisheim, P. R., Shimamoto, T., and Yamakuzi, H. (1974): Platelets, thrombosis and inhibitors. *Thromb. Diath. Haemorrh. (Suppl.)*, 60:2–15.

29. Pitt, B., Mason, J., and Cont, C. R. (1969): Observations on the plasma kallikrein system during myocardial ischemia. *Trans. Assoc. Am. Physicians*, 82:98–102.

30. Pure, E., and Needleman, P. (1979): Effect of endothelial damage on prostaglandin synthesis by isolated perfused rabbit mesenteric vasculature. *J. Cardiovasc. Pharmacol.*, 1:299–309.
31. Salmon, J. A., Smith, P. R., Flower, R. J., Moncada, S., and Vane, J. R. (1978): Further studies on the enzymatic conversion of prostaglandin endoperoxides into prostacyclin by porcine aortic microsomes. *Biochim. Biophys. Acta*, 523:250.
32. Siegel, M. J., McConnell, R. T., Abrahams, S. L., Porter, N. A., and Cuatrecasas, P. (1979): Regulation of arachidonate metabolism via lipoxygenase and cyclooxygenase by 12-HPETE, the product of human platelet lipoxygenases. *Biochem. Biophys. Res. Commun.*, 89:1278–1280.
33. Siegel, M. J., McConnell, R. T., and Cuatrecasas, P. (1979): Aspirin-like drugs interfere with arachidonate metabolism by inhibition of the 12-hydroperoxy-5,8,10,14-eicosatetraenoic acid peroxidase activity of the lipoxygenase pathway. *Proc. Natl. Acad. Sci. U.S.A.*, 76:3774–3778.
34. Sivakoff, M., Pure, E., Hsueh, W., and Needleman, P. (1979): Prostaglandins and the heart. *Fed. Proc.*, 38:78–81.
35. Turk, J., Weiss, S. J., Davis, J., and Needleman, P. (1978): Fluorescent derivatives of prostaglandins and thromboxanes for liquid chromatography. *Prostaglandins*, 16:291–310.
36. Turk, J., Wyche, A., and Needleman, P. (1980): Inactivation of vascular prostacyclin synthetase by platelet lipoxygenase products. *Biochem. Biophys. Res. Commun.*, 95:1628–34.
37. Weiss, S. J., Turk, J., and Needleman, P. (1979): A mechanism for the hydroperoxide mediated inactivation of prostacyclin synthetase. *Blood*, 53:1191–1196.

Acetylsalicylic Acid: New Uses for an Old Drug,
edited by H. J. M. Barnett, J. Hirsh, and
J. F. Mustard. Raven Press, New York © 1982.

Platelet Antiaggregants in Stroke Prevention: A Review of Rationale and Results

H. J. M. Barnett

*Department of Clinical Neurological Sciences, University of Western Ontario,
London, Ontario, Canada N6A 5A5*

More than two decades ago, observations following experimental injury to the cerebral arteries indicated that platelet thrombogenesis could cause embolization. In the retina, platelet thrombi were visualized, photographed, and examined under the microscope. Atheromatous debris emboli were also visualized in the retina, and were shown to stimulate further platelet thrombi. These observations have now been made in the cerebral arteries as well. There is strong evidence that thrombosis induced by platelets is important in producing stroke; indeed, thrombogenesis is much more prominent in the production of stroke and threatened stroke than in myocardial infarction and angina.

Following experimental injuries (mechanical, electrical and chemical) to the cerebral arteries, brain damage secondary to thrombosis by platelet antiaggregants can be prevented by acetylsalicylic acid, dipyridamole, and indomethacin as well as prostacyclin.

Four trials of platelet antiaggregants in stroke prevention have been carried out. The first, which followed a variety of stroke and stroke-threatened patients for an average of 10 months on dipyridamole, gave negative results; the study was too short and the numbers too small for final conclusions. The Canadian and American randomized trials using acetylsalicylic acid alone or with sulfinpyrazone showed a marked benefit to male patients in terms of stroke and death. A recent Swedish trial contrasting acetylsalicylic acid to coumadin reported no difference between the two, but it did not include a control group. The results were encouraging but inconclusive.

Further study is required to resolve many problems of combined drug therapy (acetylsalicylic acid with dipyridamole), appropriate dosage, and the use of enteric-coated preparations. In particular, the matter of prophylactic use of acetylsalicylic acid or other platelet anti-aggregants in populations at risk but without any evidence of vascular disease requires a careful and controlled study.

Vascular stroke is a major health problem and until recent years the prospects for its prevention did not appear promising. However, recently published statistics testify to a decrease in stroke mortality approximating 40% over two decades (20,22). There is evidence that this reduction coincides with better management of hypertension and probably with the reduced incidence of severe rheumatic disease (Fig. 1) (46). Basic medical research, technological advances, and clinical studies conducted over the past three decades encourage us to hope that further reduction in the incidence and severity of stroke is an attainable goal.

THE VARIETIES OF STROKE

Vascular stroke occurs in three major varieties: atherothrombotic stroke, stroke due to emboli from cardiac sources, and intracerebral hemorrhage. The relative incidence of these major varieties of stroke is changing (Table 1) (36,50), in part because of therapeutic advances and in part because of increased diagnostic accuracy. *Atherothrombotic stroke* is the commonest type, and yet it may be showing a slight decline. The decrease may be an artifact and simply the consequence of

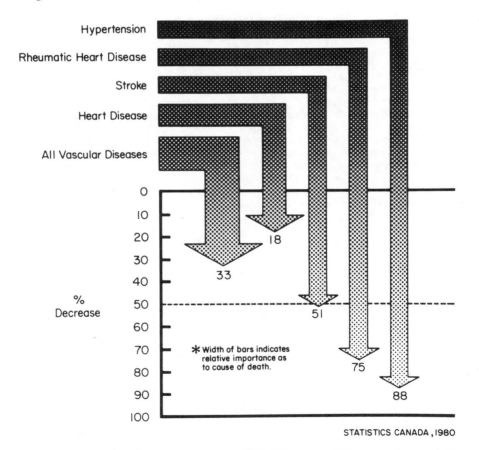

FIG. 1. Incidence of heart disease and stroke for individuals aged 65 and under over a 25-year period (1953–1978), taken from the Vital Statistics of Canada, 1980. The reduced incidence parallels a striking reduction in deaths attributed to hypertension and rheumatic heart disease.

TABLE 1. *Incidence (%) of varieties of stroke*

	Atherothrombosis	Cardiac embolism	Intracranial hematoma	Aneurysm AVM	Unknown
Mayo Clinic, 1971 (50)	75	3	10	5	7
Harvard Registry, 1978 (36)	65	19	10	6	—

the removal from this category of some cases that are now categorized as caused by cardiac emboli because of improved techniques for studying the heart valves, chambers and walls. The incidence of thromboembolic stroke of cardiac origin has increased. It is a reasonable assumption that technical advances in imaging and monitoring have been the major cause of this increased incidence. Whereas a 3% incidence was reported in 1971 (50), the prospective Boston study of 1978 estimated that this cause accounted for 19% of all strokes (36).

Cerebral angiography did more than anything else to sharpen our understanding of the atherothrombotic stroke, and more recently, CT scanning has revolutionized the diagnosis of intracerebral hemorrhage. For the first time it is possible, *ante mortem*, to detect hemorrhages of small size. Now, a significant number of them are recognized before blood appears in the cerebrospinal fluid and before the patient develops coma or is threatened by a fatal outcome. Fatal hypertensive intracerebral hemorrhage is less common, most probably because of the wide application of antihypertensive therapy. The overall figures for stroke caused by intracerebral hemorrhage have not changed (Table 1). It must be remembered, however, that the earlier figure of 10% represents cerebral hemorrhage diagnosed in an era preceding CT scanning and relates to the classic examples of massive and clinically diagnosable hemorrhage with blood in the CSF. The later figure (also 10%) includes significant numbers of patients with smaller, nonfatal hemorrhages. There remains a small, important but unchanging number of stroke deaths caused by hemorrhage from aneurysm and arteriovenous malformation. From the viewpoint of the potential prophylaxis of antithrombotic therapy, 95% of strokes are associated with atherothrombosis or thromboembolism.

The Pathogenesis of Threatened Stroke: Significance of Thrombosis in Certain Varieties of TIA

Continuing inquiry about the mechanisms that produce stroke-threatening symptoms, whether they be transient ischemic attacks (TIA), reversible ischemic neurological disability (RIND), or partial non-progressing stroke (PNS), has determined that a variety of conditions warn of a more calamitous and major stroke (5). Table 2 lists the more common stroke-threatening conditions that have been identified as related to thrombus formation and are frequently associated with recognizable platelet-induced thrombogenesis.

TABLE 2. *Varieties of transient ischemic attacks with prominent connection to platelet-induced thrombosis*

1. Artery-to-artery emboli
    Atheroma
    Fibromuscular hyperplasia

2. Emboli from the heart
    Identifiable by more traditional methods
      Subacute bacterial endocarditis
      Mitral stenosis
      Artrial fibrillation
      Myocardial infarction with mural thrombus
      Prosthetic heart valve
    Now more readily identifiable
      Nonbacterial thrombotic endocarditis
      Prolapsing mitral valve
      Mitral annulus calcification
      Akinetic segments

3. Thrombocytosis

Emboli from *the extracranial course of the cerebral arteries* or in the large arteries at the base of the brain are common. For the most part, the emboli arise in *atheromatous lesions* and pass to the cortical and penetrating branches. They are probably the commonest cause of stroke-threatening symptoms. The emboli, which are frequently composed of platelets and fibrin, may be seen in the retina and occasionally in the cortical arteries exposed at operation (Fig. 2). Atheromatous debris may produce embolization. They can be recognized in the retina as "bright plaques" and at postmortem examination by the presence of intra-arterial cholesterol clefts. Evidence from experimental studies indicates that emboli made up of atheromatous debris initiate a spreading platelet-initiated thrombosis (47).

Emboli are not common in *fibromuscular hyperplasia*, but they have been identified with increasing frequency. The continued attention focused on "threatened-stroke" patients indicates that they are more common than was originally thought.

Emboli from the heart are second only to artery-to-artery emboli in the production of stroke-threatening symptoms. Traditionally the responsible heart lesions have been mural thrombi associated with recent myocardial infarction (MI), subacute bacterial endocarditis (SBE) and mitral stenosis with or without atrial fibrillation. Atrial fibrillation from all causes is known to produce thrombi and cerebral embolization. Newer techniques have added to the varieties of cardiac lesions known to produce thromboembolism, for example, nonbacterial thrombotic endocarditis (NBTE) (Fig. 3), prolapsing mitral valve (PMV) (Fig. 4) (8) and, more recently, mitral annulus calcification (16).

The other entity in which platelets play an important role in threatened-stroke symptom production is *thrombocythemia* (52). This condition is related so obviously to platelet thrombogenesis as to require little further comment. When it has been associated with cerebral and retinal ischemic events, there has frequently been a readily recognizable tendency to spontaneous platelet aggregation in the chamber

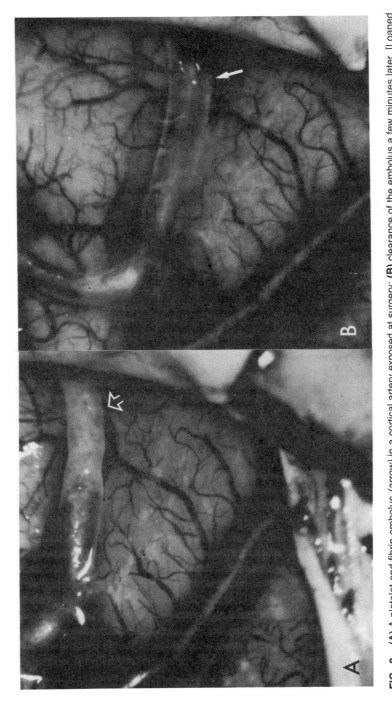

FIG. 2. **(A)** A platelet and fibrin embolus *(arrow)* in a cortical artery exposed at surgery; **(B)** clearance of the embolus a few minutes later. [Loaned by Dr. H. Reichman and from Barnett, H.J.M., in Hass, W.K., ed. (1979): *Med. Clin. North Am.,* 63:649–679. W.B. Saunders Co., Philadelphia. By permission.]

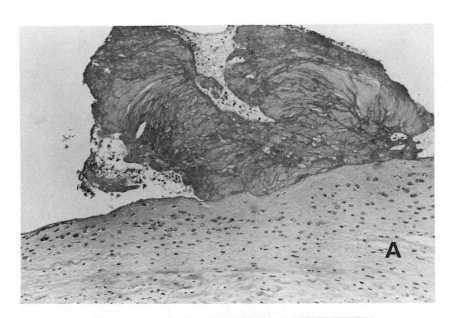

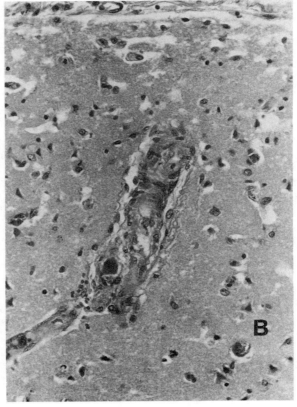

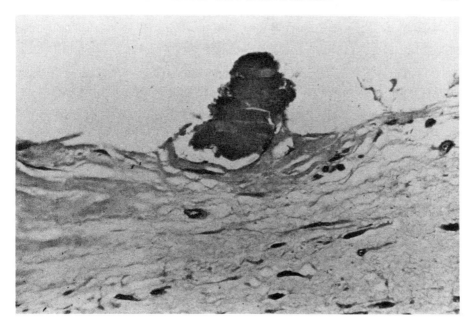

FIG. 4. A platelet-fibrin thrombosis attached to a mitral value exhibiting the characteristic myxomatous degeneration associated with prolapse. (From Hanson, M. R., et al. (1980): *Stroke*, 11:499–506. By permission.)

of the aggregometer (33,45). The symptoms respond quickly and well to measures designed to reduce the numbers of platelets or their ability to aggregate. Thus drugs cytotoxic to platelets (e.g. busulfan) or acetylsalicylic acid have proved effective in this uncommon but instructive disorder.

It is not possible to quantitate the importance of thrombosis in stroke-threatened symptoms. However, all available information indicates that thrombi in cerebral arteries are much more likely to be identified than in equally careful studies carried out on the coronary arteries in myocardial infarction.

Timing of the pathological examination in relation to the clinical events may be important. For example, thrombi are not recognized in patients with certain types of unstable angina of recent onset, or in such patients who die because of the onset of fatal ventricular arrhythmia. By contrast, thrombi are quite commonly found in the coronary arteries of patients who die after a major EKG-proven myocardial infarction superimposed on unstable angina (12,13,35,43,44).

The opposite type of data can be adduced from the examination of carotid endarterectomy specimens. Thus, if patients have had ischemic events within

---

FIG. 3. **(A)** Platelets and fibrin constitute the material in a valvular vegetation in a case of nonbacterial thrombotic endocarditis; **(B)** an embolus from the lesion in a cerebral arteriole. [From Barnett, H.J., in Hass, W.K., ed. (1979): *Med. Clin. North Am.* 63:649–679. W.B. Saunders Co., Philadephia. By permission.]

1 month of the endarterectomy, thrombi will be visible in the surgical specimens in 2 out of 3 cases (25). If a month or more has elapsed since the last ischemic event, no more than one out of five specimens will contain thrombotic material. This interesting observation suggests a pathological counterpart to the clinical observation that ischemic events have a tendency to go in flurries and to come and go spontaneously.

Cerebral angiography has quite frequently revealed obstruction of middle cerebral arteries after emboli, either from the heart or from the carotid artery in the neck, have lodged in them. The characteristic appearance is a rounded lesion in the absence of any evidence of pathological narrowing or irregularity of the artery. If the clinical event occurred several days before the angiography, the lesion is less likely to be identified. If pictures are taken soon after the event and again later, the embolus will often be found to have moved on or dissipated altogether (2).

Occlusion of a carotid artery at the level of the carotid sinus may reveal a bruit arising from a carotid stenosis. This may be followed, for a time, by cessation of transient ischemic events, and then more ischemic events may occur. These may be caused by a thrombus extending up the carotid artery into the cranium to the level of the carotid siphon (10). There may then be emboli from the white tail of the thrombus (Fig. 5). Alternatively, the stump itself may be the site of the thrombus, at times recognizable in arteriograms; it may be carried through the collateral circulation, in particular through the external carotid artery retrograde into the intracranial circulation, producing partial or complete stroke (11).

Experimental Studies on Cerebral Thromboembolism Involving Platelets

Denny-Brown (17) carried out the earliest experiments indicating the importance of platelet thromboembolism in the cerebral circulation. His experiments involved mechanical damage to cortical branches of the middle cerebral artery and the visualization of platelet emboli downstream from the sites of injury. Since these observations, many experimental models have been designed to produce thrombogenesis in cerebral arteries and test the effectiveness of platelet antiaggregants on these experimental models. In his experiments involving surgical lesions in the carotid arteries of dogs, Dyken (18) demonstrated a significant reduction in post-endarterectomy thrombosis in the animals pretreated with acetylsalicylic acid. Most recently, Weksler and Dougherty (48) induced thrombosis by an electrical injury in the extracranial cerebral arteries of rats and prevented thrombosis in a very significant number that were pretreated with indomethacin and prostacyclin.

Early Clinical Observations on TIA and Platelet Antiaggregants

Amaurosis fugax is a good clinical model for platelet thrombosis and the retina an excellent mirror in which to observe the effects of drugs. Striking reduction in recurrent amaurosis was recorded independently by Harrison and Mundall in reports on individual cases (26,39). These observations were among the most stimulating

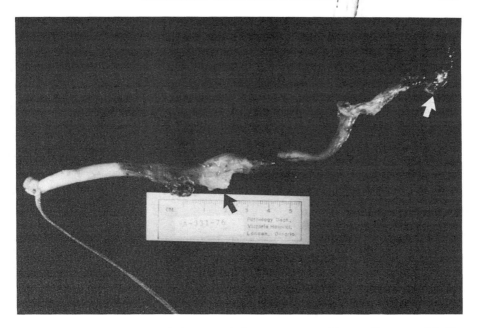

FIG. 5. Fresh thrombus 17cm in length occluding common carotid artery *(bottom end tied by string)* and region of carotid sinus of internal carotid artery *(open arrow)* and extending up to intracranial site of internal carotid artery *(closed arrow)*. (From Barnett, H. J. M., and Peerless, S. J. (1982): *The Collaborative EC/IC Bypass Study: The Rationale and a Progress Report.* Proceedings of the Williamsburg Conference 1980. Raven Press, New York, *in press.* By permission.)

to suggest the possible benefit from acetylsalicylic acid or other platelet antiaggregant therapy in threatened stroke. The natural sequel was a series of clinical trials.

Clinical Trials of Platelet Antiaggregants

A number of clinical trials have indicated the benefit or lack of benefit of particular platelet antiaggregants in a variety of stroke-threatened patients. These trials have utilized three drugs (dipyridamole, sulfinpyrazone, and acetylsalicylic acid) alone or in combination. The results are indicated in Table 3. (Trials that had no comparative groups or did not define their endpoints or entry criteria have not been included.)

The negative trial on dipyridamole conducted by Acheson, Danta, and Hutchinson (1) cannot be regarded as a final statement in respect of the usefulness of this drug. This trial was carried out on a relatively small number of patients over a short period of time and included those with threatened stroke as well as completed stroke.

In the American trial, which included subjects who had ischemic events in carotid artery territory (19), an insufficient number of cases were followed for an insufficient length of time to give definite answers as to benefit. However, by combining

TABLE 3. *Controlled trials of platelet antiaggregants in threatened stroke*

Designation of trial	Number of cases	Types of cases	Average length of follow-up	Drugs utilized	Endpoints	Positive benefit
Stoke-on-Trent trial	169	TIA RIND Stroke	24 months	Dipyridamole	TIA Stroke Death	No
American trial	179	TIA RIND PNS	6 months	ASA	TIA Stroke Death	Yes—ASA
Canadian cooperative trial	585	TIA RIND PNS	26 months	ASA Sulfinypyrazone	Stroke Death	Yes—ASA
German trial	31	TIA RIND PNS	24 months	ASA	TIA Stroke	Yes—ASA
AMIS trial	4,524	MI	3 years	ASA	Stroke	Yes—ASA
Swedish trial	156	TIA RIND	12 months	ASA Dipyridamole	TIA Stroke	Yes—both

TIA = transient ischemic attacks, RIND = reversible ischemic neurological disability, PNS = partial nonprogressing stroke, MI = myocardial infarction.

endpoints and analyzing results for a six-month period, the authors were able to show a difference in benefit for males in the acetylsalicylic acid-treated group as compared with the group receiving the placebo.

The Canadian trial involved a larger number of patients (585 patients) followed for a longer average period (26 months) and, overall, showed a reduction in stroke and death of 31% (14). In the subgroup analysis this benefit was conferred on the males but not on the females: males in the groups given acetylsalicylic acid had a 48% reduction in the endpoints of stroke and death, but there was no reduction in the groups given placebo and none in the group given sulfinpyrazone. There was no benefit to females. The trial has been criticized because of the analysis of stroke as an endpoint (49). When only stroke and stroke-death were considered, there was a 49% reduction in males in the acetylsalicylic acid-treated group compared with those not receiving acetylsalicylic acid (9). The trial has also been criticized because of the possible synergism between sulfinpyrazone and acetylsalicylic acid (32). Those who conducted and analyzed the trial, as well as most of those who have reviewed the data, have regarded it as legitimate to compare benefits to those in both the acetylsalicylic acid and the combined acetylsalicylic acid and sulfinpyrazone treatment groups with the benefit to those on placebo added to those in the group on sulfinpyrazone alone (3). The majority believe that there is no significant synergism that would negate the observations. The total lack of benefit to those on sulfinpyrazone alone was striking (Fig. 6).

The German trial (34) involved too few patients but provides interesting corroboration of the Canadian trial. The design of the Swedish trial had two major deficiencies: it had no placebo group and it utilized historical controls (40). The authors believed that there was a 10-fold reduction in what might have been expected in such patients. This conclusion is open to serious criticism because of the weakness inherent in this type of control. The AMIS study was designed to determine the benefit of acetylsalicylic acid in patients who had myocardial infarction (4). Although there was only a trend toward benefit in preventing further heart attacks, there was a reduction in stroke in the acetylsalicylic acid-treated compared with the untreated patients.

All of these studies have shortcomings, but collectively the conclusions are in the same direction: the administration of platelet antiaggregants benefits stroke-threatened individuals. Furthermore, of the three potential drugs in clinical use, acetylsalicylic acid has been studied most extensively and at the time of writing has been the most beneficial. The story is incomplete, and more clinical trials and new drugs will be emerging.

The Low-Response Groups

Treatment for threatened stroke is only beginning. Significant individual cases and groups of cases have failed to benefit from treatment useful in other more fortunate groups or individuals. Platelet antiaggregant therapy, as currently administered, offers little advantage in the following groups and individuals:

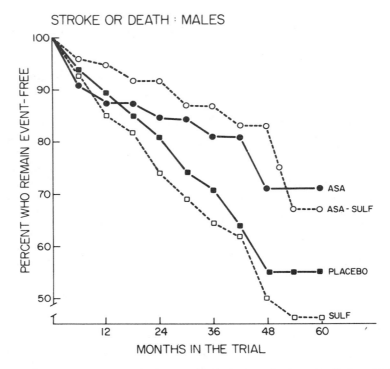

FIG. 6. The lack of benefit of sulfinpyrazone (Sulf), the benefit of acetylsalicylic acid (ASA), and the lack of synergism of antagonism between the combination of aspirin and sulfinpyrazone in the Canadian Cooperative Study. [From Barnett, H. J. M., in Hass, W. K., ed. (1979): *Med. Clin. North Am.*, 63:649–679. W. B. Saunders Co., Philadelphia. By permission.]

A. Females

It was totally unexpected that females would benefit less than males in the Canadian study. When the lack of response by stroke-threatened females was discussed at the Kalamazoo meeting, Salzman disclosed the lack of benefit from acetylsalicylic acid in the female group at risk after hip replacement and the reduction of venous thrombosis by the active therapy as compared to the placebo in males only (24). It was then recalled that in the reduction of shunt thrombosis conferred by sulfinpyrazone on dialysis patients, the improved results had been confined to the male patients (30). A retrospective review of the American Acetylsalicylic Acid Study presented evidence that in this trial as well, the outlook for females threatened with stroke was not improved (21). Finally, Linos et al. (34) have conducted an interesting survey of vascular endpoints over a 15-year period in all patients, male and female, in whom acetylsalicylic acid has been the primary therapy for rheumatoid arthritis for 10 years. Death from myocardial infarction, sudden death, development of angina, and stroke were all observed less often than expected by population life-table data in males but not in females. The experimental observations on this interesting biological phenomenon are reviewed by Kelton elsewhere in these proceedings.

B. Patients with Ruptured Plaques of Atheroma

Occasionally an atheromatous plaque ruptures into the lumen and hastens thrombosis (5). The outpouring of local thromboplastin is so massive that it is most unlikely that platelet antiaggregant treatment would have any effect on this occasional but nonpreventable process.

C. Patients with Hemorrhage into and from an Atheromatous Plaque

From time to time a carotid artery in the neck becomes painful as a prelude to clinical and radiological evidence of occlusion of the artery. The pathological counterpart to be sought in these cases is a thrombus complicating hemorrhage into an atheromatous plaque in the internal carotid artery. At times this hemorrhage breaks through into the lumen of the diseased artery (Fig. 7). Less commonly, a similar pathological process involves the basilar artery. Once again, suppression of platelet activity does not alter the stimulus to thrombosis from this process. The stimulus affects the coagulation process and appears to be overwhelming.

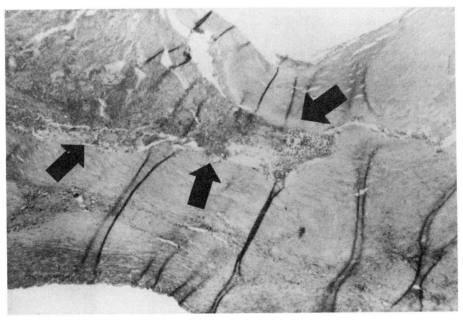

FIG. 7. Hemorrhage into arterial plaque. Patient complained of neck pain prior to contralateral hemiplegia. (From Barnett, H. J. M., in Scheinberg, P., ed. (1976): *Cerebrovascular Diseases*, pp. 1–21. Raven Press, New York. By permission.)

D. Patients with TIA Varieties that Lack Significant Platelet-induced Thrombogenesis

The varieties of threatened stroke in which thrombosis is present were outlined above. Table 4 delineates those varieties in which platelet-induced thrombosis is a minor or a secondary event. Neither individually nor collectively are they common, except for lacunar infarction, but they require consideration because the primary treatment is other than platelet antiaggregant therapy. In the case of the coagulation abnormalities, specific correction may be feasible; it may be possible to eliminate their cause (e.g., discontinue contraceptive estrogen therapy) or they may require short-term anticoagulant therapy (e.g., for postoperative conditions). In lacunar infarction, secondary thrombosis complicates the arteriolar lipohyalinosia, but most of the varieties listed in Table 4 require antihypertensive treatment. The nature of many of the non-arteriosclerotic vasculopathies (e.g., congophilic angiopathy, spontaneous carotid or basilar artery dissection, Moya-Moya disease) is obscure and no treatment is known. A number appear to respond to steroid therapy (collagen-vascular disease, granulomatous angiitis, Takayasu's arteritis) and such treatment is expected to be of greater benefit than platelet antiaggregant or other antithrombotic treatment. Mechanically induced arterial obstruction, such as chiropractic lesions of the high vertebral artery (7) and the rare examples of invasion of the vertebral artery by spondylogenic osteophytes (53), is only occasionally an indication for antithrombotic treatment.

Failure to recognize that stroke may develop in some patients, quite apart from thrombosis, could lead to erroneous treatment programs in individual cases. If these cases are overlooked, therapeutic possibilities may be misinterpreted. Their inclusion in antithrombotic trials or in the evaluation of other innovative possibilities could skew results and set the stage for false-positive or false-negative interpretation of the data.

E. Patients with Excessive Amounts of Atheromatous Disease

Subgroup analysis in the Canadian study yielded extremely disappointing results in two categories of patients in whom the available evidence indicated advanced atheromatous disease. Approximately 10% of the randomized cases had symptoms

TABLE 4. *Varieties of TIA with only a minor connection to platelet-induced thrombosis*

1. Lacunar infarction
2. Non-atherosclerotic vasculopathies
3. Hemodynamic crises
4. Mechanical arterial compressions
5. Coagulation abnormalities
6. Hyperviscosity syndromes

that were interpreted as caused by both carotid and vertebral-basilar disease. However, regardless of whether they were male or female, they did not benefit from acetylsalicylic acid. Similarly, patients whose cerebral angiograms showed recognizable atheroma in more than three arteries—whether male or female—failed to respond to acetylsalicylic acid.

Major Outstanding Problems

It appears reasonable to claim that a significant advance has been made in the reduction of stroke by the administration of acetylsalicylic acid to patients in stroke-threatened groups. However, a number of urgent problems persist and complacency would be extremely unwise. The most important ones are briefly noted below.

A. The Low-response Group

These patients form a significant segment of the population at risk. The most formidable problem is the failure to date to achieve a benefit in females. Another major source of concern is the patient who exhibits no symptoms until he presents evidence of advanced disease.

B. Failures in the High-response Group

It is disappointing, and yet a challenge to further energetic investigation, that a significant number of patients do not benefit from acetylsalicylic acid treatment, even though they are males. Of the males in the Canadian study, 20 had strokes as first-endpoint events. Admittedly, this is preferable to the 40 strokes that occurred in the patients who did not receive acetylsalicylic acid, but the number of failures is still challenging. Better treatment is required before the problem may be regarded as solved.

C. Determining the Optimal Dosage

This problem is examined in detail elsewhere in this volume. There is evidence that the inhibition of endothelial cell prostacyclin may reduce the expected benefit of its antiaggregant and vasodilating properties and that, for this reason, large doses of acetylsalicylic acid may become thrombotic. There is further evidence that as little as 160 mg/day of acetylsalicylic acid is clinically effective as an antithrombotic agent (27). The evidence for this is the disturbed state of platelet and coagulation function that obtains in uremic patients, so that this observation may not be relevant to normal patients. The problem of optimum dosage remains unsolved. Other arguments in favor of a low dosage are based on *in vitro* studies, which are less convincing than clinical trials. The best that can be stated at the moment is that no completed clinical trials have used other than 1.0 to 1.5 g/day of acetylsalicylic acid and that only this dosage range has been shown to have any benefit in stroke-threatened cases. Trials of comparative dosage schedules must be carried out before this vexed and practical question is settled. Extrapolation of data from dose-response curves is not going to give the clinical answer. These data can only be used for intelligent planning of future trials.

D. Efficacy of Combined Acetylsalicylic Acid-Dipyridamole Therapy

Since acetylsalicylic acid acts to inhibit the cyclo-oxygenase enzyme activity, and dipyridamole acts to inhibit the phosphodiesterase at the platelet membrane, one might suppose that a combination of the two would be synergistic. There is *in vitro* evidence of some potentiation (23,29,37). Clinical trials will be necessary to solve this problem, and one such collaborative study is in progress.

E. Relationship to Surgical Procedures

There is a lack of unequivocal evidence that carotid endarterectomy confers a benefit in stroke-threatened patients. The question that arises is what is the differential benefit between surgery and acetylsalicylic acid treatment, especially in males? If angiography and the subsequent surgical procedure were without risk, this question would likely not arise. A trial comparing the two modalities appears to be indicated and, in my opinion, is both ethical and necessary.

F. Acetylsalicylic Acid in the Presence of an Asymptomatic Bruit

Until recently, the majority of those who have written on the treatment of the asymptomatic bruit have favored a surgical approach, but recent studies have cast serious doubt on this view (28,31,51). In my opinion, there is insufficient evidence to justify other than a conservative approach. The need for a trial of acetylsalicylic acid or other platelet antiaggregants in this disorder is apparent. In the meantime, one might justify the empirical administration of prophylactic acetylsalicylic acid, particularly to males with an asymptomatic bruit.

G. Prophylaxis against Stroke in Normal Individuals

The question has been asked repeatedly, since the results of these stroke-prevention trials have been published, whether there is any indication for the use of acetylsalicylic acid in long-term prophylaxis against the later possibility of stroke. There are no clinical data to justify this. In this regard, the uncontrolled observations of Craven (15) may be recalled, but this report could scarcely be dignified with the descriptive term "clinical trial". There will be gastrointestinal complications, albeit infrequent, from long-term acetylsalicylic acid usage, and their occurrence in younger and middle-aged atheroma-free subjects would raise ethical questions about the rationale for acetylsalicylic acid administration.

On the other side of the coin, two interesting observations are on record. Firstly, the role of the platelet activity in atheroma production has been highlighted by the experimental observations of Moore and his colleagues (38). After the endothelial cells of rabbits' aortas had been damaged by a balloon catheter, an atherogenic diet led to the progression of a nodular and rapidly advancing variety of atheroma. The same strain, fed the same diet after the same mechanical injury but maintained in a state of chronic thrombocytopenia, did not develop significant atheromatous lesions (Fig. 7). Secondly, primates were fed an atherogenic diet and the atheromatous narrowing of their coronary arteries and abdominal aortas was analyzed quantitatively (41). Another group of the same species was studied after similar treatment, but this group of monkeys received daily prophylactic acetylsalicylic acid therapy. There was a striking reduction in the amount of coronary but not in the amount of aortic atheroma.

H. The Role of Anticoagulants in Preventing Stroke in the Era of Platelet Antiaggregant Agents

No recent hard data have emerged to settle this vexing question. On an empirical basis, many physicians will administer anticoagulants at intervals to patients afflicted with TIA who continue to have attacks despite platelet antiaggregants. Many will administer anticoagulants in the form of heparin for progressing stroke. However, no trial has ever been reported on such heparin therapy with anything approaching an acceptable control. Still, it is difficult to state without equivocation that this approach is not rational. Finally, platelet antiaggregant therapy has not been viewed as an acceptable replacement for anticoagulants in the patient who has had a minor embolic event as a sequel to myocardial infarction or mitral stenosis (with or without atrial fibrillation); also, it is not suitable as prophylaxis after prosthetic heart valve insertion. The whole area remains filled with uncertainties and unknown factors.

1. Carryover of Data from M.I. Studies

The question is whether the negative data from the myocardial infarction studies negate the early conclusions regarding stroke prevention. An affirmative answer to this question seems to be an illogical way of interpreting the results in two disparate conditions. We have abundant evidence that thrombi can be identified in less than half of those cases in which they are sought at postmortem examination after myocardial infarction. The evidence to date would place thrombosis in a more prominent position in the production of nonhemorrhagic stroke and in stroke-threatening conditions. Because of known pathological data, platelet antiaggregant therapy may well be on a more rational theoretical basis in stroke prevention than after myocardial infarction.

REFERENCES

1. Acheson, J., Danta, G., and Hutchinson, E. C. (1969): Controlled trial of dipyridamole in cerebral vascular disease. *Br. Med. J.*, 1:614–615.
2. Allcock, J. M. (1963): Occlusion of the middle cerebral artery: serial angiography as a guide to conservative therapy. *J. Neurosurg.*, 27:353–363.
3. Armitage, P. (1979): Controversy in the interpretation of clinical trials. *Ann. Neurol.*, 5:601–602.
4. Aspiring Myocardial Infarction Study Research Group (1980): A randomized controlled trial of aspirin in persons recovered from myocardial infarction. *JAMA*, 243:661–669.
5. Barnett, H. J. M. (1976): Pathogenesis of transient ischemic attacks. In: *Cerebrovascular Diseases*, edited by P. Scheinberg, pp. 1–21. Raven Press, New York.

6. Barnett, H. J. M. (1978): The role of platelets in transient ischemic attacks and cerebral vascular accidents. In: *Thrombosis: Animal and Clinical Models*, edited by H. J. Day, B. A. Molony, E. E. Nishizawa and R. H. Rynbrandt, pp. 257–264. Plenum Publishing Corp., New York.

7. Barnett, H. J. M. (1980): The Wartenburg Lecture - Progress towards stroke prevention. *Neurology (N.Y.)*, 30:1212–25.

8. Barnett, H. J. M., Boughner, D. R., Taylor, D. W., Cooper, P. E., Kostuk, W. J., and Nichol, P. M. (1980): Further evidence relating mitral-valve prolapse to cerebral ischemic events. *N. Engl. J. Med.*, 302:139–144.

9. Barnett, H. J. M., Gent, M., Sackett, D. L., and Taylor, M. D. (1979): Reply: *Ann. Neurol.*, 5:599–601.

10. Barnett, H. J. M., and Peerless, S. J. (1980): The collaborative EC/IC bypass study. Presented at the 12th Research Conference on Cardiovascular Disease, Williamsburg, Virginia, March 4.

11. Barnett, H. J. M., Peerless, S. J., and Kaufmann, J. C. E. (1978): "Stump" of internal carotid artery - a source for further cerebral embolic ischemia. *Stroke*, 9:448–456.

12. Baroldi, G. (1965): Acute coronary occlusion as a cause of myocardial infarct and sudden coronary heart death. *Am. J. Cardiol.*, 16:859–880.

13. Branwood, A. W., and Montgomery, G. L. (1956): Observations on the morbid anatomy of coronary artery disease. *Scott. Med. J.*, 1:367–375.

14. Canadian Cooperative Study Group (1978): A randomized trial of aspirin and sulfinpyrazone in threatened stroke. *N. Engl. J. Med.*, 299:53–59.

15. Craven, L. L. (1956): Prevention of coronary and cerebral thrombosis. *Miss. Valley Med. J.*, 78:213.

16. DeBono, D. P., and Warlow, C. P. (1979): Mitral-annulus calcification and cerebral or retinal ischemia. *Lancet*, 1:383–386.

17. Denny-Brown, D. (1960): Recurrent cerebrovascular episodes. *Arch. Neurol.*, 2:194–210.

18. Dyken, M. L., Campbell, R. L., Muller, J., Feuer, H., Horner, T., King, R., Kolar, O., Solow, E., and Jones, F. H. (1973): Effect of aspirin on experimentally induced arterial thrombosis during the healing phase. *Stroke*, 4:387–389.

19. Fields, W. S., Lemak, N. A., Frankowski, R. F., and Hardy, R. J. (1977): Controlled trial of aspirin in cerebral ischemia. *Stroke*, 8:301–316.

20. Garraway, W. M., Whisnant, J. P., Furlan, A. J., Phillips, L. H., Kurland, L. T., and O'Fallon, W. M. (1979): The declining incidence of stroke. *N. Engl. J. Med.*, 300:449–452.

21. Gent, M. (1979): Recent intervention studies of platelet suppressant drugs in cerebral ischemia: Methodological aspects. In: *Drug Treatment and Prevention in Cardiovascular Disorders*, edited by G. Tognoni and S. Garattini, pp. 437–448. Elsevier/North Holland Biomedical Press, Amsterdam.

22. Haberman, S., Capildeo, R., and Rose, R. C. (1978): The changing mortality of cerebrovascular disease. *Quart. J. Med.*, 47:71–88.

23. Harker, C. A., and Slichter, S. J. (1972): Platelet and fibrinogen consumption in man. *N. Engl. J. Med.*, 287:999–1005.

24. Harris, W. J., Salzman, E. W., Athanasoulis, C. A., Waltman, A. C., and DeSanctis, R. W. (1977): Aspirin prophylaxis of venous thromboembolism after total hip replacement. *N. Engl. J. Med.*, 297:1246–1248.

25. Harrison, M. J. G., and Marshall, J.' (1977): The finding of thrombus at carotid endarterectomy and its relationship to the timing of surgery. *Br. J. Surg.*, 64:511–512.

26. Harrison, M. J. G., Marshall, J., Meadows, J. C., and Ross Russell, R. W. (1971): Effect of aspirin in amaurosis fugax. *Lancet*, 2:743–744.

27. Harter, H. R., Burch, J. W., Majerus, P. W., Stanford, N., Delmez, J. A., Anderson, C. B., and Weerts, C. A. (1979): Prevention of thrombosis in patients on hemodialysis by low dose aspirin. *N. Engl. J. Med.*, 301:577–579.

28. Heyman, A., Wilkinson, W., Heyden, S., Helms, M. J., Bartel, A., Karp, H., Tyroler, H. A., and Hames, C. G. (1980): Risk of stroke in asymptomatic persons with cervical arterial bruits - a population study in Evans County, Georgia. *N. Engl. J. Med.*, 302:838–841.

29. Honour, A. J., Hockaday, T. D. R., and Mann, J. I. (1977): The synergistic effect of aspirin and dipyridamole upon platelet thrombi in living blood vessels. *Br. J. Exp. Pathol.*, 58:268–272, 1977.

30. Kaegi, A., Pineo, G. F., Shimizu, A. G., Trivedi, H., Hirsh, J., and Gent, M. (1974): The prevention of arteriovenous shunt thrombosis by sulfinpyrazone. *N. Engl. J. Med.*, 290:304–306.

31. Kagan, A., Popper, J., Rhoads, G. G., Takeya, Y., Kato, H., Goode, G. B., and Marmot, M. (1976): Epidemiologic studies of coronary heart disease and stroke in Japanese men living in Japan, Hawaii and California: Prevalence of stroke. In: *Cerebrovascular Diseases*, edited by P. Scheinberg, pp. 267–277. Raven Press, New York.
32. Kurtzke, J. F. (1979): A critique of the Canadian TIA study. *Ann. Neurol.*, 5:597–599.
33. Levine, J., and Swanson, P. D. (1968): Idiopathic thrombocytosis. A treatable cause of transient ischemic attacks. *Neurology*, 18:711–713.
34. Linos, A., Worthington, J. W., O'Fallon, W., Fuster, V., Whisnant, J. P., and Kurland, L. T. (1978): Effect of aspirin on prevention of coronary and cerebrovascular disease in patients with rheumatoid arthritis. A long-term follow-up study. *Mayo Clin. Proc.*, 53:581–586.
35. Maseri, A., L'Abbate, A., Baroldi, G., Chierchia, S., Marzilli, M., Ballestra, A. M., Severi, S., Parodi, O., Biagini, A., Distante, A., and Pesola, A. (1978): Coronary vasospasm as a possible cause of myocardial infarction. A conclusion derived from the study of "preinfarction" angina. *N. Engl. J. Med.*, 299:1271–1277.
36. Mohr, J. P., Caplan, L. R., Melski, J. W., Goldstein, R. J., Duncan, G. W., Kostler, J. P., Pessin, M. S., and Bleich, H. L. (1978): The Harvard cooperative stroke registry. A prospective registry. *Neurology*, 28:754–762.
37. Moncada, S., and Korbut, R. (1978): Dipyridamole and other phosphodiesterase inhibitors act as antithrombotic agents by potentiating endogenous prostacyclin. *Lancet*, 1:1286–1289.
38. Moore, S., Friedman, R. J., Singal, D. P., Gauldie, J., Blajchman, M. A., and Roberts, R. S. (1976): Inhibition of injury induced thromboatherosclerotic lesions by anti-platelet serum in rabbits. *Thromb. Diath. Haemorrh.*, 35:70–81.
39. Mundall, J., Quintero, P., von Kaulla, K. N., Harmon, R., and Austin, J. (1972): Transient monocular blindness and increased platelet aggregability treated with aspirin—a case report. *Neurology*, 22:280–285.
40. Olsson, J. E., Brechter, C., Bäcklund, H., Krook, H., Müller, R., Nitelius, E., and Olsson, O. (1980): Anticoagulant vs. antiplatelet therapy as prophylactic against cerebral infarction in transient ischemic attacks. *Stroke*, 11:4–9.
41. Pick, R., Chediak, J., and Glick, G. (1979): Aspirin inhibits development of coronary atherosclerosis in cynomolgus monkeys (Macaca fascicularis) fed an atherogenic diet. *J. Clin. Invest.*, 63:158–162.
42. Reuther, R., and Dorndorf, W. (1978): Aspirin in TIA platelets: a double-blind study. In: *Acetylsalicylic Acid in Cerebral Ischemia and Coronary Heart Disease*, edited by K. Breddin, W. Dorndorf, D. Loew and R. Marx, F. K. Schattauer Verlag, Stuttgart.
43. Roberts, W. C. (1974): Coronary thrombosis and fetal myocardial ischemia. *Circulation*, 49:1–3.
44. Silver, M. D., Baroldi, G., and Mariani, F. (1980): The relationship between acute occlusive coronary thrombi and myocardial infarction studied in 100 consecutive patients. *Circulation*, 61:219–227.
45. Singer, G. (1969): Migrating emboli of retinal arteries in thrombocythemia. *Br. J. Ophthal.*, 53:379–283.
46. Statistics Canada (1980): *Causes of Death 1978*. Catalogue #84–203, February 1980. Queen's Printer, Ottawa, Canada.
46a. Statistics Canada (1954): *Vital Statistics*. Catalogue #9004–505. Queen's Printer, Ottawa, Canada.
47. Warren, B. A., and Vales, O. (1974): Electron microscopy of the sequence of events in atheroembolic occlusion of cerebral arteries in the animal model. *Br. J. Exp. Pathol.*, 56:205–215.
48. Weksler, B. B., and Dougherty, J. H., Jr. (1980): Platelet function and cerebral ischemia. In: *Proceedings of the Princeton Conference*, March 4, 1980, Williamsburg, Va. Raven Press, New York.
49. Whisnant, J. P. (1978): The Canadian trial of aspirin and sulfinpyrazone in threatened stroke (letter). *N. Engl. J. Med.*, 299:953.
50. Whisnant, J. P., Fitzgibbons, J. P., Kurland, L. T., and Sayre, G. P. (1971): Natural history of stroke in Rochester, Minnesota, 1945 through 1954. *Stroke*, 2:11–22.
51. Wolf, P. A., Kannel, W. B., Gordon, T., McNamara, P. M., and Dawber, T. R. (1979): Asymptomatic carotid bruit and risk of stroke: The Framingham study. *Stroke*, 10:96.
52. Wu, K. K. (1978): Platelet hyperaggregatibility and thrombosis in patients with thrombocythemia. *Ann. Intern. Med.*, 88:7–11.
53. Yates, P. O., and Hutchinson, E. C. (1961): *Cerebral infarction: The role of stenosis of the extracranial cerebral arteries*. Medical Research Council Special Report Series No. 300. H. M. Stationery Office, London.

Acetylsalicylic Acid: New Uses for an Old Drug,
edited by H. J. M. Barnett, J. Hirsh, and
J. F. Mustard. Raven Press, New York © 1982.

The Use of Acetylsalicylic Acid in the Management of Coronary Artery Disease

J. Fraser Mustard

Faculty of Health Sciences, McMaster University, Hamilton, Ontario, Canada L8N 3Z5

A number of studies have examined the effect of acetylsalicylic acid, in dosages ranging from 300 to 1500 mg/day, on the clinical complications of patients who had had a previous myocardial infarction. At least six randomized trials with acetylsalicylic acid provide data for analysis. In five, total mortality was reduced between 15 and 30% in the patients given acetylsalicylic acid compared with the placebo group. In the largest trial (AMIS) the mortality in the acetylsalicylic acid-treated group was about 11% greater than that in the placebo group. Most of the patients in these trials were admitted months or years after the infarction. In the first study by Elwood and his colleagues, the administration of acetylsalicylic acid to patients in the first 4 to 5 weeks after myocardial infarction may have reduced the number of deaths. However, in a subsequent study in which all the patients were admitted soon after the infarction, no significant difference in mortality was demonstrated in the patients given acetylsalicylic acid. In both the AMIS and PARIS studies there was no statistically significant report on sudden death. In all the studies in which it was reported, there appeared to be a reduction in death from myocardial infarction in the acetylsalicylic acid-treated group. Unresolved questions remain concerning (a) the dose of acetylsalicylic acid that should be used in view of the assertion that high doses may inhibit PGI_2 synthesis and, in some circumstances, be thrombogenic, (b) the difference between males and females in the benefit derived from acetylsalicylic acid administration, and (c) the fact that multiple mechanisms may be involved in death in the post-myocardial infarction period and that acetylsalicylic acid may affect only some of these mechanisms. Future trials to assess the dosage of acetylsalicylic acid and other drugs in groups of patients most likely to benefit may provide more conclusive evidence about whether these drugs are beneficial in preventing complications in patients after myocardial infarction.

The role of platelets in the initiation and growth of arterial thrombi and the recognition that thromboembolism is a major cause of the clinical complications of atherosclerosis have led to considerable interest in modification of platelet function (41) and its effect on these disorders. The observations that nonsteroidal anti-inflammatory and related drugs inhibit collagen-induced platelet aggregation (19,44) and that collagen is involved in the initiation of experimental thrombi (8,23) have led to development of the concept that modification of the platelet-collagen reaction would inhibit arterial thrombosis. The evidence that thromboembolic events cause clinical complications of atherosclerosis is reasonably good (34,37), but other mechanisms are also involved (6,31). The relative importance of the different mechanisms is not yet clear.

The clinical trials of drugs that inhibit platelet function and their effect on arterial thromboembolic events were based on the assumptions that: (a) thromboembolic events are the cause of clinical complications of atherosclerosis; (b) drugs that inhibit the response of platelets to aggregating agents such as collagen will modify arterial thromboembolic events; and therefore (c) modification of thromboembolic events should lead to a corresponding reduction in the clinical complications of atherosclerosis.

MECHANISMS IN THROMBOSIS

Experimental work on thrombosis has shown that when the endothelium is lost from a normal vessel wall, subendothelial structures are exposed and the platelets adhere to the collagen, releasing the contents of some of their granules (8). Platelets also adhere to the exposed microfibrils and basement membrane, but these structures do not appear to induce the release reaction. Platelets adhering to the collagen not only release their granule contents but also undergo activation of the arachidonate pathway (46), with formation of thromboxane A_2. Both the ADP and thromboxane A_2 cause platelets that are flowing by the injury site to adhere to each other and to the platelets already adherent to the vessel wall. The platelet aggregate that forms serves as a focus for local acceleration of coagulation (38,56). Thrombin generated around the surface of the platelet mass can cause further platelet aggregation through a direct pathway and also through the release of ADP and activation of the arachidonate pathway (27,28).

In addition, thrombin causes the fibrinogen around the platelets to polymerize and adhere to the platelets. Polymerizing fibrin adhering to the platelets is believed to stabilize the aggregates and prevent the thrombus from disintegrating (39). Inhibition of thromboxane formation should diminish the extent of thrombus growth, particularly if this is a principal pathway in the initiation and growth of the thrombus. When the clinical trials to be discussed were planned, PGI_2 was unknown and thus its possible role in inhibiting thrombosis was not recognized (33). In these first-generation trials, acetylsalicylic acid, sulfinpyrazone, or dipyridamole in combination with acetylsalicylic acid were studied.

EFFECTS OF ACETYLSALICYLIC ACID, SULFINPYRAZONE, AND DIPYRIDAMOLE

When the trials were started, differences in the mode of action of acetylsalicylic acid and sulfinpyrazone had already been recognized. Acetylsalicylic acid had not been found to prolong shortened platelet survival (22), whereas sulfinpyrazone had been shown to do so (47). Although both drugs inhibited collagen-induced platelet aggregation, acetylsalicylic acid was more effective than sulfinpyrazone (19,44,55). It had also been recognized that the effect of acetylsalicylic acid on platelet aggregation and the platelet release reaction was permanent (40,53), whereas the effect of sulfinpyrazone was not (42). Subsequent studies have shown other differences in the effects of acetylsalicylic acid and sulfinpyrazone (43).

Dipyridamole was not considered to be a strong inhibitor of platelet aggregation (32,51), but in combination with acetylsalicylic acid it did reduce platelet thrombosis and embolization in damaged vessels in the microcirculation (1,20,54). It is not clear whether dipyridamole affects platelets directly or acts in some other way, such as by enhancing the effect of PGI_2 formed at an injury site (16). Because it inhibits platelet phosphodiesterase, dipyridamole can enhance the increase in cyclic AMP produced by PGI_2 (21,50). In addition, dipyridamole prolongs shortened platelet survival (22,48).

CLINICAL TRIALS

The results of the clinical trials in which acetylsalicylic acid was administered to patients who had had a myocardial infarction are summarized in Table 1. These patients were used because they have a high risk of further complications and deaths. Primary prevention trials are more difficult and expensive, because of the large number of subjects required and the problem of identifying those at greatest risk. However, a trial with patients who have had a myocardial infarction can only involve a subgroup of these patients, since a sizable number of individuals who have a myocardial infarction will have died before they can be entered into a trial. All of the large clinical trials were randomized double-blind studies, with various doses of acetylsalicylic acid used and the patients observed for different periods of time. The time between the myocardial infarction and entry into the trial varied considerably. In all of these studies except the largest one (Aspirin Myocardial Infarction Study, AMIS) (4), patients randomized to the treated group showed a reduction in mortality, in comparison with the group given placebo. In three of the studies, fatal myocardial infarction was also recorded as an endpoint (4,10,45), and in these (including the AMIS) the administration of acetylsalicylic acid reduced the incidence. However, these differences were not found to be statistically significant. The dosages of acetylsalicylic acid ranged from 300 mg/day in the first MRC trial of Elwood and his colleagues (17) to 1.5 g/day in the German/Austrian study (10).

In the first study by Elwood and his colleagues (17) patients from the Cardiff area were admitted soon after myocardial infarction. In this group, acetylsalicylic acid appeared to cause a significant reduction in mortality. Expansion of the study to include patients from other centers led to the admission of patients much longer after their myocardial infarction, and the question posed by retrospective analysis is whether the administration of acetylsalicylic acid during the early time period reduced the incidence of death. In a later trial by Elwood and Sweetnam (18) all the patients were admitted shortly after myocardial infarction and all randomized patients were counted whether or not they stayed in the study. No statistically significant beneficial effect of acetylsalicylic acid was observed, although the mortality of acetylsalicylic acid-treated patients was less than that of the placebo group. In this second study, the incidence of nonfatal myocardial infarction was signifi-

TABLE 1. *Results of clinical trials of ASA in post-myocardial infarction patients*

Trial	ASA dose (g/day)	Years observed	Entry time after M.I.	No. of patients	Nonfatal M.I.		Death					
							All causes		M.I.		Sudden	
					Rx	C	Rx	C	Rx	C	Rx	C
MRC I	0.3	2.5	1–6 months	1239	—	—	8.3	10.9	—	—	—	—
MRC II	0.9	1.0	50% within 1 wk	1682	7.1	10.9	12.3	14.8	—	—	—	—
CDPA	0.97	1–2	75% ≥ 5 yr	1529	3.7	4.2	5.8	8.3	—	—	2.6	3.2
German-Austrian	1.5	2	30–42 days	620	3.5	4.9	8.5	10.6	1.6	3.2	2.5	3.9
AMIS	1.0	3	2–60 months	4524	6.3	8.1	10.8	9.7	6.0	6.0	2.7	2.0
PARIS	0.97	3–4	2–60 months	1216	6.9	9.9	10.5	12.8	2.5	5.7	5.6	4.4
PARIS	0.97 plus 0.225 dipyridamole	3–4	2–60 months	1216	7.9	9.9	10.7	12.8	4.0	5.7	3.7	4.4

M.I. = Myocardial infarction; Rx = Treated with ASA; C = Placebo control. MRC I = Elwood et al. (17), 1974. MRCII = Elwood and Sweetnam (18), 1979. CDPA = Coronary Drug Project Aspirin® Study (13), 1976. German-Austrian Trial, Breddin et al. (10), 1979. AMIS = Aspirin Myocardial Infarction Study (4), 1980. PARIS = Persantine-Aspirin Reinfarction Study (45), 1980.

cantly reduced in the patients given acetylsalicylic acid. In the German/Austrian study (10), in which the patients started therapy within 42 days of myocardial infarction, fatal and nonfatal myocardial infarction and sudden death were reduced in those receiving acetylsalicylic acid.

The National Institutes of Health trial (AMIS) (4) showed a slightly increased percentage of deaths from all causes in the patients given acetylsalicylic acid. However, it should be pointed out that the study design and the method of analysis were very conservative. All patients randomized to the trial were included in the analysis, regardless of eligibility and whether or not they dropped out of the study. This type of statistical analysis is usually referred to as the "intent to treat" approach. Many of the patients were entered into the study months or years after the myocardial infarction, and therefore the patient population was heterogenous. No information was given about the number lost from the study. The percentage of patients reported to have had nonfatal myocardial infarcts was lower in those receiving acetylsalicylic acid, in contrast to the slightly increased mortality rates for all patients treated with acetylsalicylic acid. One could conclude that the risk of cardiovascular death while receiving acetylsalicylic acid is increased slightly. Other interpretations can be made, and the reduction of myocardial infarction seen in other studies, in which the percentage of deaths in the acetylsalicylic acid-treated group was less than that in the placebo groups, could be caused by inhibition of thrombosis by acetylsalicylic acid.

The most recent trial (Persantine-Aspirin Reinfarction Study, PARIS) (45) compares the effect of placebo, acetylsalicylic acid, and acetylsalicylic acid plus dipyridamole. Data for all patients randomized into the trial showed an 18% reduction in mortality for the group given acetylsalicylic acid and a 16% reduction in mortality in the group given acetylsalicylic acid plus dipyridamole. The difference between the group given acetylsalicylic acid and the group given dipyridamole plus acetylsalicylic acid was not statistically significant. Patients treated with acetylsalicylic acid showed a greater incidence of sudden death than patients given placebo, whereas those given acetylsalicylic acid plus dipyridamole showed a lower incidence. Secondary analysis of the data, using the combination of coronary death and nonfatal myocardial infarction as end points, showed that the "coronary incidence" was significantly less in the group given acetylsalicylic acid plus dipyridamole, and a similar but less significant trend was found for acetylsalicylic acid alone. Again, as in the AMIS (4) and Elwood and Sweetnam studies (18), the percentage of patients dying with myocardial infarction or reported to have recurrent myocardial infarction without sudden death was diminished in the subjects receiving acetylsalicylic acid.

In the PARIS study, although patients were admitted at various times after myocardial infarction, a small group was admitted within the first 6 months of infarction. The data concerning these showed a distinct trend, indicating a beneficial effect for acetylsalicylic acid or acetylsalicylic acid plus dipyridamole during the first few months. Administration of acetylsalicylic acid produced a 51% reduction in death from all causes in comparison with the placebo group, and the reduction for acetylsalicylic acid plus dipyridamole was 44%. However, this effect appeared to be primarily on the group recorded as dying a coronary death, rather than on the group classified as dying suddenly.

The impression from the smaller acetylsalicylic acid trials is that there was a trend towards reduction in overall mortality for patients receiving acetylsalicylic acid, but this was not statistically significant in any of the trials. In one large trial, AMIS (4), no effect was apparent although the number of patients was sufficient to have shown a statistically significant benefit if the trend of the other trials had occurred. The questions still remain open as to whether acetylsalicylic acid prevents myocardial infarction and whether it has a more marked effect during the early period following myocardial infarction.

It is useful to compare results from the acetylsalicylic acid studies with those of the Anturane Reinfarction Trial (2,3). The design of this study differed from that of most of the acetylsalicylic acid trials in that randomized patients subsequently found to be ineligible were excluded from analysis, and deaths were considered analyzable only if they occurred 7 days after the patients started receiving the drug, or within 7 days of cessation of therapy. This design makes it easier to test whether a drug is of benefit to the patients most at risk of dying from the specific complications the drug is supposed to affect, and this differs from the "intent to treat" approach of the other studies.

In the Anturane Reinfarction Trial (2) the patients were randomized into two groups, but 72 noneligible patients were excluded after randomization. Deaths of patients who had not received the drug for at least 7 days, or of patients who had discontinued taking the drug 7 days or longer before death, were classified as nonanalyzable. Thus in this trial there were two sources of possible bias in (a) the exclusion of noneligible patients who had been originally randomized and (b) the decision about analyzable or nonanalyzable deaths. All patients were in the study for a minimum of 1 year and all were admitted between 25 and 35 days after myocardial infarction. Table 2 shows total deaths for all subjects, including the noneligible patients and the nonanalyzable deaths. The percentage reduction in mortality for the patients given sulfinpyrazone was similar to the reduction for treated patients in the five small acetylsalicylic acid trials. Although sulfinpyrazone did not reduce death from myocardial infarction, it did reduce sudden death in the

TABLE 2. Anturane reinfarction trial—all deaths

Patients	No. of deaths	
	Sulfinpyrazone	Placebo
All randomized patients	813	816
All deaths	74	89
Eligible patients	775	783
All deaths	64	85
Analyzable deaths	44	62
Sulfinpyrazone dosage 200 mg q.i.d.		

first 6 months (3) (Table 3). The difference between the groups is striking, regardless of whether all the patients randomized to the trial are included or whether the analysis is restricted to eligible patients with analyzable deaths.

This type of retrospective analysis does not provide the same level of significance as the primary analysis based on the original protocol for the study. However, even if the probability value is discounted to take into account multiple analysis of the data, the difference is still statistically significant. The observation that sulfinpyrazone may affect the incidence of sudden death during a short period after myocardial infarction raises the question of whether acetylsalicylic acid has a similar effect.

Effect of Acetylsalicylic Acid or Sulfinpyrazone on Ventricular Fibrillation

The fact that sulfinpyrazone does not appear to inhibit the thromboembolic events associated with carotid artery disease (7) does not appear to influence death from myocardial infarction (2,3), but does change the incidence of sudden death during the early period after myocardial infarction (3), raises the possibility that its action is unrelated to an effect on platelets and thrombosis. There is experimental evidence that both sulfinpyrazone and acetylsalicylic acid inhibit ventricular fibrillation associated with myocardial ischemia, in circumstances in which platelet aggregation is not believed to be a contributing factor (9,25,36,52). An interesting question is whether prostaglandin metabolism is abnormal in the ischemic myocardium and in the healing myocardium. Since myocardial cells do not form prostaglandins, in the acute ischemic period they are probably produced by the cells in the walls of myocardial blood vessels and in the white cells and platelets of the blood. During healing, fibroblasts may be a source of prostaglandins (5).

Dosage of Acetylsalicylic Acid

One unsettled question relates to whether the dosages of acetylsalicylic acid in the postmyocardial infarction trials have been appropriate. In most of the trials, the

TABLE 3. *Anturane reinfarction trial: Sudden death up to 6 months after entry into trial*

Patients	No. of sudden deaths	
	Sulfinpyrazone	Placebo
All randomized patients	11	30
All eligible patients (includes analyzable and nonanalyzable deaths)	9	28
Eligible patients (analyzable deaths)	6	24
	Randomized Patients	
Total number	813	816
Eligible	775	783
Ineligible	38	33
Withdrew	220	195
Sulfinpyrazone dosage 200 mg q.i.d		

dosage of acetylsalicylic acid has been greater than that required to maintain a sustained inhibition of platelet function over a 24-hr period (12). Acetylsalicylic acid also inhibits PGI_2 production by the vessel wall, although the concentration required appears to be higher than that needed to inhibit platelet cyclo-oxygenase (11,33). The possibility has therefore been raised that higher doses of acetylsalicylic acid may be thrombogenic (11). However, in animal experiments, acetylsalicylic acid has been shown to be thrombogenic only in circumstances where blood flow is arrested, PGI_2 formation is strongly stimulated, and high doses of acetylsalicylic acid have been given intravenously (26). It is doubtful that this applies to patients given the oral dosages used in these clinical trials.

Two reports have appeared about the effect of acetylsalicylic acid, administered for rheumatoid arthritis, on the incidence of myocardial infarction (14,29). Both studies suffer from the problem of being case control or cohort studies and not randomized trials. In both studies the frequency of myocardial infarction tended to be greater in the control group than in the patients with rheumatoid arthritis receiving high doses of acetylsalicylic acid. Thus, these studies of individuals with rheumatoid arthritis provided no evidence that high doses of acetylsalicylic acid enhanced thrombosis. In the Mayo Clinic study (29) the effect of acetylsalicylic acid was apparent in male patients but not in females, confirming the male–female difference observed in other clinical trials (7). More recently, results from the study by McKenna and her associates (30) of venous thromboembolism in patients undergoing knee replacement operations further support the concept that high doses of acetylsalicylic acid are not thrombogenic. In this study, the majority of the patients were female, and only those receiving high doses of acetylsalicylic acid (3.9 g per day) showed a reduced incidence of venous thromboembolism. Those receiving 975 mg of acetylsalicylic acid per day showed the same incidence as the placebo group.

The effect of acetylsalicylic acid on thrombosis may involve mechanisms other than inhibition of the cyclo-oxygenase pathway. For example, in whole blood, acetylsalicylic acid or sodium salicylate activates the fibrinolytic pathway (35). It may be that the higher the dose of acetylsalicylic acid the greater the antithrombotic effect, because higher doses will both acetylate cyclo-oxygenase and increase fibrinolysis. If—as some of the experimental evidence indicates (15)—PGI_2 production by the arterial wall is not essential for limiting thrombosis, inhibition of PGI_2 formation would be of little consequence.

CONSIDERATIONS FOR FUTURE CLINICAL TRIALS

The results from the clinical trials raise a series of questions that should lead to further research into the mechanisms of thrombosis and to more refined designs for future clinical studies. Evidence about thrombus formation indicates that the process in diseased arteries may differ from that in normal vessels. When normal vessels are injured, the platelets are believed to interact with subendothelial connective tissue, particularly collagen, which causes platelet aggregation and thrombus formation (8,23). A theory has been developed that collagen plays a central role in the initiation and growth of thrombi. However, injury to the thickened intima of damaged arteries leads to the formation of thrombi that are much more dependent on the generation of thrombin for their initiation and growth (24,27,49). This could be caused by activation of the coagulation pathways and thrombin formation, leading to fibrin polymerization and platelet adherence to the polymerizing fibrin that becomes adherent to the vessel wall. It may be very difficult to inhibit the formation of this type of thrombus with drugs that inhibit cyclo-oxygenase, because thrombin-induced platelet aggregation is practically independent of thromboxane A_2 formation (28). In future studies, attempts should be made to determine which pathways are important in the initiation and growth of thrombi. This may be difficult, because different mechanisms may be operative at different times in the same individual. Several forms of therapy may be required that affect different pathways in thrombosis.

Study of the mechanisms responsible for the clinical complications of atherosclerosis should also be considered. Although thromboembolism is one of the causes of clinical complications, its importance relative to other factors is not known. Some subgroups of patients may benefit more from a certain type of therapy than others. For example, some of the clinical trials indicate that males are more likely to benefit than females. Previous clinical trials may have been relatively insensitive for demonstration that drugs that modify platelet function may inhibit thromboembolic events associated with arterial disease, because it is not possible to preselect the subgroups most likely to benefit.

In view of these uncertainties, there should be some agreement among epidemiologists about suitable protocols for these large-scale clinical trials. The "intent to treat" method is excellent for the study of mass public health use of a drug, but this approach is expensive because of the number of patients who must be involved, when only a portion of those in the trial are likely to have pathogenic mechanisms affected by the drug and up to one-quarter of the randomized subjects may withdraw from the study but still are counted. We are at a very preliminary stage in trying to understand all the mechanisms involved in the clinical complications of atherosclerosis and how to control them. Perhaps we need to compromise and design efficient randomized trials to determine whether the drugs do have an effect on thromboembolic events in the patients most likely to suffer from them, before undertaking the larger "intent to treat" trials.

REFERENCES

1. Amir, J., and Krauss, S. (1973): Treatment of thrombotic thrombocytopenia purpura with antiplatelet drugs. *Blood*, 42:27–33.
2. Anturane Reinfarction Trial Research Group (1978): Sulfinpyrazone in the prevention of cardiac death after myocardial infarction: the Anturane Reinfarction Trial. *N. Engl. J. Med.*, 298:289–295.
3. The Anturane Reinfarction Trial Research Group (1980): Sulfinpyrazone in the prevention of sudden death after myocardial infarction. *N. Engl. J. Med.*, 302:250–256.
4. Aspirin Myocardial Infarction Study Research Group (1980): A randomized controlled trial of aspirin in persons recovered from myocardial infarction. *JAMA*, 243:661–669.

5. Baenziger, N. L., Dillender, M. J., and Majerus, P. W. (1977): Cultured human skin fibroblasts and arterial cells produce a labile platelet-inhibitory prostaglandin. *Biochem. Biophys. Res. Commun.*, 78:294–301.

6. Barnett, H. J. M. (1976): Pathogenesis of transient ischemic attacks. In: *Cerebrovascular Diseases*, edited by P. Scheinberg, pp. 1–21. Raven Press, New York.

7. Barnett, H. J. M., Gent, M., Sackett, D. L., Taylor, D. W., Blakely, J. A., Hirsh, J., Mustard, J. F., and Stuart, R. K. (1978): A randomized trial of aspirin and sulfinpyrazone in threatened stroke. The Canadian cooperative study group. *N. Engl. J. Med.*, 299:53–59.

8. Baumgartner, H. R., Muggli, R., Tschopp, T. B., and Turitto, V. T. (1976): Platelet adhesion, release and aggregation in flowing blood: effects of surface properties and platelet function. *Thromb. Haemost.*, 35:124–138.

9. Beamish, R. E., Dhillon, K. S., and Dhalla, S. (1980): Arrhythmogenic activity of adrenochrome: effect of sulfinpyrazone. *Ann. Roy. Coll. Phys. Surg. Canada*, 13:113.

10. Breddin, K., Loew, D., Lechner, K., and Überlak, W. E. (1979): Secondary prevention of myocardial infarction. Comparison of acetylsalicylic acid, phenoprocoumon and placebo. A multicenter two-year prospective study. *Thromb. Haemost.*, 4:225–236.

11. Burch, J. W., Baenziger, N. L., Stanford, N., and Majerus, P. W. (1978): Sensitivity of fatty acid cyclooxygenase from human aorta to acetylation by aspirin. *Proc. Natl. Acad. Sci. U. S. A.*, 75:5181–5184.

12. Burch, J. W., Stanford, N., and Majerus, P. W. (1978): Inhibition of platelet prostaglandin synthetase by oral aspirin. *J. Clin. Invest.*, 61:314–319.

13. Coronary Drug Project Research Group (1976): Aspirin in coronary heart disease. *J. Chronic Dis.*, 29:625–642.

14. Davis, R. F., and Engleman, E. G. (1974): Incidence of myocardial infarction in patients with rheumatoid arthritis. *Arthritis Rheum.*, 17:527–533.

15. Dejana, E., Cazenave, J.-P., Groves, H. M., Kinlough-Rathbone, R. L., Richardson, M., Packham, M. A., and Mustard, J. F. (1980): The effect of aspirin inhibition of PGI_2 production on platelet adherence to normal and damaged rabbit aortae. *Thromb. Res.*, 17:453–464.

16. Di Minno, G., De Gaetano, G., and Garattini, S. (1978): Dipyridamole and platelet function. *Lancet*, 2:1258–1259.

17. Elwood, P. C., Cochrane, A. L., Burr, M. L., Sweetnam, P. M., Williams, G., Welsby, E., Hughes, S. J., and Renton, R. (1974): A randomized controlled trial of acetylsalicylic acid in the secondary prevention of mortality from myocardial infarction. *Br. Med. J.*, 1:436–440.

18. Elwood, P. C., and Sweetnam, P. M. (1979): Aspirin and secondary mortality after myocardial infarction. *Lancet*, 2:1313–1315.

19. Evans, G., Packham, M. A., Nishizawa, E. E., Mustard, J. F., and Murphy, E. A. (1968): The effect of acetylsalicylic acid on platelet function. *J. Exp. Med.*, 128:877–894.

20. Giromini, M., Bouvier, C. A., Dami, R., Denizot, M., and Jeannet, M. (1972): Effect of dipyridamole and aspirin in thrombotic microangiopathy. *Br. Med. J.*, 1:545–546.

21. Gorman, R. R., Bunting, S., and Miller, O. V. (1977): Modulation of human platelet adenylate cyclase by prostacyclin (PGX). *Prostaglandins*, 13:377–388.

22. Harker, L. A., and Slichter, S. J. (1972): Platelet and fibrinogen consumption in man. *N. Engl. J. Med.*, 287:999–1005.

23. Hovig, T. (1963): Release of a platelet aggregating substance (adenosine diphosphate) from rabbit blood platelets induced by saline "extract" of tendons. *Thromb. Diath. Haemorrh.*, 9:264–278.

24. Jørgensen, L., Packham, M. A., Rowsell, H. C., and Mustard, J. F. (1972): Deposition of formed elements of blood on the intima and signs of intimal injury in the aorta of rabbit, pig, and man. *Lab. Invest.*, 27:341–350.

25. Kelliher, G. J., Dix, R. K., Jurkiewicz, N., and Lawrence, T. L. (1980): Effect of sulfinpyrazone on arrhythmia and death following coronary occlusion in cats. In: *Cardiovascular Actions of Sulfinpyrazone: Basic and Clinical Research*, edited by M. McGregor, J. F. Mustard, M. F. Oliver, and S. Sherry, pp. 193–209. Symposia Specialists, Miami.

26. Kelton, J. G., Hirsh, J., Carter, C. J., and Buchanan, M. R. (1978): Thrombogenic effect of high-dose aspirin in rabbits. Relationship to inhibition of vessel wall synthesis of prostaglandin I_2-like activity. *J. Clin. Invest.*, 62:892–895.

27. Kinlough-Rathbone, R. L., Groves, H. M., Jørgensen, L., Richardson, M., Moore, S., Packham, M. A., and Mustard, J. F. (1980): The role of thrombin in the response of platelets to injury of the rabbit aorta. *Clin. Res.*, 28:548A.

28. Kinlough-Rathbone, R. L., Packham, M. A., Reimers, H.-J., Cazenave, J.-P., and Mustard, J. F. (1977): Mechanisms of platelet shape change, aggregation, and release induced by collagen, thrombin, or A23,187. *J. Lab. Clin. Med.*, 90:707–719.

29. Linos, A., Worthington, J. W., O'Fallon, W., Fuster, V., Whisnant, J. P., and Kurland, L. T. (1978): Effect of aspirin on prevention of coronary and cerebrovascular disease in patients with rheumatoid arthritis. A long-term follow-up study. *Mayo Clin. Proc.*, 53:581–586.

30. McKenna, R., Galante, J., Bachmann, F., Wallace, D. L., Kaushal, S. P., and Meredith, P. (1980): Prevention of venous thromboembolism after total knee replacement by high-dose aspirin or intermittent calf and thigh compression. *Br. Med. J.*, 1:514–517.

31. Maseri, A., L'Abbate, A., Baroldi, G., Chierchia, S., Marzilli, M., Ballestra, A. M., Severi, S., Parodi, O., Biogini, A., Distante, A., and Pesola, A. (1978): Coronary vasospasm as a possible cause of myocardial infarction. A conclusion derived from the study of "preinfarction" angina. *N. Engl. J. Med.*, 299:1271–1277.

32. Mills, D. C. B., and Smith, J. B. (1971): The influence on platelet aggregation of drugs that affect the accumulation of adenosine 3':5'-cyclic monophosphate in platelets. *Biochem. J.*, 121:185–196.

33. Moncada, S., and Vane, J. R. (1978): Pharmacology and endogenous roles of prostaglandin endoperoxides, thromboxane A_2, and prostacyclin. *Pharmacol. Rev.*, 30:293–331.

34. Moore, S., and Ihnatowycz, I. (1978): Vessel injury and atherosclerosis. *Adv. Exp. Med. Biol.*, 102:145–163.

35. Moroz, I. A. (1977): Increased blood fibrinolytic activity after aspirin ingestion. *N. Engl. J. Med.*, 296:525–529.

36. Moschos, C. B., Haider, B., De La Cruz, C., Jr., Lyons, M. M., and Regan, T. J. (1978): Antiarrhythmic effects of aspirin during non-thrombotic coronary occlusion. *Circulation*, 57:681–684.

37. Mustard, J. F. (1976): Function of blood platelets and their role in thrombosis. *Trans. Am. Clin. Climatol. Assoc.*, 87:104–127.

38. Mustard, J. F., Packham, M. A., and Kinlough-Rathbone, R. L. (1981): Mechanisms in thrombosis. In: *Haemostasis and Thrombosis*, edited by A. L. Bloom and D. P. Thomas, pp. 503–506. Churchill/Livingstone, Edinburgh.

39. Niewiarowski, S., Regoeczi, E., Stewart, G. J., Senyi, A. F., and Mustard, J. F. (1972): Platelet interaction with polymerizing fibrin. *J. Clin. Invest.*, 51:685–700.

40. O'Brien, J. R., Finch, W., and Clark, E. (1970): A comparison of an effect of different anti-inflammatory drugs on human platelets. *J. Clin. Pathol.*, 23:522–525.

41. Packham, M. A., and Mustard, J. F. (1977): Clinical pharmacology of platelets. *Blood*, 50:555–573.

42. Packham, M. A., and Mustard, J. F. (1975): Non-steroidal anti-inflammatory drugs, pyrimido-pyrimidine compounds and tricyclic compounds. Effects on platelet function. In: *Platelets, Drugs and Thrombosis*, edited by J. Hirsh, J. F. Cade, A. S. Gallus, and E. Schönbaum, pp. 111–123. Karger, Basel.

43. Packham, M. A., and Mustard, J. F. (1980): Pharmacology of platelet-affecting drugs. *Circulation*, 62(2):V26–41.

44. Packham, M. A., Warrior, E. S., Glynn, M. F., Senyi, A. S., and Mustard, J. F. (1967): Alteration of the response of platelets to surface stimuli by pyrazole compounds. *J. Exp. Med.*, 126:171–188.

45. Persantine-Aspirin Reinfarction Study Research Group (1980): Persantine and aspirin in coronary heart disease. *Circulation*, 62:449–461, 1980.

46. Smith, J. B., Ingerman, C., Kocsis, J. J., and Silver, M. J. (1973): Formation of prostaglandins during the aggregation of human blood platelets. *J. Clin. Invest.*, 52:965–969.

47. Smythe, H. A., Ogryzlo, M. A., Murphy, E. A., and Mustard, J. F. (1965): The effect of sulfin-pyrazone (Anturane) on platelet economy and blood coagulation in man. *Can. Med. Assoc. J.*, 92:818–821.

48. Steele, P., Rainwater, J., Vogel, R., and Genton, E. (1978): Platelet-suppressant therapy in patients with coronary artery disease. *JAMA*, 240:228–231.

49. Stemerman, M. B. (1973): Thrombogenesis of the rabbit arterial plaque. An electron microscope study. *Am. J. Pathol.*, 73:7–26.

50. Tateson, J. E., Moncada, S., and Vane, J. R. (1977): Effects of prostacyclin (PGX) on cyclic AMP concentrations in human platelets. *Prostaglandins*, 13:389–397.

51. Vigdahl, R. L., Mongin, J., and Marquis, N. R. (1971): Platelet aggregation. IV. Platelet phosphodiesterase and its inhibition by vasodilators. *Biochem. Biophys. Res. Commun.*, 42:1088–1094.
52. Vik-Mo, H., and Mjøs, O. D. (1977): Effect of sodium salicylate and acetyl salicylic acid on epicardial ST-segment elevation during coronary artery occlusion in dogs. *Scand. J. Clin. Lab. Invest.*, 37:287–294.
53. Weiss, H. J., Aledort, L. M., and Kochwa, S. (1968): The effects of salicylate on the hemostatic properties of platelets in man. *J. Clin. Invest.*, 47:2169–2180.
54. Zacharski, L. R., Walworth, C., and McIntyre, O. R. (1971): Antiplatelet therapy for thrombotic thrombocytopenic purpura. *N. Engl. J. Med.*, 285:408–409.
55. Zucker, M. B., and Peterson, J. (1970): Effect of acetylsalicylic acid, other nonsteroidal anti-inflammatory agents, and dipyridamole on human blood platelets. *J. Lab. Clin. Med.*, 76:66–75.
56. Zwaal, R. F. (1978): Membrane and lipid involvement in blood coagulation. *Biochim. Biophys. Acta*, 515:163–205.

Acetylsalicylic Acid: New Uses for an Old Drug,
edited by H. J. M. Barnett, J. Hirsh, and
J. F. Mustard. Raven Press, New York © 1982.

DISCUSSION

J. Hirsh: I think we overreact when epidemiologists tell us not to "dredge data." Data dredging can be very useful for obtaining information that can then be used to formulate hypotheses. Results of the trials in which males were randomized within 6 months of myocardial infarction are interesting in that, wherever evaluable, there was a strong trend for benefit with acetylsalicylic acid. In fact, the second study performed by Elwood and associates did report a significant difference for males, but they did not emphasize this because it was a subgroup analysis. I would suggest that this consistent trend in all three of the evaluable studies strongly supports the effectiveness of acetylsalicylic acid in this patient group.

There is solid information that sulfinpyrazone is anti-thrombotic. It prevents thrombosis in experimental animals, in AV shunts and on dialysis membranes, yet there is a tendency to forget this now and to attribute the benefits in the Anturane Reinfarction Study to an antiarrhythmic effect.

While you are considering this, I will ask Professor Ian MacDonald, Director of the Cardiac Investigation Unit at St. Vincent's Hospital of the University of Melbourne, to give us his perspectives on mechanisms leading to death and myocardial infarction in the various coronary artery syndromes.

I. MacDonald: First, I can reassure Dr. Mustard and the rest of you that cardiologists have been increasingly forced to recognize the complexities of ischemic heart disease and its clinical manifestations.

Coronary atherosclerosis is still recognized as the most important factor underlying ischemic heart disease, but we increasingly must take into consideration functional factors such as transient coronary obstruction, caused by spasm or by platelets or by some interaction of the two. Sudden cardiac death may simply be the manifestation of arrhythmia without further obstruction. We have all encountered evidence of myocardial ischemia and infarction in the absence of significant coronary artery disease as evidenced by coronary angiogram or at autopsy.

Syndromes of ischemic heart disease that are of particular interest are angina at rest, myocardial infarction, and sudden death. With respect to these, we have to consider the effects of platelet aggregates, microscopic platelet thrombi, coronary vessel spasm, the interaction of platelets and spasm, and interference with perfusion causing cardiac arrhythmias. Coronary stenosis is usually caused by an atherosclerotic plaque but can represent an area of spasm. We know a good deal about the mechanisms that provoke turbulence, shearing stresses, platelet aggregation, and activation. We can consider occlusion or narrowing of the coronary lumen as a permanent or transient phenomenon. A nonocclusive thrombus, followed by a propagated thrombus, can go proximally to pick off larger vessels or distally to obliterate collaterals. We also must consider the possibility of embolism from nonoccluding thrombi to smaller vessels, analogous to the cerebrovascular model. Also, there is the possibility of massive intravascular aggregations and distal microembolism.

Coronary spasm has a long history, going back, it is said, to Heberden in 1768, and William Osler described it clearly. In recent decades it has fallen out of fashion because of the emphasis on organic obstruction of the coronary vessels. At that time, experimental work on the coronary circulation was done in the anesthetized dog, and this underestimated the importance of coronary reflexes, while emphasizing metabolic autoregulation.

In accounting for angina, there was a shift of emphasis from localized spasm to a peripheral vasodilation, and finally, β-blockade reinforced the belief that the primary objective was to change the oxygen demand of the myocardium. There were occasional dissenters, the most important of whom was Dr. Myron Prinzmetal, who described a peculiar type, or atypical angina.

Dr. Mason Sones, the father of coronary angiography, knew all about coronary artery spasms in 1963, but did not publish his views. Clinicians have had their suspicions and have for a long time been interested in a variable effort angina—asking each other whether rest angina was always associated with increased oxygen demand by the heart.

They had noticed that on weekends, munition workers sometimes developed chest pain, myocardial infarction, and sudden death, as part of a nitrate withdrawal syndrome that they attributed to coronary spasm. All were troubled by myocardial infarction, which sometimes developed in the absence of thrombosis and even in the presence of normal coronary arteries. However, the greatest stimulus came from the angiographic demonstration that severe spasm, often total occlusion, appeared transiently in Prinzmetal's variant angina. This spasm can usually be reversed by calcium ion antagonists and sometimes by α-blockade. The injection of ergonovine in the same vessel will reproduce the same angiographic appearance. There is also evidence that other forms of rest angina are associated with less severe coronary spasm.

There is hemodynamic support for these conclusions. On catheterization of patients with rest ischemia, Dr. A. Maseri demonstrated the following: fall in coronary-sinus pO_2, rise in left ventricular diastolic pressure as evidence of myocardial embarrassment, typical EKG changes, and pain. He clearly showed that there was no increase in heart rate or blood pressure that would indicate an increased demand for oxygen. All evidence pointed to a diminished supply, and in some patients at least, the cause was coronary artery spasm.

There is also evidence of spasm in some patients with angina of effort, and Dr. Braunwald has introduced the concept of diminished coronary vasodilator reserve and an increased tendency to spasm based on use of the cold pressor test.

To date, most of this work has concentrated on the large epicardial coronary vessels—the primary conductance vessels—and we have tended to ignore the distal vessels or arterioles, where most of the adjustment for peripheral resistance takes place. There is some evidence that these vessels have α-adrenergic innervation, and there is a possibility of the distal-to-proximal reflex spread of spasm. Distal spasm can be clearly demonstrated in dogs following myocardial infarction. When the left anterior descending branch of the coronary artery is partially occluded and the atrial pacing is used to embarrass the myocardium, the left anterior descending branch may disappear angiographically. This response is relieved by calcium-ion antagonists and hence may represent distal spasm. In summary, we have direct evidence that proximal spasm plays a role in the manifestations of ischemic heart disease, but there is less evidence that distal spasm of the resistance vessel may also be important.

There is the interesting possibility of a complex interaction between platelets, spasm and coronary atherosclerosis. For example, atherosclerotic stenosis can produce turbulence that results in platelet aggregation and activation. This may cause obstruction or just embolism, but the thromboxane A_2 so released can induce spasm. In the cat basilar artery, this spasm can cause plaque rupture, hemorrhage, and distal embolism. Sudden relief of the obstruction, resolution of spasm, and disaggregation of platelets result in sudden coronory reperfusion, and, at least in the dog this chain of events can result in ventricular arrhythmias, including ventricular fibrillation and death.

The various syndromes of ischemic heart disease should be viewed against this background. Angina occurring at rest or even in bed is typified by the syndrome of Prinzmetal's angina. This is of two varieties—variant Prinzmetal's atypical angina characterized by ST-segment elevation and the nonvariant rest angina in which there is a tendency towards depression of the ST segments. Perhaps these entities represent the two ends of the same spectrum.

Prinzmetal's variant angina is a recurrent pain, occurring at rest, with ST-segment elevation indicating extensive transmural ischemia. It is often associated with severe arrhythmias. Continuous monitoring indicates that upwards of 90% of these episodes are accompanied by EKG change but not with pain, and some may result in ventricular tachycardia or ventricular fibrillation and sudden death.

There may be a diurnal variation, with attacks tending to occur in the early morning. In addition, they are cyclic in nature, sometimes related to emotional stress, and closely related to cigarette smoking. This syndrome can result in myocardial infarction, and spasm can be angiographically demonstrated in some patients. After fatal myocardial infarction, autopsy has demonstrated a thrombus that presumably is a secondary event. Where the syndrome is associated with acute coronary spasm, the patients as a group show a good response to vasodilator drugs such as nifedipine and verapamil.

Spasm can be demonstrated directly on the coronary angiogram. If it is severe, it can obliterate a large coronary branch. For example, the left anterior descending branch can "disappear" completely. Such spasm is often associated with serious coronary artery disease, but not always. If we consider "mild" disease to be less than 30% obstruction of the lumen, one-third of the patients in Australia are in that category. In these patients, anginal attacks can be provoked with ergonovine.

This phenomenon usually represents a local sensitivity of one vessel, as the rule, but may be more generalized in nature, with an associated Raynaud's phenomenon in the distal vessels of the extremities, hypertension, migraine, and spasm of the celiac artery and of the brachial artery sometimes occurring during cardiac catheterization. These responses may be precipitated by central nervous system mechanisms and we can relate platelets to this syndrome, at least in theory. Two studies have shown an increase in thromboxane B_2, with one demonstrating an increase in the coronary sinus blood during an episode of Prinzmetal's angina. Whether or not this is primary or secondary to the stasis is unknown.

With respect to the nonvariant type of rest angina with ST-segment depression, this is most likely the result of less severe spasm in association with more severe coronary disease—usually multiple-vessel involvement. To my knowledge, there is no evidence to associate thromboxane A_2 with its genesis. However, there is evidence of an increase in platelet Factor 4 after myocardial infarction but not in association with the rest angina alone. Following marked external constriction of the coronary artery in dogs, an intermittent plugging of the area with platelet aggregates has been demonstrated. This can be inhibited with acetylsalicylic acid. Exposure to cigarette smoke augmented local platelet aggregate formation that could not be prevented with acetylsalicylic acid.

Another piece of evidence relating platelets to rest ischemia involved the use of the drug triclopidine. This reduced the number of episodes of ST depression and presumably the associated ischemia occurring during ambulatory monitoring of patients with coronary artery disease.

We must also consider the lessons learned from the cerebrovascular model and the fact that nonoccluding platelet thrombi have been found at autopsy on coronary plaques and during coronary grafting. Also, distal scars are frequently found in patients dying from myocardial infarction, and we don't know if these result from distal emboli.

With regard to acute myocardial infarction and sudden death, there is some evidence for a role of spasm in its genesis. In Prinzmetal's angina, the spasm may be prolonged and end as a classical myocardial infarct.

Oliver recently reported that in 40% of cases he could reverse an occlusion in early myocardial infarction with the infusion of glyceryl trinitrate, suggesting an element of spasm. But is this primary or secondary? We don't know.

The older literature asserted that almost 90% of patients with large transmural myocardial infarcts had an occluding thrombus. More recently, it has been shown that of 100 patients with the diagnosis of transmural infarction made in a coronary care unit, only 55% had an occluding thrombus. What role does the platelet play in acute myocardial infarction? Thromboxane A_2 could contribute by inducing spasm, but this must be better defined. Thrombus formation, even as a secondary event, could increase the ischemia by blocking off local branches and preventing collateral function. We have some suggestive evidence that sulfinpyrazone and acetylsalicylic acid may interfere with this chain of events.

Finally, let us look at the mechanism of sudden death in myocardial infarction. Some patients die from massive ischemia, the so-called pump failure. Here the heart is just knocked out by the size of the infarct. In others, there is an increased risk of serious arrhythmias. The early arrhythmias are mainly related to increased sympathetic tone and circulating catecholamines, probably resulting in an increased automaticity in the heart—that is, one focus firing rapidly and repetitively.

However, patients with multiple-vessel disease who sustain severe myocardial damage with scarring demonstrate another phenomenon—namely, that of reentry where an electrical impulse goes round and round in the damaged myocardium, causing ventricular tachycardia or fibrillation. These patients show a significant tendency to ventricular arrhythmias and sudden cardiac death. Further occlusion does not have to be postulated to explain sudden death in these patients.

The typical patient experiencing sudden cardiac death is a 60-year-old male with extensive coronary artery disease. Often there has been old myocardial infarction, but much less often there is a recent occluding thrombus or microscopic infarctions. There are likely to be small scars in the myocardium, with small areas of more recent damage—although special stains may be required to demonstrate these. What events can be hypothesized to explain these findings? The patient may have died from a reentrant arrhythmia, without further coronary obstruction. This is important, because in some cases the reentrant pathway can be blocked. Also, practolol has been shown to reduce sudden death and may act through one of these mechanisms. Secondly, he could have suffered transient coronary obstruction, not seen at autopsy because it was caused by spasm or by a platelet plug that disaggregated.

Finally, there is the possibility of massive intravascular platelet aggregation, as has been demonstrated in experimental animals. We have evidence in man that increased numbers of platelet aggregates are found at autopsy, but there is no clinical evidence that massive intravascular aggregation is the primary cause.

The syndrome of angina of effort is caused by coronary artery obstruction, although in some patients there may be co-existing coronary spasm. As noted earlier, in one study of patients with angina of effort and EKG changes, there was an elevation of platelet Factor 4, indicating that the platelets had been activated.

E. Salzman: Further to Dr. MacDonald's comments, we have recently studied a group of patients with unstable angina at rest and have demonstrated that there is a highly significant elevation of plasma levels of platelet Factor 4 and β-thromboglobulin in all patients while they have pain and for 4 hr after. At other times these substances are present only in normal amounts, strongly suggesting that there is platelet activation during episodes of angina, but of course it is not known if this activation is the cause of the pain.

Hirsh: Would you like to comment on the various controlled randomized trials in myocardial infarction, either with acetylsalicylic acid or sulfinpyrazone?

Salzman: Like Dr. Mustard, I am impressed with the increasing number of trials showing a trend in favor of acetylsalicylic acid or sulfinpyrazone, although none, with the exception of the sulfinpyrazone trial, have reached levels of statistical significance. It seems to me that, in the aggregate, they strongly suggest some therapeutic effect.

M. Gent: Many people are impressed with the consistency of the acetylsalicylic acid studies. Individually, none of them reach conventional levels of statistical significance, but apart from the AMIS study, five studies showed an observed benefit in favor of acetylsalicylic acid, which varied from 17% to 30%. Indeed, Richard Peto of Oxford has already pooled the information from all of them to show that acetylsalicylic acid was significantly better than placebo.

It is particularly interesting that in three of the trials—the two Elwood studies and Breddin's German-Austrian study—patients were entered, on average, 1 month after infarction. This approximates closely the circumstances of the patients in the Anturane Reinfarction Trial. The data from these three acetylsalicylic acid studies are collectively very impressive. Also, it would be interesting to know what happened to the patients in these studies during the first 6 months of treatment. Because of the trends that developed from the Anturane Reinfarction Trial, two things are obvious: (a) patients must be entered into the study early after infarction, and (b) benefit accrues only during the first 6 months and not after. Therefore, it would be interesting to pull out these particular data from the three studies to see if they support these conclusions.

E. Genton: I would like to comment on Dr. MacDonald's view of the type of death in patients with coronary artery disease. It is correct to say that in coronary heart disease, 60% of deaths are sudden, and this is true throughout the course of the disease. Data from the the sulfinpyrazone study indicate that the patient is at high risk of sudden death only during the first few months. I don't believe this to be the case. Whatever the operative factors during those first few months of the sulfinpyrazone trial, one would expect them to carry over, unless there is a difference in the type of death related to time, following recovery from infarction. This is one area that troubles me. I think it correct to consider all sudden deaths together, after myocardial infarction. In patients with established coronary artery disease, you cannot separate sudden death from myocardial infarction. They must be related, although we are uncertain as to precisely how or why. In the acetylsalicylic acid trials, if it is correct that the drug produced a marked reduction in nonfatal infarctions, we must relate this to mortality. If, as we are told, each of the cerebrovascular studies failed to achieve statistical significance with the single endpoints of mortality or stroke, and both studies combined these endpoints in the calculations, it would seem appropriate to do the same for the M. I. studies as regards M. I. and death. It would be interesting to see what we would have if the reduction in myocardial infarction and reduction in death, both sudden and otherwise, were analyzed in a statistical manner similar to the handling of the data from the cerebrovascular studies.

Finally, with regard to platelet activation, Dr. Salzman reported changes in patients with coronary heart disease during an acute ischemic event—namely, unstable angina. We have often found β-thromboglobulin and platelet survival to be abnormal in patients with coronary disease, and this seems to bear little relationship to the clinical situation. When serial measurements are done, abnormalities are frequently found and usually return to normal. These tests are difficult to interpret and even more difficult to apply in the interpretation of drug response.

Hirsh: How do you interpret these trials? Do you believe that acetylsalicylic acid and sulfinpyrazone are useful in patients who have suffered a myocardial infarct?

Genton: The data are certainly consistent with the conclusion that acetylsalicylic acid and sulfinpyrazone alone modify the outcome, although the mechanism remain obscure. When one combines data from the acetylsalicylic acid trials, trends are so impressive and consistent that it is hard to ignore them. That is why it is necessary to examine the various endpoints together rather than dealing with them separately, as has been done to date.

Hirsh: Dr. MacDonald, do you know of any reason why the cause of sudden death should be different after 6 months than it is between 1 and 6 months?

MacDonald: Arrhythmias are important in both, but there may well be differences in their mechanism. Evidence at the moment favors the concept that catecholamines and sympathetic activity are related to the earlier very strong tendency for arrhythmia. Later episodes are fairly predictable in patients with severe chronic myocardial damage and possibly have a different electrophysiological basis, namely, reentry.

Hirsh: When you say 'later episodes', do you mean those who die after 6 months? Are the early ones those who die within 6 months?

MacDonald: No, I think that 'early', in the jargon of the platelet-suppressant trial workers, refers to the period between hospital discharge and 6 months. The term 'early', as a cardiologist uses it, means the first 5 days after infarction.

Genton: I think Elwood's patients were admitted to trial as soon as the diagnosis was made. More than 70% were admitted within 72 hours and all were entered within a few days. Breddin's study extended up to 4 or 6 weeks, but many of his came in early. Certainly all were entered early in Elwood's second study.

Salzman: One must be cautious in concluding that effectiveness is limited to the first 6 months, because the drug was continued beyond 6 months in all of these trials. In the sulfinpyrazone trial, although the drug benefit was manifest in the first 6 months, drug was continued and so we cannot conclude that the positive effect would be maintained if the drug was discontinued after 6 months.

Hirsh: Is there any logical reason why the cause of sudden death should be different after the 6 months?

MacDonald: I know of no evidence that the cause of death is different. I would guess that it probably is not. After 6 months, the most common cause is arrhythmias, not provoked by further coronary obstruction.

H. J. M. Barnett: Thrombogenesis is believed to be of greater consequence in cerebrovascular disease than in myocardial infarction. The question arises as to whether or not vasospasm, now implicated in some cases of myocardial infarction, has anything to do with the production of TIA's or partial stroke. Vasospasm has been sought in cerebral angiograms longer than it has been sought in coronary arteriograms. It is identified only in two circumstances: with blood in the subarachnoid space and very rarely during a migraine attack. When vasospasm occurs in migraine, for most people the results are inconsequential. Even if there was extensive microcirculatory vasospasm, it might be expected to be of less local consequence than in the heart, since the conduction system in the heart is more sensitive than most of the cerebral tissues that are the site of dysfunction in TIA.

H. Jick: First, I would like to point out that the conservative epidemiologists call the radical epidemiologists incompetent, and the radical epidemiologists tend to call their conservative counterparts idiotic. The fact is that in certain circumstances, one must keep excluded patients in the analysis, and in others it is clearly idiotic to do so. Obviously, each situation must be handled individually.

Second, for a number of years, when it appeared that the acetylsalicylic acid story would have a successful ending, our original article published with that of Peter Elwood was never mentioned. It was prominently mentioned for the first time in the negative AMIS study, in which they professed to regard the whole thing as an illusion. However, I am glad to see that, by one mechanism or another, these original observations have been acknowledged.

Epidemiological studies have to be taken seriously and looked at seriously. The original published data were quite impressive and worthy of further consideration. Those data applied primarily to people who had not had a first infarct—and I believe it fair to say that conditions are much different where an infarct has already occurred. After the first M. I., risk factors are quite different. Also, many of the patients involved were long-term acetylsalicylic acid users.

The AMIS study was a large trial—larger than all of the others combined. However, I have been disturbed by the distribution of risk factors between the two groups, which are strikingly different. For certain risk factors, differences between the groups are most unlikely to have occurred by chance alone. Even if they did occur by chance, they also must be taken into account in analysis of the drug-versus-placebo groups. When that is done, differences in the total deaths become essentially zero or slightly in favor of acetylsalicylic acid. Unfortunately, they did not report the same kind of analysis for the nonfatal M. I. group, which showed an impressive difference between acetylsalicylic acid and placebo. Because this was statistically on the borderline, I would guess that if they had done a multivariate analysis, taking into account all of the risk factors, they could show a statistically significant difference at the 0.01 level, which is what they demanded.

The whole organization, evaluation, and analysis of data is a complicated game. It deserves more attention than it has received, and it should get this attention from knowledgeable people who are emotionally detached from the particular issue. Many decisions have to be made in organizing such data, decisions that can be biased by either prior knowledge or an understandable clinical desire to see a particular therapy work.

With regard to these particular studies, there is strong evidence that acetylsalicylic acid has some kind of effect, and I have been impressed with the results of the sulfinpyrazone study. This type of difference rarely occurs when one gives two placebos or two drugs that have no difference in terms of treatment. Taking the sulfinpyrazone data at face value, 18 people of the treated group should have died in the first 6 months of treatment, but did not—there being a 24 to 6 difference in sudden deaths. These 24 patients are still living and constitute a different group than the one that would have remained if they had died. The fact that these subjects remain is extremely important. If this were merely a 6-month phenomenon, at the end of that period there would have been many more deaths in the sulfinpyrazone group. These things are subtle, but they are very important for the interpretation of such studies.

J. F. Mustard: Dr. Jick's message for epidemiologists seems to be to "get your house in order. Your role is to help to do critical analyses of studies that have inherent weaknesses in terms of randomization and clinical methodologies." In this regard, it is extremely important to get all the data up and out. We should not hide things. The sulfinpyrazone study with which I was associated may have accidentally hidden some information by not publishing the data for every randomized patient.

For the AMIS trial, one has no idea of important data such as withdrawals—a point that ultimately has enormous impact on the end results. Considering the cost of the study and its conservative statistical approach, all the data should be reported so that the scientific community can draw its own conclusions. It may be wrong, but at least it can provide some guidance as to where we should go in the future.

With respect to 'data dredging', clear and coherent guidelines are needed to govern retrospective analysis of data in order to distinguish differences that were not anticipated at the planning phase because the knowledge base of the time did not make it possible to do so. These studies are too big and too expensive to deny the opportunity to go back and reexamine the data. The retrospective analysis of the data may help to identify groups that are most likely to benefit from the therapy. Such information could affect the future design of trials.

The enormous expense of these studies makes it desirable to combine data from various trials, so as to conserve effort and resources. The conservative approach of analyzing total deaths is an ideal approach, but if each trial is going to cost $10 to 20 million, we should opt for more restricted trials in more specific population groups to enhance the sensitivity of the trials.

The discussion of sudden death leaves me unhappy. Did Dr. Genton mean that more people die within an hour of myocardial infarction during the first few months than later on?

Genton: I said, I believe, that sudden death is a common cause of death at all times in patients with coronary disease.

Mustard: In the placebo group in the sulfinpyrazone trial, the incidence of sudden death was about 8% during the first 3 to 6 months and about 4% after. But it depends on how you define sudden death. I agree that we do not know enough about mechanisms, but it is an area to which we must pay more careful attention. I suspect that the principal sulfinpyrazone effect may have occurred in an even tighter time frame, say in the first 2 to 3 months, rather than in 6 months. The study was not designed to determine the period of maximum benefit.

In the reinfarction trial sulfinpyrazone may not have prevented sudden death by an effect on thrombosis. In the Canadian stroke study, sulfinpyrazone did not show an effect on what we think are recurrent bouts of thromboembolism associated with carotid artery disease. If that mechanism is operative in the coronary artery, one would have expected the drug to show some positive effect. It may well turn out that sulfinpyrazone has an effect on some forms of thrombosis, because there are multiple paths to thrombosis. Indeed, Dr. Hirsh and his group have shown that in arteriovenous shunts sulfinpyrazone reduces the extent of thrombosis. However, in that condition, the thrombotic mechanism may be different from that in the coronary artery.

Dr. Needleman raised the important point of what is going on in the myocardium when it is repairing itself after an acute infarct. He talked about reentry, but that is an electrical description. We still must consider cellular control mechanisms. Is abnormal prostaglandin metabolism in the myocardium involved during the first few months after a myocardial infarction? Do prostaglandins have other effects that we should give credence to? Others have shown that if PGI_2 is infused into the ischemic dog myocardium at a certain critical stage, ventricular fibrillation is precipitated. Does something like this go on in the human myocardium?

My final point is to emphasize Dr. Jick's concern. The real challenge is to prevent myocardial infarction in people at risk—before they have a myocardial infarction. Therapy in these people may give a totally different result than when used in post-myocardial-infarction patients. Obviously, those with a diseased myocardium who survive a myocardial infarction represent a different population group than individuals who are yet to develop a myocardial infarct.

Acetylsalicylic Acid: New Uses for an Old Drug,
edited by H. J. M. Barnett, J. Hirsh, and
J. F. Mustard. Raven Press, New York © 1982.

Effect of Acetylsalicylic Acid in Conditions Associated with Platelet Aggregation or Thrombosis in the Systemic Circulation

Edward Genton

Faculty of Health Sciences, McMaster University, Hamilton, Ontario, Canada L8N 3Z5

Acetylsalicylic acid has been evaluated as a prophylactic antithrombotic agent for prosthetic heart valves and in hemodialysis shunts, as well as in spontaneous platelet aggregation, the symptoms of ischemia in the extremities resulting from thrombocytosis, and aortocoronary bypass grafts.

Even modern prosthetic heart valves are associated with thromboembolism, which can be reduced but not prevented by oral anticoagulants (A/C). The combination of A/C plus platelet suppressants, either acetylsalicylic acid alone or with dipyridamole, has been evaluated. In two studies, 0.5 and 1.0 g of acetylsalicylic acid plus oral A/C decreased the incidence of embolism by more than 75%. Acetylsalicylic acid without A/C was not effective except in doses exceeding 3 g. Bleeding complications were increased with combination therapy, but consideration should be given to the use of acetylsalicylic acid in patients with prosthetic heart valves on A/C therapy, especially if they have suffered breakthrough embolism.

Thrombosis is frequent in patients with hemodialysis shunts, and continuous A/C therapy is hazardous. Acetylsalicylic acid, in a low dosage of 160 mg daily, reduced the incidence of thrombosis by 75% as compared to placebo therapy. This substantiates the antithrombotic effect of small doses of acetylsalicylic acid and indicates the value of such treatment in shunt patients.

Thrombocytosis is occasionally associated with a syndrome of spontaneous platelet aggregation and symptoms of ischemia involving the fingers and toes and occasionally the cerebrum. In such cases, acetylsalicylic acid even in low dosage may dramatically reverse the spontaneous aggregation and relieve the symptoms, with the benefit of even a single dose persisting for days.

Platelet mitogenic-factor stimulus may contribute to aortocoronary bypass occlusion by inducing intimal proliferation within the graft. In two randomized trials, acetylsalicylic acid was administered to patients after bypass surgery and graft patency confirmed by follow-up angiography. In one study an insignificant reduction in graft occlusion was noted with acetylsalicylic acid treatment (from 28 to 20%). In the second trial, no evidence of benefit was observed for acetylsalicylic acid/dipyridamole-treated patients, as compared with a control group or with patients receiving A/C therapy alone.

The use of acetylsalicylic acid in selected conditions associated with arterial thrombosis provides evidence for the antithrombotic effect of the drug as used alone in certain cases or in combination with other drugs.

Drugs that alter platelet reactivity have been evaluated in coronary artery and cerebrovascular disease, in addition to several other conditions associated with arterial thromboembolism. These studies not only clarify the therapeutic potential of platelet-suppressant drugs but also provide a new perspective on their mechanism of action. The conditions reviewed in this chapter include aortocoronary bypass grafts, prosthetic heart valves, arteriovenous hemodialysis shunts, thrombocytosis–ischemic extremities syndrome and peripheral artery thrombosis.

AORTOCORONARY ARTERY BYPASS GRAFTS

The majority of aortocoronary saphenous vein grafts remain patent, but between 15 and 35% become occluded within 2 years (7,9,23,24,26,29,32,38). Grafts may be occluded early, that is within the first few days of placement, or several months after operation. This early closure is caused by a mixed platelet-coagulation thrombus and is usually associated with some "technical" factor, such as poor distal circulation, suboptimal anastomosis or damage to the vein graft (7–9,15,16,25). Between 10 and 15% of vein grafts are occluded early (7–9,12,15,16,24,25,38). Late occlusion of bypass grafts is associated with lumen narrowing from intimal hyperplasia. Some degree of hyperplasia affects all vein grafts, but in some it is sufficient to greatly narrow or actually obstruct the lumen. This may occur within a few months, but usually takes up to 12 months to become complete (4,36). Evidence suggests that the intimal hyperplasia is produced by smooth muscle cells migrating from the media of the saphenous vein, perhaps stimulated by mitogenic factor protein released from the blood platelets.

Thus, blood platelets may be involved in the closure of saphenous vein grafts through their contribution to the thrombotic occlusion that occurs early, and by stimulating the intimal proliferation that leads to late occlusion. It also appears that abnormalities of platelet function may contribute to graft occlusion in patients with aortocoronary bypass. Steel and his colleagues (33) have reported that platelet survival is more frequently shortened in patients with occluded aortocoronary grafts than in those who have coronary disease of similar severity but have maintained a patent graft. Experiments in dogs have demonstrated that combined dipyridamole/acetylsalicylic acid treatment reduces the degree of intimal narrowing resulting from intimal hyperplasia (14).

Two clinical studies have evaluated the effect of platelet-suppressant drugs after aortocoronary bypass. In both, patients with angiographically documented coronary artery disease who had undergone aortocoronary bypass surgery were randomized within a few days after operation to placebo, a platelet-suppressant agent, or warfarin. Patency of the grafts was determined 6 or more months later by repeat angiography (27,30). In the study comparing acetylsalicylic acid, warfarin, and placebo, warfarin produced a significant decrease in graft occlusion. Although the study also showed a trend that favored acetylsalicylic acid treatment, this was not statistically significant (Table 1). In the second study, the authors used a dipyridamole/acetylsalicylic acid combination for platelet suppression, and could dem-

TABLE 1. *Platelet suppressant therapy—aortocoronary bypass*

Drug	No. of patients	Grafts	Occlusion (%)
Placebo	52	74	28
ASA	47	81	20
Warfarin	56	65	16

Adapted from McEnany, M.T., et al. (27).

TABLE 2. *Platelet suppressant therapy—aortocoronary bypass*

Drug	No. of patients	Grafts	Occlusion[a] (%)
Control	24	61	18
Dipyridamole/ASA	13	33	18
Warfarin	13	37	21

[a]Determined by angiography 6 months after operation.
Adapted from Pantely, G.A., et al. (30).

onstrate no difference between the control group and the two treatment groups (Table 2). Neither of these studies included observations that would establish the "early" status of the grafts, that is, within the first few weeks of operation. It is therefore possible that many or most of the occlusions occurred early, and hence no conclusions can be drawn that depend on a distinction between early and late closure. This observation may be important because different mechanisms may underlie early and late graft occlusion and since early occlusion is related chiefly to technical factors and may occur within the first few hours or days after operation, treatment started after surgery may be ineffective. Also, the data do not allow any conclusions concerning the effect of acetylsalicylic acid on the process of intimal hyperplasia. At this time, and based on the available data, we cannot recommend either acetylsalicylic acid or acetylsalicylic acid/dipyridamole in combination for use in coronary bypass patients. However, a number of trials are presently under way that address this question specifically.

PROSTHETIC HEART VALVES

Tremendous progress has been made in the surgical management of valvular heart disease, primarily in the continuous improvement in prosthetic valve design. In great part, this progress has related to success in reducing thrombogenicity, and at present, the valves being inserted are far less reactive than those introduced in the early 1960s. Unfortunately, even current prosthetic valves still have significant thrombogenicity, and there is general agreement that all patients should be given lifelong antithrombotic therapy. Oral anticoagulants have been effective in preventing embolization in the majority of patients; however, breakthrough emboli are seen even with optimal anticoagulant therapy, and alternatives to anticoagulants are of continued interest. The consequences of valve thrombosis may be "local", resulting from interference with valve function, or perhaps more frequently, distal, resulting from organ dysfunction from embolization. Even with anticoagulant therapy, approximately 5% of patients with mitral and 3% with aortic valves develop emboli each year. For a number of reasons, therefore, the use of platelet suppressant drugs after the implantation of prosthetic heart valves is rational.

Histologically, the genesis of thrombus on the prosthetic valve surface begins with platelets, and the resultant thrombus contains an abundance of platelets mixed with fibrin. In addition, patients with valvular heart disease show a number of alterations in platelet tests: elevation of platelet-specific proteins such as platelet Factor 4 and β-thromboglobulin (17,18) and reduced platelet-survival time in the presence of a prosthetic heart valve. Here, there is some correlation between the incidence of embolization with a particular prosthetic valve and the degree of reduction of platelet survival. In addition, among patients with a particular prosthetic valve, those with prior thromboembolism tend to have shorter platelet survival than patients without embolic complications.

Several randomized trials have compared the incidence of embolization in patients treated with oral anticoagulants and in those on a combination of oral anticoagulants and a platelet-suppressant drug (Table 3) (1,3,10,34,35). Two of the trials have been properly randomized (10,34). The results in both have been reasonably consistent and suggest a greater reduction in embolization with the combination treatment than with the oral anticoagulants alone. Acetylsalicylic acid or a combination of acetylsalicylic acid with dipyridamole produced consistent lowering of emboli-

TABLE 3. Platelet-suppressant therapy in patients with prosthetic heart valves

	No. of patients	Observed (months)	Emboli (%)
Sullivan et al. (34)			
Oral A/C + dipyridamole (400)	79	12	1.3
Oral A/C	84	12	14.0
Arrants and Hairston (3)			
Oral A/C + dipyridamole (200)	39	10	2.5
Oral A/C	20	24	40.0
Taguchi et al. (35)			
Dipyridamole (450) + ASA (3)	35	14	2.9
Untreated	34	14	14.7
Altman et al. (1)			
Oral A/C + ASA (0.5)	57	24	5.2
Oral A/C	65	24	20.3
Dale et al. (10)			
Oral A/C + ASA (1)	75	42	2.6
Oral A/C + placebo	73	42	13.7

zation. Taguchi et al. (35) reported similar benefits with platelet-suppressant drugs alone. However, they employed a very high dosage, and most of the patients withdrew from the study because of side effects. Others have evaluated the effect of platelet-suppressant drugs without oral anticoagulants, usually with negative results. In one study, untreated patients were compared with those receiving 1 g of acetylsalicylic acid/100 mg dipyridamole and a group receiving dicumarol. In this trial, the platelet-suppressant group had the same high incidence of embolization as the untreated group, and this frequency was far greater than that seen with dicumarol (6). Another group studied a small number of patients from whom anticoagulants were withdrawn 2 to 12 months after operation and replaced by 1,200 mg of acetylsalicylic acid per day. These were compared with another group continued on oral anticoagulants. Nearly 20% of the acetylsalicylic acid-treated patients developed emboli, in contrast to less than 3% of the patients receiving anticoagulants (21).

Thus, the evidence is reasonably persuasive that platelet suppressants—either acetylsalicylic acid or dipyridamole or the two together—in combination with oral anticoagulants provide more effective antithrombotic therapy than oral anticoagulants alone. Unfortunately, the side effects encountered with combination treatment are greater than with oral anticoagulants alone. In one study there was a substantial incidence of side effects. For example, 15% of patients developed G.I. bleeding during a 2-year period of observation, compared with 3% in those treated with oral anticoagulants alone (10). It can be concluded that platelet-suppressant drugs potentiate the antithrombotic effects of oral anticoagulants in patients with prosthetic heart valves, but their use is associated with a higher incidence of bleeding complications, and therefore they are probably not indicated on a routine basis. However, for patients who have breakthrough embolization while on optimal anticoagulant therapy, the addition of acetylsalicylic acid alone or in combination with dipyridamole seems reasonable. Only in patients in whom oral anticoagulants are absolutely contraindicated does it seem appropriate to rely upon these drugs alone, and larger dosages may be required. The endpoints used in the study of patients with prosthetic valves were the results of thrombosis, and the significant reduction in frequency of these complications provides strong evidence that acetylsalicylic acid is antithrombotic.

ARTERIOVENOUS HEMODIALYSIS SHUNTS

Although Silastic shunts are used less frequently for chronic hemodialysis than are A-V fistulas, many patients have such shunts and these are often complicated by thrombosis. The thrombi usually form at the junction of the Silastic material and entrance to the vein—a point at which there is often evidence of intimal hyperplasia. The thrombosis may be localized or may extend in a retrograde and antegrade fashion. Obstruction to shunt flow is caused chiefly by thrombosis, which can be observed directly, and often the thrombus can be extracted and flow restored. This model is well suited for tests of the antithrombotic effect of various agents, and two such trials of platelet-suppressant drugs have been reported (19,22). In one, the effectiveness of sulfinpyrazone (600 mg daily) was documented in a crossover trial in which patients were given active drug or placebo, each for 6 months (Table 4). An 86% incidence of thrombosis was observed during the placebo phase compared to an incidence of 50% during sulfinpyrazone treatment. The frequency of thrombi was reduced from 0.64/month during the placebo phase to 0.21/month in the sulfinpyrazone phase. In this study, males obtained considerably greater benefit than did females. The trial evaluating acetylsalicylic acid used a similar design, with patients randomized into a placebo group or one given acetylsalicylic acid in a dosage of 160 mg/day. This study, which was designed to determine whether a low dosage of acetylsalicylic acid would be effective, demonstrated a significant reduction in the incidence of thrombosis—from 72% to 32%. The number of thrombi/patient-month was reduced from 0.46 in the placebo group to 0.16 in the acetylsalicylic acid group. Although this study used only a small number of patients, it showed no apparent difference in the response of males and females.

These interesting trials again provide evidence that both sulfinpyrazone and acetylsalicylic acid exert an antithrombotic effect in the presence of prosthetic materials and indicate that even a small dosage of acetylsalicylic acid has this potential. This experience suggests that the effect on platelet aggregation, as mediated through inhibition of the prostaglandin pathway, does reduce the response to thrombogenic stimuli.

THROMBOCYTOSIS–ISCHEMIC EXTREMITIES SYNDROME

On rare occasions, patients with thrombocytosis develop a syndrome whose major manifestations are symptoms of ischemia involving the toes and sometimes fingers, resulting in burning or aching pain, cyanosis, and occasionally ulceration or even gangrene of the involved digits. The platelet count has ranged from 0.7 to 1.3 million/mm^3, and spontaneous platelet aggregation may be demonstrated when citrated platelet-rich plasma is gently agitated. These patients may manifest such thromboembolic phenomena as transient ischemic attacks, stroke, myocardial infarction, or episodes of deep-vein thrombosis. In most cases the thrombocytosis has been primary, but the syndrome may be a secondary manifestation of malignant disease or myeloproliferative disorders. Several studies of this interesting condition have shown a dramatic and consistent response to acetylsalicylic acid therapy. Although other drugs, including dipyridamole, have not produced clinical benefit, the administration of acetylsalicylic acid, in a dosage ranging from 0.3 to 2.4 g/day,

TABLE 4. *Platelet-suppressant prophylaxis in patients with A-V hemodialysis shunts[a]*

Author	Drug	Dose (mg/day)	Thrombosis (%)	
			Rx	Control
Kaegi et al. (22)	Sulfinpyrazone	600	50	86
Harter et al. (19)	ASA	160	32	72

[a]Followed for an average of 5 to 6 months.

has been associated with an abrupt cessation of symptoms, often within a few hours of the first dose (5,28,31,37) (Table 5). The symptomatic relief persists for several days after a single dose and may be sustained by continued treatment. Symptomatic improvement is usually associated with a cessation of spontaneous platelet aggregation, even while the platelet count remains elevated. Permanent relief may be achieved by reduction of the platelet count with cytotoxic agents. Experience with this condition provides strong evidence that the symptoms are related to platelet aggregation and that inhibition of such aggregation by acetylsalicylic acid, presumably by alterations in the prostaglandin pathway, is responsible for the improvement. The dosage range that achieves benefit is consistent with cyclo-oxygenase inhibition, and the fact that a large dose is equally effective provides some evidence against the concept that high doses produce prostacyclin inhibition and may induce a paradoxical platelet aggregation.

Regardless of the drug's mechanism of action, these patients usually have a dramatic improvement on acetylsalicylic acid, and the drug seems to prevent ischemic damage to the various organs. Thus, acetylsalicylic acid is indicated and should be administered in a dosage titrated to control the symptoms.

PERIPHERAL ARTERIAL LESIONS

A number of studies have examined the effect of acetylsalicylic acid in patients after arterial "invasion" or surgery. Invasion of an artery leads to damage of the endothelium and vessel wall and predisposes to thromboembolic phenomena. After cardiac catheterization, such damage occurs not only at the site of insertion but anywhere the catheter comes into contact with the endothelium. Evidence of partial or totally occlusive thrombi or emboli in the microcirculation of a catheterized extremity is common. Two studies have evaluated the efficacy of acetylsalicylic acid in preventing post-catheterization thromboembolic complications (Table 6). In one study (20), treatment was started 12 to 15 hrs before catheterization, using 325 to 600 mg of ASA. Here, the endpoint was a palpable decrease in pulse following catheterization or the recovery of thrombus on a balloon catheter passed at the end of the procedure. In the other study, infants or children were given 5 doses of acetylsalicylic acid beginning the evening before and continuing through to the morning following the procedure, and oscillometry was done to detect reduced blood flow (13). In neither of the studies was there evidence of reduction in end-

TABLE 5. *Platelet-suppressant therapy in patients with thrombocytosis and arterial ischemic syndrome*

Author	No. of patients	Drug/dose	Effect
Vreeken and van Aken (37)	1	ASA 0.3	
Biermé et al. (5)	3	ASA 0.5 +	Rapid in onset
Preston et al. (31)	6	ASA 0.6 +	Sustained
Mundall et al. (28)	1	ASA 2.4	Correlates with platelet effect

TABLE 6. *Platelet-suppressant therapy in the presence of peripheral arterial lesions*

Author	Dose ASA (mg)	Condition	No. of patients	Thrombi (%) Rx	Thrombi (%) Control
Hynes et al. (20)	650	Cardiac cath.	150	23	18
Freed et al. (13)	15/kg	Cardiac cath.	95	21	24

TABLE 7. *ASA therapy in artery surgery: Randomized trials*

	Dose (mg)	No. of patients	Condition	Thrombosis Rx	Thrombosis Control
Zekert et al. (39)	1500	61	Bypass graft (iliofemoral)	7	30 (14 days)
		237	Endarterectomy	13	16
Ehresmann et al. (11)	1500	428	Reconstruction	11	22[a] (1 year)
Andrassy et al. (2)	1500	92	A-V fistula	4	23 (28 days)

[a]$p < 0.05$.

points. Thus, it appears that acetylsalicylic acid in moderate dosage does not prevent the interaction between platelets and the catheter or damaged endothelium, at least to the degree required to prevent thromboembolic complications.

The use of acetylsalicylic acid in patients who have had operations involving arteries has been evaluated in several studies. One double-blind trial employed acetylsalicylic acid to reduce the early thrombosis in arteriovenous fistulae created for chronic hemodialysis (Table 7) (2). After procedures for the surgical reconstruction of arteries, acetylsalicylic acid in a dosage of 1500 mg/day reduced the arterial occlusion in patients with chronic obliterative peripheral vascular disease (11). Another study found that acetylsalicylic acid treatment reduced the occlusion rate following iliac- or femoral-artery bypass grafts, but the same author found no reduction in the incidence of occlusion in endarterectomized arteries with acetylsalicylic acid treatment (39).

In relation to arterial surgery, we can conclude that acetylsalicylic acid may reduce occlusion, on both an acute and a chronic basis, but that the precise dosage remains to be determined—although moderate dosages have been shown to be effective.

SUMMARY

Evaluation of acetylsalicylic acid treatment in a number of clinical conditions has shown a beneficial effect and provides considerable insight into the mechanisms of action and dose response. Completed trials in patients following aortocoronary bypass surgery have not confirmed the hypothesis that acetylsalicylic acid, by suppressing the release of mitogenic factor from platelets, might reduce or prevent intimal hyperplasia. The design of these studies did not permit a critical assessment of this hypothesis, because early occlusion of grafts was not assessed and hence their closure may not have been related to intimal hyperplasia. Results in patients with prosthetic heart valves and with Silastic A-V shunts clearly indicate that acetylsalicylic acid is antithrombotic, even in a small dosage, as has been demonstrated in studies of hemodialysis patients. The effectiveness of high dosage in patients with prosthetic valves suggests that acetylsalicylic acid does not exert a paradoxical effect in this dosage range. In fact, 3.6 g of acetylsalicylic acid/day was effective when used alone, whereas 1.0 g/day was not.

REFERENCES

1. Altman, R., Boullon, F., Rouvier, J., Raca, R., de la Fuente, L., and Favaloro, R. (1976): Aspirin and prophylaxis of thromboembolic complications in patients with substitute heart valves. *J. Thorac. Cardiovasc. Surg.*, 72:127–129.
2. Andrassy, K., Malluche, H., Bornefeld, H., Comberg, M., Ritz, E., Jesdinsky, H., and Möbring, K. (1974): Prevention of p.o. clotting of a.v. cimino fistulae with acetylsalicylic acid. Results of a prospective double blind study. *Klin. Wochenschr.*, 52:348–349.
3. Arrants, J. E., and Hairston, P. (1972): Use of Persantine in preventing thromboembolism following valve replacement. *Am. Surg.*, 38:432–435.
4. Batayias, G. E., Barboriak, J. J., Korns, M. E., and Pintar, K. (1977): The spectrum of pathologic changes in aortocoronary saphenous vein grafts. *Circulation*, 56 (Suppl. 2): II–18–II–22.
5. Biermé, R., Boneu, B., Guiraud, B., and Pris, J. (1972): Aspirin and recurrent painful toes and fingers in thrombocythaemia (letter). *Lancet*, 1:432.
6. Bjork, V. O., and Henze, A. (1975): Management of thrombo-embolism after aortic valve replacement with the Bjork-Shiley tilting disc valve. *Scand. J. Thorac. Cardiovasc. Surg.*, 9:183–191.
7. Bonchek, L. I., Rahimtoola, S. H., Chaitman, B. R., Rosch, J., Anderson, R. P., and Starr, A. (1974): Vein graft occlusion. Immediate and late consequences and therapeutic implications. *Circulation*, 49,50 (Suppl. 2): 11–84–II–97.
8. Bourassa, M. G., Lespérance, J., Campeau, L., and Simard, P. (1972): Factors influencing patency of aortocoronary vein grafts. *Circulation*, 45-46 (Suppl. 1): I–79–I–85.
9. Campeau, L., Crochet, D., Lesperance, J., Bourassa, M. G., and Grondin, C. M. (1975): Postoperative changes in aorto-coronary saphenous vein grafts revisited: angiographic studies at two weeks and at one year in two series of consecutive patients. *Circulation*, 52:369–377.
10. Dale, J., Myhre, E., Storstein, O., Stormorken, H., and Efskind, L. (1977): Prevention of arterial thromboembolism with acetylsalicylic acid. A controlled clinical study in patients with aortic ball valves (review). *Am. Heart J.*, 94:101–111.
11. Ehresmann, V., Alemany, J., Loew, D. (1977): Prophylaxe von Rezidivverschlussen nach Revaskularisation –eingriffen mit Acetylsalicylsaure. *Med. Welt*, 28:1157–1162.
12. FitzGibbon, G. M., Burton, J. R., and Leach, A. J. (1978): Coronary bypass graft fate: angiographic grading of 1400 consecutive grafts early after operation and of 1132 after one year. *Circulation*, 57:1070–1074.
13. Freed, M. D., Rosenthal, A., and Fyler, D. (1974): Attempts to reduce arterial thrombosis after cardiac catheterization in children: Use of percutaneous technique and aspirin. *Am. Heart J.*, 87:283–286.
14. Fuster, V., Dewanjee, M. K., Kaye, M. P., Josa, M., Metke, M. P., and Chesebro, J. H. (1979): Noninvasive radio-isotopic technique for detection of platelet deposition in coronary artery bypass grafts in dogs and its reduction with platelet inhibitors. *Circulation*, 60:1508–1512.
15. Grondin, C. M., Castonguay, Y. R., Lespérance, J., Bourassa, M. G., Campeau, L., and Grondin, P. (1972): Attrition rate of aorta-to-coronary artery saphenous vein grafts after one year. A study in a consecutive series of 96 patients. *Ann. Thorac. Surg.*, 14:223–231.
16. Grondin, C. M., Lepage, G., and Castonguay, Y. (1971): Aortocoronary bypass graft: initial blood flow through the graft and early postoperative patency. *Circulation*, 44:815–819.
17. Han, P., Turpie, A. G. G., and Genton, E. (1977): The effect of antiplatelet drugs on plasma β-thromboglobulin in coronary artery disease (abstract). *Thromb. Haemost.*, 42:59.
18. Handin, R. I., McDonough, M., and Lesch, M. (1978): Elevation of platelet factor four in acute myocardial infarction: measurement by radioimmunoassay. *J. Lab. Clin. Med.*, 91:340–349.

19. Harter, H. R., Burch, J. W., Majerus, P. W., Stanford, N., Delmez, J. A., Anderson, C. B., and Weerts, C. A. (1979): Prevention of thrombosis in patients on hemodialysis by low-dose aspirin. *N. Engl. J. Med.*, 301:577–579.
20. Hynes, K. M., Gau, G. T., Rutherford, B. D., Kazmier, F. S., and Frye, R. L. (1973): Effect of aspirin on brachial artery occlusion following brachial arteriotomy for coronary arteriography. *Circulation*, 47:554–557.
21. Isom, O. W., Williams, C. D., Falk, E. A., Spencer, F. C., and Glassman, E. (1973): Evaluation of anticoagulant therapy in cloth-covered prosthetic valves. *Circulation*, 47–48 (Suppl. 3) III–48–50.
22. Kaegi, A., Pineo, G. F., Shimizu, A., Trivedi, H., Hirsh, J., and Gent, M. (1975): The role of sulfinpyrazone in the prevention of arterio-venous shunt thrombosis. *Circulation*, 52:497–499.
23. Kloster, F. E., Kremkau, E. L., Ritzmann, L. W., Rahimtoola, S. H., Rösch, J., and Kanarek, P. H. (1979): Coronary bypass for stable angina: a prospective randomized study. *N. Engl. J. Med.*, 300:149–157.
24. Lawrie, G. M., Lie, J. T., Morris, G. C. Jr., and Beazley, H. L. (1976): Vein graft patency and intimal proliferation after aortocoronary bypass: early and long-term angiopathologic correlations. *Am. J. Cardiol.*, 38:856–862.
25. Lespérance, J., Bourassa, M. G., Biron, P., Campeau, L., and Saltiel, J. (1972): Aorta to coronary artery saphenous vein grafts. Preoperative angiographic criteria for successful surgery. *Am. J. Cardiol.*, 30:459–465.
26. Mathur, V. S., Guinn, G. A., Anastassiades, L. C., Chahine, R., Korompai, F. L., Montero, A. C., and Luchi, R. J. (1975): Surgical treatment for stable angina pectoris: prospective randomized study. *N. Engl. J. Med.*, 292:709–713.
27. McEnany, M. T., DeSanctis, R. W., Harthorne, J. W., Mundth, E. D., Weintraub, R. M., Austin, W. G., and Salzman, E. W. (1976): Effect of antithrombotic therapy on aortocoronary vein graft patency rates. *Circulation*, 54 (Suppl. 2):II–124.
28. Mundall, J., Quintero, P., von Kaulla, K. N., Harmon, R., and Austin, J. (1972): Transient monocular blindness and increased platelet aggregability treated with aspirin. A case report. *Neurology*, 22:280–285.
29. Murphy, M. L., Hultgren, H. N., Detre, K., Thomsen, J., and Takaro, T. (1977): Participants of the Veterans Administration Corporate Study: Treatment of chronic stable angina: A preliminary report of survival data of the randomized Veterans Administration Cooperative Study. *N. Engl. J. Med.*, 297:621–627.
30. Pantely, G. A., Goodnight, S. H. Jr., Rahimtoola, S. H., Harlan, B. J., DeMoto, H., Calvin, L., and Rösch, J. (1979): Failure of antiplatelet and anticoagulation therapy to improve patency of grafts after coronary-artery bypass: A controlled randomized study. *N. Engl. J. Med.*, 301:962–966.
31. Preston, F. E., Emmanuel, I. G., Winfield, D. A., and Malia, R. G. (1974): Essential thrombocythaemia and peripheral gangrene. *Br. Med. J.*, 3:548–552.
32. Sheldon, W. C., Rincon, G., Effler, D. B., Proudfit, W. L., and Sones, F. M. Jr. (1973): Vein graft surgery for coronary artery disease. Survival and angiographic results in 1,000 patients. *Circulation*, 47-48 (Suppl. 3): III–184–III–189.
33. Steele, P., Rainwater, J., Vogel, R., and Genton, E. (1978): Platelet-suppressant therapy in patients with coronary artery disease. *JAMA*, 240:228–231.
34. Sullivan, J. M., Harken, D. E., and Gorlin, R. (1971): Pharmacologic control of thromboembolic complications of cardiac-valve replacement. *N. Engl. J. Med.*, 284:1391–1394.
35. Taguchi, K., Matsumura, H., Washizu, T., Hirao, M., Kato, K., Kato, E., Mochizuki, T., Takamura, K., Mashimo, I., Morifuji, K., Nakagaki, M., and Suma, T. (1975): Effect of arthrombogenic therapy, especially high dose therapy of dipyridamole, after prosthetic valve replacement. *J. Cardiovasc. Surg.*, 16:8–15.
36. Unni, K. K., Kottke, B. A., Titus, J. L., Frye, R. L., Wallace, R. B., and Brown, A. L. (1974): Pathologic changes in aortocoronary saphenous vein grafts. *Am. J. Cardiol.*, 34:526–532.
37. Vreeken, J., and van Aken, W. G. (1971): Spontaneous aggregation of blood platelets as a cause of idiopathic thrombosis and recurrent painful toes and fingers. *Lancet*, 2:1394–1397.
38. Wertheimer, M., and Liddle, H. V. (1975): Results of direct coronary artery graft reconstruction: a five-year clinical and arteriographic appraisal. *Ann. Thorac. Surg.*, 20:538–549.
39. Zekert, F., Kohn, P., Vormittag, E., Piza, F., and Thien, M. (1975): Zur acetylsalicylsaure–prophylaxe von Sofortverschlussen nach gefasschirurgischen Eingriffen. In: *Colfarit Symposium III*, pp. 109–119. Bayer, Cologne.

Acetylsalicylic Acid: New Uses for an Old Drug,
edited by H.J.M. Barnett, J. Hirsh, and
J.F. Mustard. Raven Press, New York © 1982.

Acetylsalicylic Acid for Prevention of Venous Thromboembolic Disease in Surgical Patients

*Edwin W. Salzman and William H. Harris

Departments of Surgery and Orthopedics, Harvard Medical School, Beth Israel Hospital, and Massachusetts General Hospital, Boston, Massachusetts 02215

Rationale for the use of drugs that alter platelet function to prevent venous thrombosis and pulmonary embolism rests on the involvement of platelets in the initial events in venous thrombosis, the role of substances secreted by platelets in the symptomatology of thromboembolism, and the less severe derangement of hemostasis induced by these drugs as compared with anticoagulants. Of the agents available, acetylsalicylic acid and dextran have been evaluated the most extensively. The literature with regard to acetylsalicylic acid is conflicting, with strongest evidence for its effectiveness in orthopedic patients. Acetylsalicylic acid appears more effective in men than in women; this feature of its behavior and the use of excessive acetylsalicylic acid dosage in reported trials have done much to confuse the early literature. The sex difference in the antithrombotic effect of acetylsalicylic acid may be caused by differences in platelet reactivity in the two sexes. The combination of acetylsalicylic acid with other forms of prophylaxis deserves further assessment.

Although conventional dogma holds that platelets play a secondary role in the pathogenesis of venous thromboembolism, as opposed to their primary role on the arterial side, the possibility that acetylsalicylic acid might protect against the development of postoperative venous thrombosis (DVT) was among the first potential applications explored, shortly after its activity in inhibiting platelet function was described. In addition, the frequency of postoperative venous thrombosis makes this condition an attractive endpoint for a clinical trial of antithrombotic agents, in contrast to the many practical difficulties of studying thrombotic events in the arterial tree. In 1971, we reported that acetylsalicylic acid reduced the frequency of venous thrombosis following vitallium-mold arthroplasty of the hip (33). Today we recognize that this study suffers from serious methodologic shortcomings, the most important

---

*Mailing address: Dr. E.W. Salzman, Department of Surgery, Beth Israel Hospital, 330 Brookline Avenue, Boston, Massachusetts 02215

of which is the necessity for a *clinical* diagnosis of DVT, since today's more sensitive and objective diagnostic methods only became available after completion of the trial. Nonetheless, the report served to kindle interest in the use of acetylsalicylic acid for prophylaxis against venous thromboembolism in high-risk patients, and it was followed by a legion of other studies.

There is of course no objection to the observation that the bulk of the venous thrombus consists of fibrin with entrapped erythrocytes. Many authorities believe that, for the most part, venous thrombi develop because of the combination of a hematologic predisposition to thrombosis (hypercoagulability) and venous stasis (23). There is some evidence, however, that platelets may be of primary importance in the initiation of venous thrombosis, at least in some patients, and that the typical sequence may be the "white head" of platelet thrombus followed by a red fibrin tail. Among 100 unselected autopsies in patients dying of all causes, Freiman (personal communication) found isolated platelet thrombi in the lower extremities of 60%. Thus it is possible that drugs that inhibit the formation of the initial thrombotic deposit by inhibiting platelet function may have a salutary effect on the subsequent progression to the familiar red stasis thrombus characteristic of the lower extremity veins.

Further evidence that platelets participate in the pathogenesis of venous thrombi is found in reports of elevated circulating plasma levels of the platelet-derived protein β-thromboglobulin in patients with overt venous thrombosis (36). Harker and Slichter (8) reported that platelet survival was shortened in patients with clinically evident venous thrombosis, although we were not able to confirm this in patients with less extensive subclinical thrombi detected by labeled fibrinogen scanning (4).

It has been suggested that platelets are hyperreactive in patients who develop venous thrombosis, with such an effect contributing to the thrombotic tendency in patients receiving oral contraceptives and in the postoperative state. Walsh et al. (42) found that measurement of platelet coagulant activity helped to predict which patients would develop venous thrombi after operation. Hirsh and McBride (12) found increased platelet retention in glass-bead columns ("platelet adhesiveness"), in patients with recurrent venous thrombosis. Wu et al. (45) reported the presence of circulating platelet aggregates in patients with venous thrombosis, who also had more active platelet aggregation *in vitro* than did a control group.

None of the foregoing observations can be taken as indicating that abnormal platelet function causes venous thrombosis. Only Walsh described abnormalities that preceded the development of the venous thrombi and therefore could not be viewed as the *effects* of venous thrombosis, rather than its cause. Taken as a group, however, the reports support the hypothesis that platelets participate in venous thromboembolism and that the use of platelet-active drugs may help to prevent venous thrombosis and pulmonary embolism.

Further support for this thesis is offered by Thomas et al. (39), who suggested that vasoactive substances such as serotonin, which are released by platelets under the influence of thrombin, may contribute to the hemodynamic changes of pulmonary embolism. This suggestion does not offer much encouragement for the use of acetylsalicylic acid to influence the course of pulmonary embolism, since thrombin–platelet interactions are not inhibited by this agent. However, the studies do draw attention to hemodynamic changes associated with pulmonary embolism, which may be relevant to some of the effects of acetylsalicylic acid.

Several platelet-active drugs have been studied in postoperative patients to prevent venous thrombosis and pulmonary embolism; these include dextran, acetylsalicylic acid, pnenylbutazone, ibuprofen, hydroxychloroquine, and dipyridamole. Experience with these agents has been reviewed elsewhere (30,32), and this report will consider only the use of acetylsalicylic acid.

Prospective trials of acetylsalicylic acid for prophylaxis of venous thromboembolism in postoperative patients are summarized in Tables 1–4. Although there are exceptions, the majority of the studies in both general surgical and orthopedic patients show that acetylsalicylic acid has a beneficial effect. The studies vary widely in the number of patients and other details. In the aggregate, the reports of acetylsalicylic acid's effect in orthopedic cases seems to show the clearest evidence of its efficacy.

The study of Harris et al. in 1977 (10) was a double-blind prospective placebo-controlled randomized trial employing phlebography to make the diagnosis in every patient. The frequency of postoperative venous thrombosis following total hip replacement was halved through the use of acetylsalicylic acid. An unexpected finding in this study was a striking sex difference in the antithrombotic effect of acetylsalicylic acid (Table 5). Reexamination of the results of an earlier study by the same group (9) revealed that the sex difference had been present there as well, although it had not been appreciated in the initial analysis of the data. The use of acetylsalicylic acid provided protection against thrombosis only in male patients. Subsequently, the Canadian Cooperative Study Group (3) reported a similar sex difference in patients with extracranial cerebrovascular disease. Once again, the frequency of transient ischemic attacks and strokes was reduced only in male

TABLE 1. *Effect of ASA on deep venous thrombosis (DVT) in general surgery*

	Treatment		Control		
	No. of pts.	% DVT	No. of pts.	% DVT	F/M-ASA
Clinical diagnosis					
Weber, 1971 (43)	510	2.0	527	5.1	—
Loew, 1974 (19)	454	1.3	448	4.2	314/196
	964	1.7	975	4.7	
Objective diagnosis					
O'Brien, 1971 (26)	38	74	20	65	—
MRC, 1972 (24)	153	27	150	22	112/41
Clagett, 1975 (4)	49	6	49	20	35/21
Loew, 1977 (18)	63	30	57	19 (heparin)	45/18
Buttermann, 1977 (2)	79	26	175	36	—
Adolf, 1978 (1)	79	18	75	29	154/0
Plante, 1979 (28)	38	8	66	21	18/20
	499	26	592	28	

F/M = female/male.

TABLE 2. *Effect of ASA on DVT in orthopedic operations*

	Treatment		Control		
	No. of pts.	% DVT	No. of pts.	% DVT	F/M-ASA
Clinical diagnosis					
Salzman, 1971 (33)	43	14	67	34	22/21
Hey, 1973 (11)	160±	5	160±	12	—
Zekert, 1973 (46)	120	5	120	13	—
	323	6	347	17	
Objective diagnosis					
Wood, 1973 (44)	9	78	9	56	7/2
Harris, 1974 (9)	51	35	20	73 (heparin)	29/21
Soreff, 1975 (37)	21	47	18	36	—
Schöndorf, 1976 (35)	30	53	15	60	18/12
Harris, 1977 (10)	44	25	51	45	21/23
Tscherne, 1978 (40)	95	34	61	54	—
Hume, 1978 (15)	58	31	54	39	26/32
Hull, 1979 (13)	8	38	21	76	—
McKenna, 1980 (22) -low	9	76	12	75	9/0
			291	53	
-high	12	8			11/1
	337	36			
Stamatakis, 1978 (38)	30	80	—	—	12/18

F/M = female/male.

TABLE 3. *Effect of ASA on pulmonary embolism (PE)*

	Treatment		Control	
	No. of pts.	% PE	No. of pts.	% PE
General surgery				
Loew, 1974 (19)	510	0.8	527	3.2
Buttermann, 1977 (2)	79	5	175	23
Orthopedics				
Salzman, 1971 (33)	43	9	67	10
Hey, 1973 (11)	160±	1	160±	8
Zekert, 1973 (46)	120	<1	120	7 (fatal PE)
Harris, 1974 (9)	51	0	20	5 (heparin)
Harris, 1977 (10)	44	0	51	2
Hume, 1978 (15)	58	0	54	7
	476	1.5	472	7.2

patients. Thus, the sex difference in the antithrombotic effect of acetylsalicylic acid is expressed on both the arterial and venous sides of the circulation.

Appreciation that acetylsalicylic acid exerts its antithrombotic effect predominantly, if not exclusively, in males makes it necessary to reinterpret the results of many of the clinical trials listed in the tables. The results of negative trials must be regarded with suspicion when the study population contains a great preponderance of women, for example, those of the Medical Research Council (24), Loew et al. (18), Schöndorf and Hey (35) and Morris and Mitchell (25). Needless to say, the

TABLE 4. Combination of ASA and another agent in deep venous thrombosis (DVT)

		Control		ASA		Other		ASA & Other		F/M-ASA
	Type	No.	% DVT	No.	% DVT	No.	% DVT	No.	% DVT	
Heparin										
Loew 1977 (18)	General	—	—	63	30	57	19	57	9	45/18–33/24
Flicoteaux, 1977 (7)	Hip	—	—	—	—	20	20	20	20	13/7
Schöndorf, 1978 (34)	Hip	15	60	—	—	30	33	30	27	—
Vinazzer, 1980 (41)	General	—	—	365	3.9	378	2.4	350	0.3	50%/50%
Dipyridamole										
O'Sullivan, 1972 (27)	General	75	47	—	—	—	—	75	18	—
Dechavanne, 1975 (5)	Hip	20	40	—	—	—	—	20	50	11/9
McBride, 1975 (21)	Hip	22	37	—	—	—	—	21	38	—
Renney, 1976 (29)	General	85	28	—	—	—	—	85	14	—
Morris, 1977 (25)	Hip Fx.	56	67	—	—	24	63	20	63	28/4
Tscherne, 1978 (40)	Hip	—	—	—	DHE/hep	63	25	95	34	—
Plante, 1979 (28)	General	66	21	—		—	—	33	8	16/17
		324	39			349		26		
RA 233										
Den Ottolander 1972, (6)	CHF	14	50	—	—	—	—	14	21	—
Wood, 1973 (44)	Hip Fx.	9	67	—	—	12	92	9	100	7/2
Hydroxychloroquine										
Hume, 1977 (14)	Hip	20	50	21	33	20	50	20	25	—
EPC										
Hull, 1979 (13)	Knee	8	100	21	52	8	0	20	8	39/22 (total)

F/M = female/male.
EPC = external pneumatic compression.
DHE = dehydroergotamine.

TABLE 5. *Total hip replacement*

Harris, 1977 (10)	Placebo	ASA
Number of patients	51	41
Thromboembolism	23 (45%)	11 (25%)
Males	14/25	4/23 ($p < 0.01$)
Females	9/26	7/21 (NS)
Harris, 1974 (9)		
Thromboembolism		
Males	—	3/15
Females	—	15/27 ($p < 0.03$)
Both sides		
Males	14/25	7/38
Females	9/26	22/48
	(NS)	($p < 0.02$)

influence of this effect should be taken into account in future studies of acetylsalicylic acid as an antithrombotic agent.

The explanation of this sex difference is not clear. In a study of 14 men and 18 women receiving acetylsalicylic acid for prophylaxis following total-hip replacement (Coppe D, submitted for publication), we observed no difference in the pharmacokinetics of acetylsalicylic acid in the two sexes, in acetylsalicylic acid-induced whole-blood fibrinolysis or in the effect of acetylsalicylic acid on bleeding time. However, the platelets of women showed significantly greater *in vitro* aggregation in response to collagen, ADP, and epinephrine. Although both sexes developed a defect in platelet function upon ingestion of acetylsalicylic acid, a sex difference in platelet aggregation persisted after acetylsalicylic acid. There was no correlation of platelet aggregation with hematocrit; thus these results do not appear to be based on an artifactual effect of sex differences in red cell mass, as suggested by Kelton et al. (17). Whether this difference in platelet reactivity of the two sexes accounts for the difference in antithrombotic activity is of course not known.

In clinical trials of acetylsalicylic acid for prevention of venous thrombosis, surveillance by labeled fibrinogen scanning of the extremities is customary. It is difficult to assess the effect of a drug on pulmonary embolism in the same trial, since early diagnosis of venous thrombi, as a result of the surveillance, leads to earlier treatment than in a conventional clinical setting. Earlier diagnosis leads to a reduction in the rate of pulmonary embolism in both the treated and control groups. The investigator is therefore under an obligation to examine the effect of the drug on pulmonary embolism in a separate study conducted without sensitive surveillance for venous thrombosis. Jennings et al. (16) reported such a survey for acetylsalicylic acid in 528 patients (55% female) who underwent total hip replacement without a fatal pulmonary embolism. In an unprotected group of similar patients, the mortality from pulmonary embolism averaged 2% (31), so it seems likely that acetylsalicylic acid exerts a protective effect, even in women. Our own experience (Harris, personal communication) now comprises 420 patients, approximately half of whom are women. All received acetylsalicylic acid prophylactically following hip reconstruction and none experienced pulmonary emboli. There is a strong suggestion that acetylsalicylic acid's ability to prevent fatal pulmonary embolism may exceed its effectiveness against venous thrombosis. One suspects that acetylsalicylic acid has some action aside from its antiplatelet/antithrombotic effect, possibly on the production of arachidonic acid metabolites in the lung. This appears to be a fruitful area for further investigation.

It is not certain that conventional acetylsalicylic acid dosage, around 1 g/day—the dose used in most of the studies cited—is optimal for prevention of venous thromboembolism. Inhibition of vessel wall prostacyclin formation by too much or too frequent acetylsalicylic acid might compromise the antithrombotic effect of suppression of platelet thromboxane production by acetylsalicylic acid (20). In a study now in progress, we have thus far found no significant difference in antithrombotic effectiveness between 1.2 and 3.6 g/day of acetylsalicylic acid, among patients undergoing total hip replacement, but a clear answer will require more patients. An even lower dose might be preferable. On the other hand, McKenna and associates (22) recently described significantly better results in patients following operations on the knee, with 3,900 mg rather than 975 mg daily. At the present time, the issue must be regarded as unsettled.

An attractive feature of the use of acetylsalicylic acid to prevent venous thromboembolism in high-risk patients is its low cost, which compares favorably with that of the other agents in common use. Analysis of cost/effectiveness of the various approaches to prophylaxis suggests that, at least in males, the use of acetylsalicylic acid (on the average) will result in the saving of 18 lives/1000 patients undergoing total hip replacement, at a cost of $148,000 (31). This figure is approximately $200,000 less than the estimated cost to society of the complications expected in a similar patient group operated upon without prophylactic measures.

Although acetylsalicylic acid affords impressive protection, it is not complete, and there is still a significant frequency of thrombotic complications even in patients in whom acetylsalicylic acid's protective effect is clearly manifest. Therefore, the combination of acetylsalicylic acid with other prophylactic measures has been proposed, and a limited number of studies have been reported on these combinations (Table 4). Our preliminary impression is that there is something to be gained by the combination of acetylsalicylic acid with other antithrombotic measures, including pneumatic compression of the calves. However, combining acetylsalicylic acid with other antithrombotic drugs increases the frequency of bleeding side effects, which may dilute the benefit obtained by increasing the antithrombotic efficiency. Additional experience is required to provide perspective on this issue.

Acknowledgment

We gratefully acknowledge support of grants no. HL 13754 and no. HL 18738 from the National Heart, Lung, and Blood Institute.

REFERENCES

1. Adolf, J., Buttermann, G., Weidenbach, A., and Gmeineder, F. (1978): Optimierung der postoperativen Thromboembolieprophylaxe in der Gynakologie. *Geburstshilfe Frauenheilkd.*, 38:98–104.

2. Buttermann, G., Theisinger, W., Weidenbach, A., Hartung, U., Welzel, D., and Pakt, H. W. (1977): Quantitative Betwetung der postoperativen Thromboembolieprophylaxe. *Med. Klin.*, 72:1624–1638.

3. Canadian Cooperative Study Group (1978): A randomized trial of aspirin and sulfinpyrazone in threatened stroke. *N. Engl. J. Med.*, 299:53–59.

4. Clagett, G. P., Schneider, P., Rosoff, C. B., and Salzman, E. W. (1975): The influence of aspirin on post-operative platelet kinetics and venous thrombosis. *Surgery*, 77:61–74.

5. Dechavanne, M., Ville, D., Viala, J. J., Kher, A., Faivre, J., Pousset, M. B., and Dejour, H. (1975): Controlled trial of platelet anti-aggregating agents and subcutaneous heparin in prevention of postoperative deep vein thrombosis in high risk patients. *Haemostasis*, 4:94–100.

6. Den Ottolander, G. J. H., van der Maas, A. P. C., and Veen, M. R. (1972): The preventive value against venous thrombosis by treatment with acetylsalicylic acid and RA 233 in patients with decompensated heart disease. Abstract, 3rd Congress, International Society for Thrombosis and Haemostasis, Washington, p. 414.

7. Flicoteaux, H., Kher, A., Jean, N., Blery M., Judit, T., Honnent, F., and Casteyer, J. (1977): Comparison of low dose heparin and low dose heparin combined with aspirin in prevention of deep vein thrombosis after total hip replacement. *Pathol. Biol. (Paris)*, 25:55–58.

8. Harker, L. A., and Slichter, S. J. (1972): Platelet and fibrinogen consumption in man. *N. Engl. J. Med.*, 287:999–1005.

9. Harris, W. H., Salzman, E. W., Athanasoulis, C., Waltman, A. C., Baum, S., and De Sanctis, R. W. (1974): Comparison of warfarin, low-molecular-weight dextran, aspirin, and subcutaneous heparin in prevention of venous thromboembolism following total hip replacement. *J. Bone Joint Surg. (Am.)*, 56A: 1552–1562.

10. Harris, W. H., Salzman, E. W., Athanasoulis, C. A., Waltman, A. C., and De Sanctis, R. W. (1977): Aspirin prophylaxis of venous thromboembolism after total hip replacement. *N. Engl. J. Med.*, 297:1246–1249.

11. Hey, D., Heinrich, D., and Burkhardt, H. (1973): Zur prophylaxe thromboemolischer Komplikationen bei grossen Hüftgelenkseingriffen. Eine vergleichende kontrollierte Studie mit subkutanem Kalzium-heparinat und Acetylsalicylsaure. *MMW*, 115:1967–1970.

12. Hirsh, J., and McBride, J. A. (1965): Increased platelet adhesiveness in recurrent venous thrombosis and pulmonary embolism. *Br. Med. J.*, 2:797–799.

13. Hull, R., Delmore, T. J., Hirsh, J., Gent, M., Armstrong, P., Lofthouse, R., MacMillan, A., Blackstone, I., Reed-Davis, R., and Detwiler, R. C. (1979): Effectiveness of intermittent pulsatile elastic stockings for the prevention of calf and thigh vein thrombosis in patients undergoing elective knee surgery. *Thromb. Res.*, 16:37–45.

14. Hume, M., Bierbaum, B., Kuriakose, T. X., and Surprenant, J. (1977): Prevention of postoperative thrombosis by aspirin. *Am. J. Surg.*, 133:420–422.

15. Hume, M., Donaldson, W. R., and Suprenant, J. (1978): Sex, aspirin, and venous thrombosis. *Orthop. Clin. North Am.*, 9:761–767.

16. Jennings, J. J., Harris, W. H., and Sarmiento, A. (1976): A clinical evaluation of aspirin prophylaxis of thromboembolic disease after total hip arthroplasty. *J. Bone Joint Surg. Am.*, 58A:926–928.

17. Kelton, J. G., Powers, P., Julian, J., Boland, V., Carter, C. J., Gent, M., and Hirsh, J. (1980): Sex-related differences in platelet aggregation: influence of the hematocrit. *Blood*, 56:38–41.

18. Loew, D., Brucke, P., Simma, W., Venazzer, H., Dienstl, E., and Boehme, K. (1977): Acetylsalicylic acid, low dose heparin, and a combination of both substances in the prevention of postoperative thromboembolism - a double blind study. *Thromb. Res.*, 11:81–86.

19. Loew, D., Wellmer, H. K., Baer, U., Merguet, H., Rumpf, P., Petersen, H., Bromig, G., Persch, W. F., Marx, F. J., and von Basy, J. M. (1974): Postoperative Thromboembolie-prophylaxe mit Acetylsalicylsaure. *Dtsch. Med. Wochenschr.*, 99:565–572.

20. Marcus, A. J. (1977): Aspirin and thromboembolism—a possible dilemma. *N. Engl. J. Med.*, 297:1284–1285.

21. McBride, J. A., Turpie, A. G. G., Kraus, V., and Hiltz, C. (1975): Failure of aspirin and dipyridamole to influence the incidence of leg scan detected venous thrombosis after elective hip

surgery. Abstract, Vth Congress, International Society for Thrombosis and Haemostasis, Paris, p. 244.

22. McKenna, R., Galante, J., Bachmann, F., Wallace, D. L., Kaushal, S. P., and Meredith, P. (1980): Prevention of venous thromboembolism after total knee replacement by high-dose aspirin or intermittent calf and thigh compression. *Br. Med. J.*, 280:514–517.

23. McLachlin, A. D. (1969): Venous thrombosis and pulmonary embolism. In: *Recent Advances in Surgery*, edited by S. Taylor, pp. 339–360. Little, Brown, Boston.

24. Medical Research Council (Report of the Steering Committee) (1972): Effect of aspirin on postoperative venous thrombosis. *Lancet*, 2:441–444.

25. Morris, G. K., and Mitchell, J. R. A. (1977): Preventing venous thromboembolism in elderly patients with hip fractures: studies of low-dose heparin, dipyridamole, aspirin, and flurbiprofen. *Br. Med. J.*, 1:535–537.

26. O'Brien, J. R., Tulevski, V., and Etherington, M. (1971): Two in-vivo studies comparing high and low aspirin dosage. *Lancet*, 2:399–400.

27. O'Sullivan, E. F., and Renney, J. T. G. (1972): Antiplatelet drugs in the prevention of postoperative deep-vein thrombosis. Abstract, 3rd Congress, International Society for Thrombosis and Haemostasis, Washington, p. 484.

28. Plante, J., Boneu, B., Vaysse, C., Barret, A., Gouzi, M., and Bierme, R. (1979): Dipyridamole-aspirin versus low doses of heparin in the prophylaxis of deep venous thrombosis in abdominal surgery. *Thromb. Res.*, 14:399–403.

29. Renney, J. T. G., O'Sullivan, E. F., and Burke, P. F. (1976): Prevention of postoperative deep vein thrombosis with dipyridamole and aspirin. *Br. Med. J.*, 1:992–994.

30. Salzman, E. W. (1978): Antiplatelet drugs as antithrombotic agents. In: *Mechanisms of Hemostasis and Thrombosis*, edited by C. H. Mielke and R. Rodvien, pp. 269–294. Symposia Specialists, Inc., Miami.

31. Salzman, E. W., and Davies, G. C. (1980): Prophylaxis of venous thromboembolism - analysis of cost effectiveness. *Ann. Surg.*, 191:207–218.

32. Salzman, E. W., and Harris, W. H. (1976): Prevention of venous thromboembolism in orthopaedic patients. *J. Bone Joint Surg. (Am.)*, 58A:903–913.

33. Salzman, E. W., Harris, W. H., and De Sanctis, R. W. (1971): Reduction in venous thromboembolism by agents affecting platelet function. *N. Engl. J. Med.*, 284:1287–1292.

34. Schöndorf, T. H. (1978): Thromboembolieprophylaxe mit Heparin bei elektiven Hüftgelenksoperationen. *Dtsch. Med. Wochenschr.*, 103:1877–1881.

35. Schöndorf, T. H., and Hey, D. (1976): Combined administration of low dose heparin and aspirin as prophylaxis of deep vein thrombosis after hip joint surgery. *Haemostasis*, 5:250–257.

36. Smith, R. C., Duncanson, J., Ruckley, C. V., Webber, R. G., Allan, N. C., Dawes, J., Bolton, A. E., Hunter, W. M., Pepper, D. S., and Cash, J. D. (1978): β thromboglobulin and deep vein thrombosis. *Thromb. Haemost.*, 39:338–345.

37. Soreff, J., Johnson, H., Diener, L., and Göransson, L. (1975): Acetylsalicylic acid in a trial to diminish thromboembolic complications after elective hip surgery. *Acta Orthop. Scand.*, 46:246–255.

38. Stamatakis, J. D., Kakkar, V. V., Lawrence, D., Bentley, P. G., Nairn, D., and Ward, V. (1978): Failure of aspirin to prevent postoperative deep vein thrombosis in patients undergoing total hip replacement. *Br. Med. J.*, 1:1031.

39. Thomas, D. P., Tenabe, G., Kahn, M., and Stein, M. (1965): Humoral factors mediated by platelets in experimental pulmonary embolism. In: *Proceedings from the Symposium on Pulmonary Embolic Disease*, edited by A. A. Sasahara and M. Stein, pp. 59–64. Grune, New York.

40. Tscherne, H., Westermann, K., Trentz, O., Pretschner, P., and Mallmann, J. (1978): Thromboembolische Komplikationen und ihre Prophylaxe beim Hüftgelenksersats (English abstr.). *Unfaltheilkunde*, 81:178–187.

41. Vinazzer, H., Loew, D., Simma, W., and Brücke, P. (1980): Prophylaxis of postoperative thromboembolism by low dose heparin and by acetylsalicylic acid given simultaneously. A double blind study. *Thromb. Res.*, 17:177–184.

42. Walsh, P. N., Rogers, P. H., Marder, V. J., Gagnatelli, G., Escovitz, E. S., and Sherry, S. (1976): The relationship of platelet coagulant activities to venous thrombosis following hip surgery. *Br. J. Haematol.*, 32:421–437.

43. Weber, W., Wolff, K., and Bromig, G. (1971): Postoperative Thromboembolie-Prophylaxe mit Colfarit. *Ther. Ber.*, 43:229–232.

44. Wood, E. H., Prentice, C. R. M., McGrouther, D. A., Sinclair, J., and McNicol, G. P. (1973): Trial of aspirin and RA 233 in prevention of post-operative deep vein thrombosis. *Thromb. Diathes. Haemorrh.*, 30:18–24.
45. Wu, K. K., Barnes, R. W., and Hoak, J. C. (1976): Platelet hyperaggregability in idiopathic recurrent deep vein thrombosis. *Circulation*, 53:687–691.
46. Zekert, F., Kohn, I., and Vormittag, E. (1973): Prophylaxis of thromboembolic diseases in traumatologic patients—a randomised double blind study with acetylsalicylic acid. Abstract, IVth Congress, International Society for Thrombosis and Haemostasis, Vienna, p. 481.

Acetylsalicylic Acid: New Uses for an Old Drug,
edited by H. J. M. Barnett, J. Hirsh, and
J. F. Mustard. Raven Press, New York © 1982.

DISCUSSION

J. F. Mustard: Dr. Needleman, you showed us that the principal sites of prostaglandin production are the vascular cells in the myocardium, but most of your data relate to normal hearts. If the myocardium is made ischemic, does the heart muscle release arachidonic acid? Does cardiac muscle have the enzyme pathways to convert arachidonic acid to prostaglandins? Finally, are other products formed in the ischemic myocardium, in addition to PGE_1 and PGI_2?

P. Needleman: The heart is loaded with arachidonic acid and membrane lipids. When various fatty acids are used to label the phospholipid pool in the heart, hormone stimulation releases arachidonic acid. Bradykinin and angiotensin have been shown in the kidney and heart, and Bills, Smith, and Silver (1) showed in platelets, for example, that thrombin selectively releases only arachidonic acid. However, it appears that ischemia releases any fatty acid from heart tissue, with no selectivity whatsoever. But ischemic release of fatty acid is not associated with a high level of prostaglandin synthesis, and probably represents a nonspecific release to provide fuel for energy metabolism.

I am not aware that anyone has been able to show the existence in the heart of an enzyme that converts arachidonic acid to thromboxane or other products. The heart does not seem to "turn on" some other system. So at the moment, work with labeled fatty acids in isolated cell cultures and with myocardial homogenates from various species indicates that cardiac muscle is, at best, a weak synthesizer of prostaglandin.

Mustard: My second question relates to the healing zone in myocardial infarction—that area between normal and ischemic tissue. Has anyone studied prostaglandin synthesis in such healing tissue—for example, in proliferating fibroblasts? I am thinking about the heart's instability and the possible effect of prostaglandins in the zone between healthy and ischemic tissue.

Needleman: We are very interested in the fibrosis that occurs after infarction, because fibroblasts are little prostaglandin factories. However, that is a different story, in that it represents invasion of a tissue. It can be shown in the kidney, for example, that an ischemic event brings in a tissue that is initially compatible with normal tissues, but may then make a prostaglandin that induces resistance to normal function.

Mustard: Are you saying that the fibroblasts that come in during normal healing of the heart could produce harmful effects?

Needleman: Yes.

Mustard: My third question concerns eicosapentaenoic acid, which can be incorporated in membrane phospholipids and can be released but is not converted to PGI_2 and thromboxane A_2. Indeed, it inhibits cyclo-oxygenase. When subjects ingest increased amounts of eicosapentaenoic acid, do we have any knowledge about their inflammatory response or the action of drugs such as acetylsalicylic acid?

Needleman: There are hardly any good data on this subject. Studies with Eskimos are based on very limited populations, and all we learn from Eskimos is that a major dietary substitution of eicosapentaenoic acid (EPA) for arachidonic acid is possible. If you pool their platelets, it can be demonstrated that the membrane phospholipids are very high in EPA. Recently, a small study reported in the *Lancet* (3) described seven patients who were fed a high mackerel diet in order to raise their level of EPA. They increased their normal

235

levels fivefold and decreased arachidonic acid levels by about 40%, and their platelets did not aggregate. You can show that thrombin released both eicosapentaenoic acid and arachidonic acid. It blocked thromboxane synthesis with inhibition of aggregation—all of which fits my bias, but I'm not prepared to eat 2 lb of mackerel/day, until the study is larger.

Needleman: I would like to ask Dr. Salzman a question. What is the rationale for not using the lowest possible acetylsalicylic acid dose producing platelets that won't aggregate with exogenous arachidonic acid in an aggregometer?

Salzman: What you say is rational, but it has not been demonstrated in any clinical trial that such a dose will have an antithrombotic effect in patients or in subjects with normal platelet function. Until this information becomes available from a trial, we have to be sceptical.

E. Genton: Several studies have shown that when a low dose of acetylsalicylic acid (although much greater than that required to completely inhibit the prostaglandin pathway) has failed to be effective, higher doses will work. In one of the prosthetic valve studies, in which acetylsalicylic acid was used alone, 1.0 g did not protect a patient while 3.6 g did. The point is that the platelet aggregometer measures one simple effect of acetylsalicylic acid, but there is no clear-cut evidence that this is the mechanism by which the drug exerts its antithrombotic action or that this is the dose which will provide antithrombotic clinical benefits.

At this time, I can see no other basis for the beneficial action of acetylsalicylic acid beyond its effect of inhibiting arachidonic acid metabolism in the platelet. One has to determine what happens in clinical situations when platelets do not metabolize arachidonic acid. And when one uses higher doses that evoke other mechanisms, the whole basis of the study is destroyed. Why not test the hypothesis directly? What does a dose that blocks arachidonic acid metabolism do, in carefully controlled studies?

Genton: The question asked in the clinical trials was whether or not acetylsalicylic acid was antithrombotic—not whether acetylsalicylic acid used in a dose that inhibits platelet aggregation was antithrombotic. That has not been the question, and I suspect it will not be for some time.

Sulfinpyrazone can be examined in the same light. If it was antithrombotic, the dosage would have been quite different. But even here we are not certain, using available tests, that the drug is a potent platelet suppressant.

Needleman: Pharmacologists are therapeutic nihilists, because as soon as the dose is increased, there is an increase in side effects. If you push the dose of indomethacin, you will inhibit phosphodiesterase, affect calcium metabolism, and perhaps affect peroxidase. As soon as you push high doses of acetylsalicylic acid, you must be acetylating every protein that it comes in contact with. We know it is possible, for example, to take enough acetylsalicylic acid to acetylate all the cyclo-oxygenase in an isolated organ like the kidney.

J. G. Kelton: Dr. Needleman said in his talk that vessel wall cyclo-oxygenase was "sluggish." What is meant by this?

Needleman: Under the best of circumstances, in studies of vessel wall the substrate concentration of exogenous arachidonic acid is varied; the conversion rate does not exceed 5 or 10%. When we compare that to, let us say, kidney cells or GI smooth muscle, cyclo-oxygenase activity is much lower.

Kelton: Dr. Salzman, in 1970 Hardisty and co-workers reported that female platelets aggregated to a greater degree than male platelets, and that there was an inverse relationship between the hematocrit and degrees of aggregation (2). Did you test this correlation in your studies?

Salzman: No, we did not correct our samples for hematocrit, but we did look for a correlation between the aggregation results and hematocrit values. There was no correlation.

J. W. D. McDonald: I would like to ask Dr. Barnett if neurologists are now combining classes of drugs, as with anticoagulants, for example?

H. J. M. Barnett: Most neurologists do not combine the drugs because they worry about the value of anticoagulants. These agents were studied in stroke-threatened patients 20 years ago, before we knew how to design a proper study. There is some evidence that anticoagulants are useful in patients with a recent myocardial infarction, and they may be useful in mitral stenosis with arterial fibrillation and in those who, despite platelet-depressant drugs, have a flurry of TIAs or a progressive stroke. These patients are frequently given anticoagulants, but the neurologist hopes they can be put on safer drugs in the foreseeable future. In any event, a combination of drugs is unusual, except in situations such as those involving a prosthetic heart valve.

Genton: Certainly there are instances in which these agents should be used together, but unless they are specifically needed, the combination only increases the risk of bleeding.

J. Hirsh: It is often stated that if you combine acetylsalicylic acid with an anticoagulant it produces bleeding, but the only way this could be proved is with a randomized study.

Genton: Dale used acetylsalicylic acid alone without the oral anticoagulant, because with the combination he experienced a 25% incidence of complications, including a 15% incidence of gastrointestinal bleeding. His anticoagulant-only treated group had an incidence of only 3% over the same period.

Hirsh: Dale's study is one of the few that have specifically addressed this point. I believe he did demonstrate more bleeding with combined therapy.

Rotem: I am a cardiologist and do many cardiac catheterization studies. I do not think that many of these drug trials are useful, because they are dealing with a variety of disturbances of quite different etiologies. We call a chest pain event a myocardial infarction if it meets certain EKG and enzyme criteria, but we are not really looking at a unitary or single disease. These patients may have hypertension, diabetes, familial hyperlipoproteinemia, and they may or may not smoke. They are not always of the same sex. Each disease entity has a different prognosis and therefore the effect of drugs may be quite different. In addition, as a "catheter pusher" I know that the underlying anatomic pathology is quite different. We all see patients who do not seem to have coronary artery disease and yet present with infarction. There are people who have not had angina before their first myocardial infarction. Others have unstable angina for weeks and accumulate tiny areas of myocardial damage that we are not able to identify by EKG or enzyme studies. Patients have single, double, or triple vessel disease. I urge those who design drug studies to consider this wide spectrum of disease. It is unreasonable to attempt in a single study to demonstrate that any agent or procedure is effective in 3 or 6 months in *all* of these circumstances.

Hirsh: You have made a very important point, which perhaps brings us back to the matter of "data dredging" in clinical trials. If the reduction in sudden death in the sulfin-pyrazone trial is real, we are influencing only sudden death and reducing the overall mortality of myocardial infarction by 2%, in a population where most die before they get their infarct.

Rotem: That is right. I am proposing that in the future, for example, we should do coronary angiography to better sort out patients into the various groups and then have a statistician examine the comparison groups to determine if they are indeed comparable.

Mustard: Dr. Rotem's point is valid. I have emphasized the heterogeneity of the pathological mechanisms that cause the clinical complications of atherosclerosis. This heterogeneity has probably diluted the results of the studies in which attempts were made to demonstrate specific drug effects on thrombosis. I doubt that coronary angiography will provide a more specific approach because of the high cost and scarcity of technical resources. However, when the noninvasive techniques for studying vessels and thrombosis become more sophisticated, it may be possible to determine the sites where thrombi have formed and their size. It should also be possible to determine whether drugs specifically modify the process.

REFERENCES

1. Bills, T. K., Smith, J. B., and Silver, M. J. (1976): Metabolism of 14C-arachidonic acid by human platelets. *Biochem. Biophys. Acta*, 424:303.
2. Hardisty, R. M., Hutton, R. A., Montgomery, D., Rickard, S., and Trebilcock, H. (1970): Secondary platelet aggregation: A quantitation study. *Br. J. Haematol.*, 19:307.
3. Siess, W., Roth, P., Scherer, B., Bohlig, B., Kurzmann, I., and Weber, P. (1980): Platelet-membrane fatty acids, platelet aggregation, and thromboxane formation during a mackerel diet. *Lancet*, 1:441–444.

Acetylsalicylic Acid: New Uses for an Old Drug,
edited by H. J. M. Barnett, J. Hirsh, and
J. F. Mustard. Raven Press, New York © 1982.

Adverse Effects of Acetylsalicylic Acid

*Hershel Jick

Boston Collaborative Drug Surveillance Program, Boston University Medical Center, Boston, Massachusetts 02154

The potentially more serious adverse effects of acetylsalicylic acid include gastrointestinal bleeding, gastric ulcer, and deafness. The more common side effects involve minor gastrointestinal complaints. These have been assessed over a period of 12 years by the Boston Collaborative Drug Surveillance Program (BCDSP), and every indication is that serious side effects associated with acetylsalicylic acid use are quite rare. Even without this formal study, the fact that millions of patients take the drug each day, on a regular basis in the United States alone, attests to its relative lack of serious toxicity.

The BCDSP is based on a standardized monitoring of medical inpatients, and of 2,391 patients who had received plain acetylsalicylic acid on an acute basis, minor GI symptoms were reported in 2.1% and central nervous system effects in 1.2%. There was a good correlation between side effects and the average daily dose, and adverse reactions were statistically more common among females. Although interview history revealed an incidence of allergy of 1 in 200, there was an absence of allergic reactions in the monitored inpatients. There was an overall incidence of deafness in 1.1% of patients, with a direct correlation to unit dose—reaching 15% in patients receiving 1,200 mg or more. Acute major gastrointestinal bleeding requiring blood transfusion occurred in 0.3% of exposed patients without predisposing disease and minor bleeding in 1.6%. Of the patients admitted to hospital with gastrointestinal bleeding, 16% gave a history of heavy regular acetylsalicylic acid use compared with 6.9% of controls. No statistically significant difference was attributed to light use. There was a statistically significant greater use of acetylsalicylic acid among patients presenting with benign gastric ulcer. The present data, based on a large observational study, indicate that whereas the acute side effects of acetylsalicylic acid occur in about 5% of patients, they are rarely serious and virtually all are short-term and reversible. Long-term effects are quite rare and primarily involve gastrointestinal bleeding and ulceration of the stomach.

This review of the clinical toxicity of acetylsalicylic acid is based on information collected by the Boston Collaborative Drug Surveillance Program (BCDSP) over a period of 12 years in some 50,000 hospitalized medical and surgical patients. In considering the magnitude of the acetylsalicylic acid toxicity problem, it is important

---

*Mailing address: Dr. H. Jick, Boston Collaborative Drug Surveillance Program, 400 Totten Pond Road, Waltham, Massachusetts 02154

to keep in mind that tens of millions of people in the United States alone take acetylsalicylic acid on any given day. Although most take the drug for a brief period, there are millions who take it on a regular basis, i.e., virtually every day. In view of this, it should be apparent even without the formal collection of data that serious side effects from acetylsalicylic acid must be quite rare. If this were not the case, we would have a continuous epidemic of acetylsalicylic acid toxicity.

The toxicity of acetylsalicylic acid may be considered under two major headings: acute toxicity or that appearing shortly after the drug is first used and long-term toxicity or that occurring after continuous use for weeks, months or years.

The information on acute toxicity is based on careful, standardized monitoring of medical inpatients, and the results, strictly speaking, apply only to this population.

ACUTE ACETYLSALICYLIC ACID TOXICITY

The type and frequency of acute adverse reactions attributed to acetylsalicylic acid in 2,391 medical patients who received plain acetylsalicylic acid are given in Table 1 (6). Minor gastrointestinal symptoms were reported in 2.1% and central nervous system effects in 1.2%. Other reactions—excluding gastrointestinal bleeding, which will be reported separately—were uncommon. There was good corre-

TABLE 1. *Adverse reactions attributed to ASA[a]*

Adverse reaction	No. of patients	%
Minor gastrointestinal disturbances (heartburn, nausea, cramps, indigestion, vomiting, anorexia, loss of taste, flatulence)	51	2.1
Central nervous system effects (tinnitus, temporary deafness, vertigo)	29	1.2
Prolonged prothrombin time values	3	0.1
Drug fever	2	0.1
Leukopenia	2	0.1
Epistaxis	2	0.1
Diaphoresis	1	0.04
Metabolic acidosis	1	0.04
Petechiae and purpura	1	0.04
Palpitations and dyspnea	1	0.04
Stomatitis	1	0.04
Hypothermia	1	0.04
Elevated serum uric acid level	1	0.04
Total	96	4.0

[a]Gastrointestional bleeding is described separately.

lation between the frequency of adverse reactions and average daily dose; this was particularly impressive for central nervous system side effects. Reported adverse reactions were also more common among females (6.3%) than among males (3.5%) ($p < 0.002$). There was no important correlation between the frequency of acetylsalicylic acid side effects and age, body weight, or renal function. It is of interest that none of the recipients were reported to have developed an allergic reaction to acetylsalicylic acid.

Three special analyses were carried out to quantify more precisely the frequency of allergy, deafness, and gastrointestinal bleeding attributable to acetylsalicylic acid.

Allergy

As noted above, none of the monitored patients were reported to have been allergic to acetylsalicylic acid. Our interview history included a question about previous drug allergy, and on review, we found that about 1 in 200 patients gave a history of acetylsalicylic acid allergy. It seems likely, therefore, that the vast majority of acetylsalicylic acid-allergic patients become aware of their allergy before age 40 and subsequently avoid the drug. If this is correct, it explains the absence of acetylsalicylic acid allergy among monitored patients, almost all of whom are over 40 years of age.

Deafness

We have previously reported our experience with acetylsalicylic acid-induced deafness among 32,842 consecutively monitored patients, of whom 2,974 received acetylsalicylic acid in some form (7). The results are shown in Tables 2 and 3. The frequency of deafness attributed to acetylsalicylic acid was 33 of 2,974 patients (1.1%) (Table 2). This frequency strongly correlated with unit dose; the rates were extremely low for patients receiving less than a 900 mg unit dose but reached 15% in those receiving a dose of 1200 mg or more (Table 3).

TABLE 2. Drug-induced deafness by drugs implicated

Drug	No. of patients developing deafness	No. of patients exposed
Acetylsalicylic acid	33	2,974
Neomycin	7	802
Kanamycin[a]	5	372
Gentamicin	4	1,125
Ethacrynic acid (intravenous)[a]	2	184
Paromomycin	1	75
Quinidine	1	1,024
Propranolol	1	853

[a]In one patient, deafness developed after treatment with ethacrynic acid and again after treatment with kanamycin.

TABLE 3. *Unit doses of ASA received by patients with and without deafness*

Dose (mg)	No. of patients with deafness	No. of patients exposed	Rate/1000
< 600	0	312	0
600–899	3	2,273	1
900–1199	12	269	45
1200 +	18	120	150

TABLE 4. *Major[a] gastrointestinal bleeding in patients with no known predisposing illness*

Drug(s)	No. of patients with major GI bleeding[b]	No. of patients exposed	%
Heparin alone[c]	7 (3)	575	1.2
Steroids alone	7 (3)	1,484	0.5
Acetylsalicylic acid alone	6 (4)	2,081	0.3
Ethacrynic acid alone	5 (5)	111	4.5
Warfarin alone	1 (0)	423	0.2
Heparin + warfarin	3 (0)	457	0.7
Steroids + acetylsalicylic acid	3 (1)	389	0.8
Steroids + ethacrynic acid	2 (2)	22	9.1
Heparin + ethacrynic acid	1 (1)	26	3.8
Heparin + acetylsalicylic acid	1 (0)	136	0.7
Heparin + warfarin + steroids	1 (0)	34	2.9
Other combinations	0 (0)	271	0.0
None of the above	20 (17)	10,637	0.2
Total	57 (36)	16,646	0.3

[a]Major is defined as requiring transfusion.

[b]The numbers in parentheses refer to those whose bleeding was not drug-attributed by the attending physician.

[c]"Alone" refers to the absence of the other four drugs identified as associated with gastrointestinal bleeding.

Gastrointestinal Bleeding

The frequency of acute gastrointestinal bleeding attributable to acetylsalicylic acid has been carefully studied and previously reported (2). We considered that the frequency of acute major gastrointestinal bleeding, defined as bleeding requiring blood transfusion, was about 0.3% in hospitalized medical patients with no known predisposing disease (Table 4). The frequency of minor gastrointestinal bleeding in such patients was estimated to be 1.6%.

LONG-TERM ACETYLSALICYLIC ACID TOXICITY

We have previously reported on the frequency of gastrointestinal bleeding and gastric ulcer requiring hospitalization among chronic acetylsalicylic acid users (3).

Gastrointestinal Bleeding

During the first 10 months of 1972, the BCDSP carried out a survey of some 25,000 consecutive medical and surgical admissions to 24 Boston-area hospitals to evaluate the relationship between a variety of drugs taken regularly before admission and a number of diseases. This survey provided an opportunity to examine the relationship of regular acetylsalicylic acid ingestion to hospital admission for major upper gastrointestinal bleeding.

Shortly after admission, the patients were asked, among other questions, whether they had regularly taken medications during the previous 3 months for any of 26 indications (e.g., high blood pressure, diabetes, headache, or "pain"). "Regular" use was defined as taking a drug at least once a week during the preceding 12 weeks. Whenever a positive history was obtained, the patient was asked how many days/week, on the average, the drug was taken. Duration of use was also determined, but exact dosage was not.

At the time of interview, the monitors routinely collected limited information concerning medical histories of a number of diseases, including peptic ulcer. After discharge, diagnoses up to six in number were recorded, in the same order they were written in the hospital discharge summaries.

For the purposes of this study, all drugs containing acetylsalicylic acid were divided into three categories: preparations containing acetylsalicylic acid only, buffered acetylsalicylic acid, and compound preparations containing other drugs in addition to acetylsalicylic acid. Any person regularly taking any one of these preparations was classified either as a "heavy acetylsalicylic acid user" (4 or more days/week) or a "light acetylsalicylic acid user" (1–3 days/week).

The group of cases selected for analysis consisted of patients admitted to the hospital for acute, major upper-gastrointestinal bleeding in the absence of known predisposing conditions.

All 467 patients with discharge diagnoses of upper gastrointestinal bleeding were identified from the computer files, and their discharge summaries were reviewed without knowledge of drug intake. Excluded from further analyses were the following categories of patients: those with a history of peptic ulcer or gastric surgery; those who had cancer, cirrhosis, alcoholism, or blood dyscrasias, and those who had been receiving anticoagulants, steroids, phenylbutazone, indomethacin, or cytotoxic agents before admission.

In addition, we excluded all the patients in whom bleeding occurred after admission and those who had no major evidence of acute gastrointestinal bleeding, such as frank hematemesis, melena, or both.

The control cases consisted of all patients who were admitted to hospital either for conditions that were unlikely to be associated with acetylsalicylic acid consumption or with disorders predisposing to upper gastrointestinal bleeding or peptic ulcer disease.

Where relevant, all exclusion criteria used for the cases were applied to the controls.

With the above specifications, the final material consisted of 96 patients with major upper gastrointestinal bleeding in the absence of known predisposing conditions and 16,226 controls.

Heavy Regular Acetylsalicylic Acid Use

In this section, in the comparisons that follow, all patients giving a history of light regular acetylsalicylic acid use have been omitted.

Among the 88 patients who bled in the absence of known predisposing conditions, 14 gave a history of heavy regular acetylsalicylic acid use before admission (16%), whereas among the 14,813 controls, 1,015 gave such a history (6.9%).

The frequencies of acetylsalicylic acid use among the cases and controls, subdivided by age and sex, are given in Table 5. Upon control of these factors, the summary X^2 value with one degree of freedom (4) is 7.1 ($p < 0.01$), and the estimate of the standardized morbidity ratio (5) is 2.1.

Division of the patients according to hospital of entry, smoking habits, or month of admission did not materially affect the comparisons.

Light Regular Acetylsalicylic Acid Use

In this section, in the comparisons that follow, all patients giving a history of heavy regular acetylsalicylic acid use have been omitted.

The frequencies of light regular acetylsalicylic acid use were as follows. Among 82 cases of major upper gastrointestinal bleeding in absence of predisposing conditions, there were eight users (9.8%), and among 15,211 controls, there were 1,413 users (9.3%). These differences are not statistically significant.

TABLE 5. *Frequencies of heavy regular ASA use[a] among patients admitted to hospital for upper gastrointestinal bleeding and among controls*

Age (years)	Patients with bleeding		Controls	
	ASA users	Total	ASA users	Total
Men:				
20–39	0 (0.0%)	8	51 (2.8%)	1,794
40–59	2 (14.3%)	14	132 (4.6%)	2,867
60–75	2 (10.5%)	19	102 (5.4%)	1,874
Women:				
20–39	0 (0.0%)	6	150 (5.4%)	2,781
40–59	4 (30.8%)	13	290 (9.4%)	3,085
60–75	6 (21.4%)	28	290 (12.0%)	2,412
Totals	14 (15.9%)	88	1,015 (6.9%)	14,813

Standardized morbidity ratio = 2.1
$X^2_1 = 7.1$ ($p < 0.01$)
[a]Regular use at least four days per week for at least three months.

Estimates of Incidence

It is estimated that the 24 collaborating hospitals serve a population of about 1,300,000 in the greater metropolitan Boston area, which has a population of approximately 2,800,000 (1). Census data (8) indicate that persons between the ages of 20 and 75 years represent 60% of the total population. Thus, it is estimated that 780,000 people would have been eligible for admission to the surveyed hospitals. On the basis of the control series, the age-adjusted and sex-adjusted number of persons who did not take acetylsalicylic acid regularly in that population is estimated to be about 666,000. From the above data, the 10-month incidence rate of hospital admissions for major upper gastrointestinal bleeding in persons without known predisposing conditions or evidence of duodenal ulcer, and not taking acetylsalicylic acid regularly, is estimated to be 11/100,000 (74 per 666,000)—or 13/100,000/year. With use of the estimated standardized morbidity rate (2.1), the incidence rate in heavy regular users taking acetylsalicylic acid for 4 or more days/week is approximately 28/100,000/year, and the incidence rate of hospital admissions for major upper gastrointestinal bleeding attributable to heavy regular use of the drug is about 15/100,000/year.

Benign Gastric Ulcer

Among the 26 patients with newly diagnosed benign gastric ulcer, five gave a history of heavy regular acetylsalicylic acid use (19%) as compared with 6.9% among the controls. The frequencies of acetylsalicylic acid use among cases and controls, subdivided according to age and sex, are given in Table 6. Upon control of these factors, the summary X^2 value with one degree of freedom (4) is 4.2 ($p < 0.05$) and the estimate of the standardized morbidity ratio (5) is 3.4.

TABLE 6. *Frequencies of heavy regular ASA use[a] among patients admitted to hospital for gastric ulcer and among controls*

Age (years)	Gastric ulcer		Controls	
	ASA users	Totals	ASA users	Totals
Men:				
20–39	0 (0.0%)	0	51 (2.8%)	1,794
40–59	1 (20.0%)	5	132 (4.6%)	2,867
60–75	2 (28.6%)	7	102 (5.4%)	1,874
Women:				
20–39	0 (0.0%)	5	150 (5.4%)	2,781
40–59	1 (20.0%)	5	290 (9.4%)	3,085
60–75	1 (25.0%)	4	290(12.0%)	2,412
Totals	5 (19.2%)	26	1,015 (6.9%)	14,813

Standardized morbidity ratio = 3.4
$\chi^2_1 = 4.2$ ($p < 0.05$)
[a] Regular use at least 4 days/week for at least 3 months.

Evaluation of the data in terms of hospital of entry, smoking habits, or month of admission did not materially affect the comparisons.

Other Long-Term Effects

We have observed no other episodes of toxicity attributed to or attributable to acetylsalicylic acid.

COMMENT

Since the data presented are nonexperimental, i.e., observational in nature, a few words about their interpretation are necessary.

Inferences about the cause-and-effect relationships between a drug and a symptom or illness are sometimes virtually certain, but usually they are uncertain. For example, the development of severe hypoglycemia shortly after the administration of insulin can be attributed with certainty to the drug. There is a close and obvious time relationship between the drug and the event, because the event represents the result of a pharmacological action of the drug and because the event virtually never occurs in the absence of the drug. Similarly, deafness that develops acutely in a patient taking high doses of acetylsalicylic acid is almost surely caused by acetylsalicylic acid.

At the other extreme, the development of gastrointestinal bleeding or benign gastric ulcer can rarely, if ever, be attributed with absolute certainty to a drug in a given patient. The event occurs reasonably often in the absence of drug use and, as opposed to acute hypoglycemia, it is "non-specific" in that it is not a well-defined, unique, pharmacologic endpoint for any drug.

The question of whether a given drug produces gastrointestinal bleeding, therefore, becomes quite complicated. Since this event is uncommon, its association with a specific drug cannot be studied using randomized clinical trials. We are, therefore, left with the technique of large observational studies to try to estimate whether a drug such as acetylsalicylic acid does indeed cause clinically important gastrointestinal bleeding.

Unfortunately, hopelessly insoluble methodologic problems preclude the study of acetylsalicylic acid and gastrointestinal bleeding or benign ulcer in patients who have conditions that predispose to gastrointestinal bleeding, and any inferences we have been able to draw relate to people who have no known upper gastrointestinal disease and in whom acetylsalicylic acid is not contraindicated. The risks given in this chapter on acetylsalicylic acid-induced gastrointestinal problems provide our best estimates based on carefully collected and analyzed nonexperimental data.

In general, the present data indicate that whereas acute side effects to acetylsalicylic acid are reasonably common (about 5%), they are rarely serious. No deaths attributable to acetylsalicylic acid have been reported and virtually all of the reported side effects have been short-term and reversible. Long-term side effects of acetylsalicylic acid appear to be quite rare and primarily involve bleeding and ulceration of the stomach.

REFERENCES

1. Boston Collaborative Drug Surveillance Program (1973): Oral contraceptives and venous thromboembolic disease, surgically confirmed gallbladder disease, and breast tumours. *Lancet*, 1:1399–1404.
2. Jick, H., and Porter, J. (1978): Drug-induced gastrointestinal bleeding. *Lancet*, 2:87–89.
3. Levy, M. (1974): Aspirin use in patients with major upper gastrointestinal bleeding and peptic-ulcer disease. A report from the Boston Collaborative Drug Surveillance Program. *N. Engl. J. Med.*, 290:1158–1162.
4. Mantel, N., and Haenszel, W. (1959): Statistical aspects of the analysis of data from retrospective studies of disease. *J. Natl. Cancer Inst.*, 22:719–748.
5. Miettinen, O. S. (1972): Standardization of risk ratios. *Am. J. Epidemiol.*, 96:383–388.
6. Miller, R. R., and Jick, H. (1977): Acute toxicity of aspirin in hospitalized medical patients. *Am. J. Med. Sci.*, 274:271–279.
7. Porter, J., and Jick, H. (1977): Drug-induced anaphylaxis, convulsions, deafness, and extrapyramidal symptoms *Lancet*, 1:587–588.
8. United States Bureau of the Census (1971): Final Report (PC [1]-B23), p. 66. Government Printing Office, Washington, D. C.

Acetylsalicylic Acid: New Uses for an Old Drug,
edited by H. J. M. Barnett, J. Hirsh, and
J. F. Mustard. Raven Press, New York © 1982.

DISCUSSION

J. W. D. McDonald: It appears that the incidence of toxic effects is defined in terms of patients admitted to hospital. However, you do not have a good "handle" on numbers unless you know how many patients with gastric ulcer or dyspepsia on chronic heavy-dose acetylsalicylic acid are not admitted to hospital. Surely a great many factors determine whether an individual patient is admitted to hospital?

H. Jick: Strictly speaking, we do not have any information on the toxicity of acetylsalicylic acid in outpatients who are not hospitalized. With regard to gastrointestinal bleeding, it must be assumed that we are interested only in GI bleeding serious enough to lead to hospital admission. Minor gastrointestinal bleeding with acetylsalicylic acid is common— possibly occurring in 100% of patients.

J. Hirsh: Can we get some better idea of outpatient experience from the various acetylsalicylic acid studies? Although there is no control group, we do know the incidence of the various GI side effects. In the Canadian stroke study and in various other studies, the number of patients complaining about GI bleeding was very low.

Jick: Let me make an epidemiological point. In a randomized controlled trial, bias is not eliminated but simply distributed equally between study groups. In almost all clinical trials involving anticoagulants or acetylsalicylic acid, the proportion of bleeding is usually high because the clinician specifically looks for the evidence. Therefore, these clinical trials almost always show a higher incidence of such adverse effects than the usual clinical situation.

H. J. M. Barnett: Concerning data on gastrointestinal bleeding in hospitalized patients, it is difficult to interpret these without knowing the length of hospital stay and whether the acetylsalicylic acid was started in hospital or prior to admission. This distinction might eliminate patients who had other conditions leading to GI bleeding.

Jick: The patients we studied were well defined. They were general medical patients, and only 5 or 10% were on acetylsalicylic acid when admitted to hospital. Spontaneous massive gastrointestinal bleeding in medical patients without a history of GI disease is quite uncommon—in 33,000 there were perhaps only 50 cases, and these rare events tend to be associated with the combination of corticosteroids and anticoagulants or acetylsalicylic acid and ethacrynic acid.

J. F. Mustard: To conclude that gastrointestinal bleeding is uncommon when these drugs are combined, even on the best data, can be misleading if extrapolated to chronic administration, even though treatment was started in hospital. The incidence could be quite different when the patient is sent home on the combination of drugs.

Jick: Right. Based on available data, giving acetylsalicylic acid to patients on anticoagulants is contraindicated, except under specific conditions. We described the toxicity of acetylsalicylic acid in otherwise healthy people not receiving anticoagulants or antitumor agents. The incidence of adverse reactions to acetylsalicylic acid in patients with other illnesses cannot be separated out because of all the other factors. All we can say is that the drug is probably contraindicated in anybody who has any tendency to bleed from the GI tract.

Mustard: Do you have data on patients with rheumatoid arthritis who take acetylsalicylic acid in fairly high dose over a long period of time? I realize they may also be taking other drugs.

Jick: It is a general principle of clinical pharmacology that if a drug is toxic, it will not be tolerated by large numbers of individuals. Yet hundreds of thousands, if not millions, of patients with rheumatic diseases take large doses of acetylsalicylic acid every day, and only the rare individual experiences long-term toxicity. Obviously, it is an extraordinarily "benign" drug.

Unidentified: My field is clinical rheumatology. How do you contrast your data to that of others who have shown a high incidence of asymptomatic gastric ulcers?

Jick: I am not familiar with those data, but if an ulcer is asymptomatic, we don't know about it. Certainly we must be careful in interpreting the data from our study.

Unidentified: Can you give me a reference for "drop-out" data on long-term, high-dose acetylsalicylic acid treatment? Buchanan in Glasgow and Hutchison have reported drop-out rates of 30 to 70%/year for patients taking uncoated acetylsalicylic acid therapy, primarily related to dyspepsia—although there is poor correlation between dyspepsia and pathology.

Jick: Interview data from patients suggest that about 5% cannot tolerate acetylsalicylic acid because of GI distress. However, our rheumatic population ingests massive doses, so it would not surprise me if 30% could not tolerate the drug. But those who do tolerate it can apparently take it without much risk.

P. Needleman: What about your data on the relationship of acetylsalicylic acid and anticoagulants?

Jick: We have a report coming out that presents an elegant analysis of the risk of gastrointestinal bleeding from heparin. Patients receiving acetylsalicylic acid at the same time as heparin had a strikingly higher incidence of both minor and major "bleeds." These data are very convincing. One should not mix acetylsalicylic acid with heparin. On the other hand, serious warfarin bleeds are uncommon in hospital, and many of these patients must be using acetylsalicylic acid. But we do not seem to have major problems when giving acetylsalicylic acid with warfarin.

We have disturbing data on the incidence of side effects, particularly of the GI system, in patients taking enteric-coated acetylsalicylic acid. It is hard to interpret these data because by definition, if a patient is on enteric-coated acetylsalicylic acid, he already has a GI problem. We have not said much about this, but a careful evaluation of a large number of patients on enteric-coated acetylsalicylic acid would be worthwhile.

Stuart: Do patients develop tolerance to acetylsalicylic acid? When long-term acetylsalicylic acid is administered, do some cells begin to produce a variant cyclo-oxygenase or adapt in some way?

Jick: There is overwhelming evidence against such tolerance.

Needleman: There is no reason to postulate a special adaptation of cyclo-oxygenase with chronic inhibition. This is determined by the rate of protein synthesis in the cells, and has been studied in endothelial cells by looking at the rate of enzyme turnover.

Stuart: I was fascinated by Dr. Jick's dose-response curve. The plot of acetylsalicylic acid dosage versus level of side effects certainly shows that one part of the curve has a lower incidence of side effects.

Acetylsalicylic Acid: New Uses for an Old Drug,
edited by H. J. M. Barnett, J. Hirsh, and
J. F. Mustard. Raven Press, New York © 1982.

Some Unresolved Methodological Problems in Long-Term Clinical Trials

*Michael Gent and Cedric J. Carter

Faculty of Health Sciences, McMaster University, Hamilton, Ontario, Canada L8S 3Z5

The results obtained in some recent major secondary prevention trials in myocardial infarction and cerebral ischemia suggest that platelet-suppressing drugs may have little or only marginal benefit. At the same time, two other studies, the Canadian Stroke Study and the Anturane Reinfarction Trial, have claimed quite dramatic benefits, but such conclusions were based on strategies that excluded certain patients and outcome events from the primary analysis of efficacy and also involved issues relating to the multiple challenges of data and their consequent effect on conventional levels of statistical significance. Even though the criteria for the eligibility of patients, the analyzability of outcome events, and the identification of clinically cogent subgroups of patients were laid down prospectively, they have given rise to considerable controversy about the validity of the conclusions of these studies. Some of the pros and cons of such strategies are discussed, as are the essential components for assessing the overall strength of evidence.

A number of clinical trials (1,3,5,7–9,13,14,16,37) for the evaluation of various platelet-suppressing drugs in the secondary prevention of myocardial infarction and cerebral ischemia have ended in the past two or three years (Table 1). It had been the hope of many that promising drugs such as sulfinpyrazone, acetylsalicylic acid (ASA), and dipyridamole would have been shown by now to be clearly beneficial and capable of considerable impact on two of the three major causes of death in the western world. Failing this, it might have been hoped that they would be shown to be of no value, allowing efforts to be redirected to other opportunities.

Unfortunately, the findings from these studies have not led to uniform agreement. On the contrary, they have led to heated debates, particularly about the design methodology and analysis of some of the studies. The results from the acetylsalicylic acid myocardial infarction studies have been equivocal and at best of only marginal significance, and the claimed benefit for sulfinpyrazone is based on rather controversial interpretations that exclude certain deaths. Although the results of the two stroke

---

*Mailing address: Dr. Michael Gent, Department of Clinical Epidemiology & Biostatistics, McMaster University, 1200 Main Street, West Hamilton, Ontario L8S 3Z5.

TABLE 1. *Secondary prevention studies in myocardial infarction and cerebral ischemia*

Myocardial infarction studies	Year	Drug
Elwood et al. (13)	1974	ASA
CDP (A)	1975	ASA
German-Austrian	1977	ASA
Elwood and Sweetnam (14)	1979	ASA
ART	1978/1980	Sulfinpryazone
AMIS	1980	ASA
PARIS	1980	ASA + dipyridamole
Cerebral ischemia studies		
AITIA	1977	ASA
RRPCE	1978	ASA + sulfinpyrazone

studies are more generally accepted, there is still some reservation on the part of many.

Because of this, there is growing skepticism about the randomized controlled clinical trial, in that it might not be the research tool claimed and that perhaps there is a need for alternative research designs—including nonrandomized studies. However, such a conclusion would be a serious error. Randomization is an essential element in the evaluation of therapeutic and prophylactic procedures, and any deviation from this principle would only increase difficulties in interpretation. Particularly in myocardial infarction and cerebral ischemia, long-term trials are complex and extremely time-consuming, and there is a need for considerable care in their design, execution, and analysis if there is to be general credibility and acceptance of the findings.

A series of methodological standards have been developed for this field, which most agree are important prerequisites (20,21,40). These include:

a) the definition of precise and appropriate patient inclusion/exclusion criteria;

b) the ensurance that sufficient patients are available and included in the study to enable valid conclusions to be drawn;

c) the allocation of patients to their respective treatment groups by means of randomization following appropriate stratification, so as to generate patient groups that are likely to be comparable with respect to important clinical and demographic prognostic factors;

d) the provision of a concurrent control group with an identical-appearing placebo;

e) the conduct of the study in a double-blind fashion; and

f) the provision of all treatment groups with identical care and attention, except for the drug agent(s) being studied. The protocol must be strictly monitored and enforced, in order to minimize any possible bias in study execution. Finally, statistical analyses must include and appropriately assess the various outcome measures.

None of the studies listed in Table 1 are above criticism, but they do seem to meet most of these methodological requirements. For example, all the studies were randomized and double-blind, with appropriate controls, and generally included large numbers of patients, although in some cases these were still insufficient. However, concerns have still been raised about these studies in correspondence and editorials and at various scientific meetings, and no studies have received more scrutiny and criticism, as well as defense, than the Canadian Stroke Study and the Anturane Reinfarction Trial (3,6,10–12, 15,17,22,29–31,34,40,44–47). Constructive criticism is healthy and some of the concerns about these studies are certainly valid. However, many are questionable and some simply reflect a lack of understanding of basic methodological and statistical principles as well as confusion about the principal research question. It is of value to consider specific examples from these studies, since they represent more general methodological issues.

MULTIPLE ANALYSES OF DATA

The term "statistically significant" is frequently used in the scientific literature, yet its true meaning is still not widely understood. When, in a well-designed and carefully executed clinical trial, a greater mean response to treatment is observed with Drug A than with Drug B, then either Drug A is truly superior or else the random variation in response—i.e., the sampling error—accounts for the observed difference. "Statistically significant" at the 5% level ($p < 0.05$) simply means that, based on the null hypothesis that there really is no difference in benefit between the two treatments, the probability of the observed difference resulting from chance alone is less than 0.05. Hence, by convention, we then infer in such circumstances that the evidence is sufficiently persuasive to conclude that there is a real difference.

When making inferences from the analysis of data from these large, long-term studies, one needs to be careful, since there is the strong possibility of spurious statistical significance occurring as a result of the many questions that must necessarily be asked of the data. It can be shown that if one makes a number of independent analyses of the data—for example, ten—then the significance level at which each test should be carried out is approximately 0.005 (i.e., 0.05/10) in order to ensure maintaining an *overall* level of statistical significance equal to 0.05. Of course, one needs to be even more careful about making inferences from analyses which have been stimulated by examination of the data!

In these large clinical trials, multiple challenges of the data can result from (a) repeated examination of the accumulating data over time, (b) the existence of several treatment groups to be compared, (c) analysis of specific subsets or clusters of various outcome measures, and (d) the analysis of clinically cogent subgroups of patients.

In such long-term trials, there is an important ethical requirement that the data be assessed periodically as they accumulate, in order to identify a superior treatment as quickly as possible, or, perhaps even more important, to identify whether a particular test treatment is harmful. Clearly, these are not statistically independent examinations of the data, but adjustments needed to be taken into account in the calculation of the final p-value.

With four treatment groups in the Canadian Stroke Study and the particular factorial arrangement employed, there were three principal questions that were almost statistically independent. These related to the overall effect of acetylsalicylic acid, the overall effect of sulfinpyrazone, and possible synergism–antagonism between the two drugs. This must be taken into account in considering the p-values for specific treatment hypotheses.

Most long-term trials include several outcome events of interest, which may be fatal or nonfatal. Total mortality should always be reported, but it is often appropriate also to analyze cause-specific mortality, such as cardiac deaths or sudden deaths. Nonfatal events that are clinically relevant include myocardial infarction and stroke, but one should be careful not to examine these without also considering fatal events at the same time (17,19,42). Another important subset of outcome events might relate to a specific time period. For example, in the Anturane Reinfarction Trial the most striking treatment benefit appeared to be during the first 6 months of treatment, when these patients are known to be still at particularly high risk.

Such subgroup analyses are often referred to as "retrospective analyses." In general, this is really not the case, since they represent questions that were specifically identified at the start of the trial, and therefore the only concern is to allow for multiple tests in the assessment and interpretation of resulting p-values. Retrospective analysis is an appropriate description only when it applies to a test that was stimulated by an examination of the data. In such circumstances, these are hypothesis-generating and not hypothesis-testing situations.

It is worth pointing out that the potential for bias exists when only a subset of the outcome events is considered for a particular analysis and when those who decide whether a given patient has suffered such an event are also privy to the patient's trial therapy. Even where the trial is double-blind, precise operational definitions for all outcomes of interest must be developed beforehand and applied consistently throughout the study. In multicenter trials, there should be a central adjudicating committee with this specific responsibility.

A number of issues relating to subgroup analyses and the subsequent identification of highly responsive subgroups among patients with transient ischemic attacks have been discussed by Gent and Hirsh (18). They point out two approaches that can be used to identify potentially highly responsive patients. The first relates to an examination, within a particular study, of statistically significant differences in response between complementary groups, as for example between males and females, or between patients with and without a history of hypertension. The second approach is to look for consistency of such differences in other trials, since this would considerably strengthen the evidence obtained from a single study.

One potential pitfall in the identification of complementary patient groups with different response to therapy can be demonstrated by an example from the Canadian Stroke Study. There appeared to be a difference in response to acetylsalicylic acid depending on whether or not the patient had a history of hypertension at entry to the trial. For patients with a history of hypertension, the risk reduction for stroke or death was only 9%, whereas for those without a history of hypertension, the risk reduction was 47%. This latter reduction is statistically significantly different from zero ($p < 0.01$), and it would be tempting to conclude that only those without a history of hypertension were responsive to acetylsalicylic acid. However, to really establish this point, it would be necessary to test the hypothesis that the response to acetylsalicylic acid was different in these two subgroups—in other words, that the observed difference in benefit between a risk reduction of 47% and one of 9% is statistically significantly different from zero, which it is not in this particular case.

As with any large follow-up trial, it was intended in the Canadian study to examine potential interactions between clinically cogent subgroups of patients and the trial drugs. Some 10 different subgroups were defined, for example, those with single versus multiple attacks before entry, and the presence or absence of neurological residua. The most striking difference in response to acetylsalicylic acid was found between male and female patients ($p < 0.003$), that is, the drug was of no benefit in reducing stroke or death among the women but was associated with an observed risk reduction of 48% among the men. Even allowing for the fact that several subgroups were examined, the p-value of 0.003 alone provides quite convincing evidence of a true difference in the response to acetylsalicylic acid between males and females.

The conclusion that males represent a highly responsive subgroup for acetylsalicylic acid is considerably strengthened by the findings of several other studies. In the United States study of cerebral ischemia (16), the observed risk reduction for stroke or death with acetylsalicylic acid was 47% for men, whereas there was no observed reduction for women. The difference in response to acetylsalicylic acid in this study was not of itself statistically significant, because of the small numbers of patients, but the data are remarkably similar to, and therefore supportive of, those from the Canadian study. Harris et al. (23) also observed that only men showed a beneficial response when acetylsalicylic acid was used for the prevention of thromboembolism following total hip replacement. Analysis of these data demonstrates a risk reduction of 69% for males, but only 4% for females. Linos et al. (32), in a long-term follow-up study of patients with rheumatoid arthritis who received acetylsalicylic acid treatment, found that the occurrence of myocardial infarction, angina pectoris, cerebral infarction, and sudden death was 37% less than that expected from population statistics for men, whereas it was 25% higher for females. Hirsh et al. (24) have demonstrated a differential effect of acetylsalicylic acid on bleeding time between the two sexes. A possible sex-related difference with a different drug was described by Kaegi et al. (26), who found sulfinpyrazone to have a greater effect in men than in women in reducing thrombosis in arteriovenous shunts. Johnson et al. (25) demonstrated statistically significant sex differences in human platelet sensitivity to aggregating stimuli.

The one study to show a benefit for acetylsalicylic acid in females was that reported by McKenna et al. (33). This demonstrated a significant reduction in deep vein thrombosis following surgery for knee replacement, but it is worth noting that the dosage of acetylsalicylic acid was about 4 g/day, which is very much higher than that used in the other cited studies.

Following completion of the Canadian Stroke Study, and stimulated by the observed sex difference in response to acetylsalicylic acid, Kelton et al. (28), investigating the antithrombotic effect of acetylsalicylic acid, showed in their particular animal model that it resulted in a significant reduction in thrombosis in male rabbits but no observed reduction among female animals.

This concept of "highly responsive subgroups" of patients has several important implications. In addition to clearly influencing recommendations for patient management, the identification of such groups may provide invaluable insight both into the study of underlying mechanisms of action for antiplatelet agents and into the pathogenesis of the thrombotic process in a number of thromboembolic disorders.

This concept will also have to be taken into account in the design and analysis of future studies in myocardial infarction and cerebral ischemia. For example, in practice a certain benefit may be postulated for a test treatment, but suppose that in a given study only an identifiable two-thirds of the patients are really responsive to therapy. Inclusion of the nonresponsive one-third of the study population would seriously mask the true benefit of the drug, thus making it more difficult to demonstrate an overall treatment effect.

DISQUALIFICATION OF PATIENTS AND EVENTS

Despite care in the planning and conduct of such trials, there will always be protocol failures. From time to time, some patients will be entered into the study, only to be subsequently found not to meet entrance criteria. On occasion there will be unplanned interruptions in treatment, which may be patient- or physician-initiated. Other patients may drop out of the trial for reasons that may or may not be related to treatment of the clinical conditions. These reasons include loss of interest, a geographic move from the immediate area, difficulty in maintaining the follow-up schedule, occurrence of side effects (real or apparent), deterioration of physical condition, or, finally, attainment of some intermediate endpoint for which either the patient or the physician decides the patient should withdraw from the study.

These problems raise a number of methodological questions (4,19,42,43). One school of thought states that once a patient has been identified and randomized, he/she must be retained in the study, and all outcome events that occur from the point of randomization to the end of the study must be accounted for (27,36). The problem with this strategy is that "noise" is introduced into the study because of (a) the inclusion of patients who do not qualify—and even in the best-run studies some patients get in by mistake and do not meet entrance eligibility criteria; (b) noncompliers who do not take the treatment as prescribed or—and this is a particular problem in trials of platelet-suppressant drugs—do not avoid contaminating therapy that may include the many commonly available products that contain acetylsalicylic acid; and (c) patients who drop out for reasons not related to their clinical condition and/or the trial medication.

The consequence of this all-inclusive policy is that, although there is no resulting bias, there is a resulting loss of sensitivity in the statistical analysis because of the extra "noise." This results in the need for greater numbers of trial patients, and this is of particular concern in these large and very expensive studies. For example, the

Aspirin Myocardial Infarction Study cost $17 million. This conservative approach can be justified if one is asking about the impact of a treatment policy or "the intention to treat" and this may be fully appropriate on occasion but often is not.

In order to increase the efficiency of their studies, both the Anturane Reinfarction Trial Research Group and the Canadian Cooperative Study Group took a rather different approach. It was declared before the studies started that only patients satisfying specific inclusion/exclusion criteria would be counted and that any patients getting into the trials by mistake would be ruled ineligible. In addition, specific rules were defined for which outcome events would be counted when the efficacy of the test treatment was to be assessed. The expected consequence of this policy was that outcome events that could not be influenced by treatment would be excluded, and that these would occur with equal frequency in the different treatment groups. Hence the studies would be more sensitive and require relatively fewer patients. On the other hand, the opportunity for bias was increased because of possible differences between treatment groups in such factors as compliance and dropout rates.

Clearly, the exclusion of patients before randomization cannot bias treatment comparisons, but exclusion after randomization increases the potential for bias. Even though precise inclusion/exclusion criteria are established beforehand, some patients who do not meet these criteria will find their way into even well-executed trials. One example of such entry error occurred several times in the Anturane Reinfarction Trial and concerned the time elapsed from the qualifying myocardial infarction. For some entrants this was 37 days or 39 days even though the protocol clearly specified the acceptable range to be 25 to 35 days inclusive.

Although some deviations may seem relatively minor, strict adherence to the protocol is essential. It is important to apply the inclusion/exclusion criteria rigorously because of a particular confusion related to randomized trials. Many think that a randomized trial implies a randomly selected group of patients, but this is not true. A randomized trial is one in which patients are randomly allocated to treatment groups but are, in fact, highly selected. It is important to define and apply very precise eligibility criteria because the population to which the resultant findings will be generalized are those patients with the characteristics described in the protocol.

Another point of contention in both the Anturane Reinfarction Trial and the Canadian Stroke Study was the issue of "analyzability" of outcome events. In both studies it was agreed that for an event to qualify in the assessment of efficacy, it should occur at least 7 days after the initiation of test treatment. In other words, any event that took place during the first 7 days of treatment was ignored. The rationale for this was based on earlier work by Kaegi et al. (27), who demonstrated in patients with arteriovenous shunts that the antithrombotic effect of sulfinpyrazone occurred within 7 days and this effect was lost within 7 days following withdrawal of therapy. This latter finding prompted inclusion in the Anturane Reinfarction Trial of a second rule, to the effect that if a patient withdrew from study treatment, outcome events that took place more than 7 days after withdrawal would not be included in the primary analysis—except for those occasions when one could clearly relate the event to something that took place while the patient was actually on therapy.

In the same way, specific rules were set up to deal with patients who withdrew from test treatment during the course of the Canadian Stroke Study. Recognizing that withdrawal of patients from the trial might be precipitated by deterioration in neurological status and that exclusion from subsequent analysis might bias the results in favor of their particular study treatment, all events that occurred within the first 6 months following withdrawal were charged against the corresponding study treatment. The selection of 6 months was arbitrary, but it was felt that any bias resulting from this particular maneuver would be against showing a benefit for the treatment (Type II error) rather than a bias in favor of it (Type I error).

The effect of this, in terms of increased sensitivity, can be demonstrated by results of the Anturane Reinfarction Trial (ART). The total number of deaths among eligible patients in the placebo group was 85, with the corresponding total in the sulfinpyrazone group numbered at 64. It turned out—and in a way validated the initial postulation—that 23 deaths were excluded as being nonanalyzable in the placebo group and 20 deaths in the sulfinpyrazone group. Therefore, in terms of statistical assessment of efficacy, the ART group compared the 62 analyzable deaths on placebo with the 44 analyzable deaths on sulfinpyrazone, and not the 85 versus 64 total deaths. Statistically, this is a much more sensitive comparison.

Similarly, as a result of this policy, events experienced by 23 patients in the Canadian Stroke Study were not counted in the primary efficacy analysis. These included 7 strokes that occurred during the first 7 days of therapy and 4 strokes and 12 deaths that occurred more than 6 months after withdrawal from the study regimen. This decision to exclude 23 events did not produce a bias in favor of acetylsalicylic acid. On the contrary, it produced a more conservative result, since they were divided 9 and 14 in favor of acetylsalicylic acid. If all events had been included in the analysis, the overall risk reduction for stroke or death with acetylsalicylic acid would have increased to 32% ($p = 0.024$).

It is also worth noting what happened to the dropouts in two other secondary prevention trials in myocardial infarction. In one study with practolol (36), there were 83 deaths among those who withdrew from study treatment. Of these, 41 were in the placebo group and 42 were on practolol. In the acetylsalicylic acid study of Elwood and Sweetnam (14), 228 were withdrawn from each treatment group and of these, only 27 from the acetylsalicylic acid group died compared with 36 from the placebo group.

Clearly, in none of these studies did the disregarding of deaths among study withdrawals introduce bias in favor of the test treatment. Indeed, in the Canadian Stroke Study the observed difference was of sufficient magnitude in the other direction that inclusion of these events would have *improved* the statistical significance of the findings. In the three myocardial infarction studies, the omission of such deaths among dropouts did not result in any observed bias, bud did result in a significant increase in sensitivity of the statistical assessment of efficacy.

In closing, two important principles relating to the design, execution, and analysis of such large controlled clinical trials should be emphasized. The careful development of a detailed protocol, incorporating the methodological standards discussed above, is a first essential. A second, and perhaps more difficult, requirement is the maintenance of high dedication and discipline in execution of the trial, in order to maximize the completeness and quality of accumulated data. To help achieve this, it is important to:

   a. increase awareness both of potential bias and of the loss of sensitivity that can result from the incomplete study of individual patients;
   b. reduce such consequences by increased efforts to
     i. maximize patient drug compliance,
     ii. minimize co-interventions, and
     iii. improve overall adherence to the protocol, both by physicians and patients;
   c. include an explicit declaration of criteria for the disqualification of patients and events, as a mandatory section of both the original protocol and subsequent publications.

STRENGTH OF EVIDENCE

Assessment of the overall strength of evidence, as it relates to conclusions drawn from any given study, must be as objective as possible but also may involve some personal judgments. In a particular study, the conviction for conclusions drawn is dependent on the quality of the study design, the discipline of its execution, and the level of statistical significance for any observed benefit of treatment. However, in making the overall assessment of credibility of the findings, one must also take into account a number of extraneous considerations, some of which may not be readily synthesized into a single quantitative evaluation.

These extraneous considerations include existing knowledge of the pathogenesis of disease, the mode of action of the drug, and the biological compatibility of the two. They also include results from any previous related animal studies and/or clinical studies that must have formed part of the background information and rationale on which the major intervention study was based.

Additional evidence may be available from similar independent and even concurrent studies, and this must be included in the final equation. For example, although none of the individual observed benefits were statistically significant in the six acetylsalicylic acid secondary prevention studies in myocardial infarction, appropriate statistical techniques demonstrate that not only are these findings consistent, but when combined, the overall benefit is highly statistically significant. Another illustration would be the finding of a consistent sex differential, in response to acetylsalicylic acid, across a variety of studies.

It is also possible that small trials may be designed to confirm particular results from a major intervention study. In the case of the sex-related response to acetylsalicylic acid, the study of Kelton et al. (28) was subsequently undertaken with the specific purpose of verifying the initial observation from the Canadian Stroke Study.

Similarly, when the dramatic effect of sulfinpyrazone on sudden death was observed in the Anturane Reinfarction Trial, it raised the possibility of sulfinpyrazone having antiarrhythmic properties. The credibility of this observed benefit on sudden death was strengthened by subsequent studies by Moschos (35), which demonstrated an antiarrhythmic effect of sulfinpyrazone in animals.

In summary, final judgment on the true benefit of a particular treatment regimen cannot be based entirely on the statistical significance of an observed result from a single major trial but must appropriately incorporate evidence available from other related studies.

REFERENCES

1. Anturane Reinfarction Trial Research Group (1978): Sulfinpyrazone in the prevention of cardiac death after myocardial infarction. The Anturane Reinfarction Trial. *N. Engl. J. Med.*, 298:289–295.
2. The Anturane Reinfarction Trial Research Group (1980): Sulfinpyrazone in the prevention of sudden death after myocardial infarction. *N. Engl. J. Med.*, 302:250–256.
3. Armitage, P. (1979): Controversy in the interpretation of clinical trials. *Ann. Neurol.*, 5:601–602.
4. Armitage, P. (1979): Trials of antiplatelet drugs: some methodological considerations. *Rev. Epidémiol. et Santé Publique*, 27:87–90.
5. Aspirin Myocardial Infarction Study Research Group (1980): A randomized, controlled trial of aspirin in persons recovered from myocardial infarction. *JAMA*, 243:661–669.
6. Barnett, H. J. M., Gent, M., Sackett, D. L., and Taylor, D. W. (1979): Controversy in neurology: the Canadian study on TIA and aspirin. A critique of the Canadian TIA study. Reply. *Ann. Neurol.*, 5:599–601.
7. Breddin, K. (1979): Multicenter two-year prospective study on the prevention of secondary myocardial infarction by acetylsalicylic acid in comparison with phenprocoumon and placebo. In: *Essais contrôles multicentres: Principles et problèmes*, edited by J. P. Boissel and C. R. Klimt, pp. 79–92. Institut National de la Santé et de la Recherche Médicale, Paris.
8. Canadian Cooperative Study Group (1978): A randomized trial of aspirin and sulfinpyrazone in threatened stroke. *N. Engl. J. Med.*, 299:53–59.
9. The Coronary Drug Project Research Group (1976): Aspirin in coronary heart disease. *J. Chronic Dis.*, 29:625–642.
10. Editorial (1980): The FDA says no to anturane. *Science*, 208:1130–1132.
11. Editorial (1978): Sulfinpyrazone and prevention of myocardial infarction. *FDA Drug Bull.*, 8:3.
12. Editorial (1978): Sulfinpyrazone, cardiac infarction, and the prevention of death: a successful trial or another tribulation? *Br. Med. J.*, 1:941–942.
13. Elwood, P. C., Cochrane, A. L., Burr, M. L., Sweetnam, P. M., Williams, G., Welsby, E., Hughes, S. J., and Renton, R. (1974): A randomized controlled trial of acetylsalicylic acid in the secondary prevention of mortality from myocardial infarction. *Br. Med. J.*, 1:436–440.
14. Elwood, P. C., and Sweetnam, P. M. (1979): Aspirin and secondary mortality after myocardial infarction. *Lancet*, 2:1313–1315.
15. Evans, D. W. (1978): Anturane Reinfarction Trial (letter). *Lancet*, 2:366–367.
16. Fields, W. S., Lemak, N. A., Frankowski, R. F., and Hardy, R. J. (1977): Controlled trial of aspirin in cerebral ischemia. *Stroke*, 8:301–314.
17. Gent, M. (1979): Recent intervention studies of platelet suppressant drugs in cerebral ischemia: methodological aspects. In: *Drug Treatment and Prevention in Cerebrovascular Disorders*, edited by G. Tognoni and S. Garattini, pp. 437–448. Elsevier/North-Holland Biomedical Press, Amsterdam.
18. Gent, M., and Hirsh, J. (1979): Definition of high risk/high response population for stroke in patients with transient ischemic attacks. *Thromb. Haemost.*, 41:43–59.
19. Gent, M., and Sackett, D. L. (1979): The qualifications and disqualifications of patients and events in long-term cardiovascular clinical trials. *Thromb. Haemost.*, 41:123–134.

20. Genton, E., Barnett, H. J. M., Fields, W. S., Gent, M., and Hoak, J. C. (1977): XIV. Cerebral ischemia: the role of thrombosis and of antithrombotic therapy. Study group on antithrombotic therapy. *Stroke*, 8:150–175.

21. Genton, E., Gent, M., Hirsh, J., and Harker, L. A. (1975): Platelet-inhibiting drugs in the prevention of clinical thrombotic disease. *N. Engl. J. Med.*, 293:1174–1178, 1236–1240, 1296–1300.

22. Harnes, J. R. (1978): Sulfinpyrazone after myocardial infarction (letter). *N. Engl. J. Med.*, 298:1258.

23. Harris, W. H., Salzman, E. W., Athanasoulis, C. A., Waltman, A. C., and DeSanctis, R. W. (1977): Aspirin prophylaxis of venous thromboembolism after total hip replacement. *N. Engl. J. Med.*, 297:1246–1249.

24. Hirsh, J., Blajchman, M., and Kaegi, A. (1978): The bleeding time. In: *Platelet Function Testing*, pp. 1–12. Publication no. (NIH) 78–1087. Department of Health, Education, and Welfare, Washington, D. C.

25. Johnson, M., Ramey, E., and Ramwell, P. W. (1975): Sex and age differences in human platelet aggregation. *Nature*, 253:355–357.

26. Kaegi, A., Pineo, G. F., Shimizu, A., Trivedi, H., Hirsh, J., and Gent, M. (1974): Arteriovenous-shunt thrombosis. Prevention by sulfinpyrazone. *N. Engl. J. Med.*, 290:304–306.

27. Kaegi, A., Pineo, G. F., Shimizu, A., Trivedi, H., Hirsh, J., and Gent, M. (1975): The role of sulfinpyrazone in the prevention of arterio-venous shunt thrombosis. *Circulation*, 52:497–499.

28. Kelton, J. G., Hirsh, J., Carter, C. J., and Buchanan, M. R. (1978): Sex differences in the antithrombotic effects of aspirin. *Blood*, 52:1073–1076.

29. Kurtzke, J. F. (1979): Controversy in neurology; the Canadian study of TIA and aspirin. A critique of the Canadian TIA study. *Ann. Neurol.*, 5:597–599.

30. Kurtzke, J. F. (1979): Critique of the Canadian "TIA" study. In: *Cerebrovascular Diseases*, edited by T. R. Price and E. Nelson, pp. 243–250. Raven Press, New York.

31. Lilienfeld, A. M. (1979): Critique of "A randomized trial of aspirin and sulfinpyrazone in threatened stroke". In: *Cerebrovascular Diseases*, edited by T. R. Price and E. Nelson, pp. 239–241. Raven Press, New York.

32. Linos, A., Worthington, J. W., O'Fallon, W., Fuster, V., Whisnant, J. P., and Kurland, L. T. (1978): Effect of aspirin on prevention of coronary and cerebrovascular disease in patients with rheumatoid arthritis. A long-term follow-up study. *Mayo Clin. Proc.*, 53:581–586.

33. McKenna, R., Galante, J., Backmann, F., Wallace, D. L., Kaushal, S. P., and Meredith, P. (1980): Prevention of venous thromboembolism after total knee replacement by high-dose aspirin or intermittent calf and thigh compression. *Br. Med. J.*, 1:514–517.

34. Millikan, C. H. (1979): Does taking aspirin prevent stroke in the general population, TIA patients, completed stroke patients? In: *Drug Treatment and Prevention in Cardiovascular Disorders*, edited by G. Tognoni and S. Garattini, pp. 347–357. Elsevier/North Holland Biomedical Press, Amsterdam.

35. Moschos, C., Escobinas, A., Jorgensen, O., and Regan, T. (1979): Effect of sulfinpyrazone on survival following experimental non-thrombotic coronary occlusion (abstract). *Am. J. Cardiol.*, 43:372.

36. Multicentre International Study (1977): Reduction in mortality after myocardial infarction with long-term beta-adrenoceptor blockade. Multicentre International Study: supplementary report. *Br. Med. J.*, 2:419–421.

37. The Persantine-Aspirin Reinfarction Study Research Group (1980): Persantine and aspirin in coronary heart disease. *Circulation*, 62:449–461.

38. Peto, R., Pike, M. C., Armitage, P., Breslow, N. E., Cox, D. R., Howard, S. V., Mantel, N., McPherson, K., Peto, J., and Smith, P. G. (1976): Design and analysis of randomized clinical trials requiring prolonged observation of each patient. I. Introduction and design. *Br. J. Cancer*, 34:585–612.

39. Peto, R., Pike, M. C., Armitage, P., Breslow, N. E., Cox, D. R., Howard, S. V., Mantel, N., McPherson, K., Peto, J., and Smith, P. G. (1977): Design and analysis of randomized clinical trials requiring prolonged observation of each patient. II. Analysis and examples. *Br. J. Cancer*, 35:1–39.

40. Sackett, D. L. (1975): Design, measurement and analysis in clinical trials. In: *Platelets, Drug and Thrombosis*, edited by J. Hirsh, J. F. Cade, A. S. Gallus, and E. Schönbaum, pp. 219–225. Karger, Basel.

41. Sackett, D. L., for the Canadian Cooperative Study Group (1978): The Canadian trial of aspirin and sulfinpyrazone in threatened stroke (letter). *N. Engl. J. Med.*, 299:955.

42. Sackett, D. L., and Gent, M. (1979): Controversy in counting and attributing events in clinical trials. *N. Engl. J. Med.*, 301:1410–1412.
43. Schwartz, D., and Lellouch, J. (1967): Explanatory and pragmatic attitudes in therapeutic trials. *J. Chron. Dis.*, 20:637–648.
44. Sherry, S., Gent, M., Mustard, J. F., McGregor, M., Lilienfeld, A., and Yu, P. (1978): Sulfinpyrazone after myocardial infarction (letter). *N. Engl. J. Med.*, 289:1259.
45. Thompson, J. E. (1978): The Canadian trial of aspirin and sulfinpyrazone in threatened stroke (letter). *N. Engl. J. Med.*, 299:954.
46. Whisnant, J. P. (1978): The Canadian trial of aspirin and sulfinpyrazone in threatened stroke (letter). *N. Engl. J. Med.*, 299:953.
47. Whisnant, J.P. (1980): The Canadian trial of aspirin and sulfinpyrazone in threatened stroke. *Am. Heart J.*, 99:129–130.

Acetylsalicylic Acid: New Uses for an Old Drug,
edited by H. J. M. Barnett, J. Hirsh, and
J. F. Mustard. Raven Press, New York © 1982.

DISCUSSION

E. Salzman: I would like to ask Drs. Hirsh and Kelton about the various acetylsalicylic acid doses used in the rabbit thrombosis model. It seems to me that sodium salicylate is not a proper control for acetylsalicylic acid at 200 mg/kg, because it does not control for the acetylating effects. Do you have any studies of intermediate dose ranges between 10 and 200 mg/kg? Also, did you do a direct correlation of the rate of thrombus formation with the ability of vessel segments to produce prostacyclin in the presence of varying acetylsalicylic acid doses?

J. G. Kelton: With respect to the thrombogenic effect, we studied acetylsalicylic acid doses up to and including 100 mg/kg and did not see an increase in thrombogenicity. We looked at PGI_2 inhibition by vessel wall segments but did not have a sufficiently sensitive assay at the time. We observed that about 10 mg/kg acetylsalicylic acid gave some degree of PGI_2 inhibition. In fact, we did not test higher doses, but with that assay system, it would have been likely to see PGI_2 shut down before we could measure thrombogenicity. But my conclusion from this is, in fact, that thrombogenicity may be a more sensitive index of PGI_2 shutdown than PGI_2 or PGI_2-like production from vessel wall segments. I agree that massive doses of acetylsalicylic acid acetylate lots of things. Also, we did observe thrombogenicity with tranylcypromine, which is also a PGI_2 synthetase inhibitor.

J. F. Mustard: I understand that you use a segment of vein in your vessel wall preparation and that this is subjected to a certain amount of surgical trauma. Is this not a stimulus to PGI_2 production? And are not ligatures used to reduce blood flow?

Hirsh: The answer is yes on both counts. Without a partial stenosis, we do not see thrombosis in the preparation.

Mustard: It is important to understand that the thrombus that would be formed is a powerful stimulus for PGI_2 production, and, under these circumstances, PGI_2 would be helping to reduce thrombus formation.

Arteries have high-flow systems and we do not have an arrest in flow. In addition, a diseased vessel wall may not produce much PGI_2. It remains to be determined if PGI_2 produced by an artery is able to diffuse back into the lumen and have much effect on the process of arterial thrombosis. In hip surgery, it seems you have conditions much like John Kelton's jugular vein in rabbits. There, high-dose acetylsalicylic acid seems to work.

Buchanan continues to work in the field, using a slightly different experimental approach. He uses an artery and ^{51}Cr-labeled platelets, damages the vessel, and treats the animal with various doses of acetylsalicylic acid. Then he takes a vessel from the other side, does a PGI_2 assay, and correlates inhibition of PGI_2 formation within the rabbit, with accumulation of platelets. This work suggests that PGI_2 may be important in protecting the rabbit, because he found a rough correlation between PGI_2 production and massive platelet adherence, based on the ^{51}Cr assay. It was quite clear that in some rabbits acetylsalicylic acid caused no inhibition of PGI_2 formation and very little thrombogenicity or increase in thrombosis. Thus, the rabbits could be divided roughly into two groups. When he could not detect PGI_2, he observed a significant increase in the number of platelets accumulating on the damaged vessel. He was subsequently able to demonstrate this with doses of acetylsalicylic acid as low as 10 mg/kg.

It should also be emphasized that all of these studies are being done in normal animals with normal vessels, which may not bear much relationship to what is happening in diseased arteries in humans.

Unidentified: I would like to say something about methodology in clinical trials. Much basic research has been done on platelets and some clinical trials have now been carried out to determine its relevance to the real world of patients. Although some investigators seem impressed by the data presented to date, I am less so. After six or seven attempts to demonstrate some effect for acetylsalicylic acid in myocardial infarction, no one has consistently demonstrated a statistically significant difference. There are trends, but more often there is no difference at all between placebo and the acetylsalicylic acid groups. I am extremely skeptical of the sulfinpyrazone trial. Last week, J. Richard Crout of the Food and Drug Administration said of the study, "The data is not of sufficient scientific quality to justify release of the drug for this indication in the United States."

Concerning the PARIS reinfarction study, Professor Mustard showed us the data at 44 months. There were "look-ins" every 4 months for 2 years and again at 36 months, making a total of 8 different "look-ins". A disease score of 2.6 was used to assess statistical significance. This is equivalent to a p-value of .0047. At every instance from 4 months to 2 years, the dipyridamole group had a significant difference compared to placebo. At 8 and 24 months, the acetylsalicylic acid group had a significant difference compared to placebo. If one uses the less stringent criterion of $p = 0.05$, the acetylsalicylic acid group was significant in 4 of the 7 "look-ins". There was no difference at the end of the trial, but certainly there were differences in the drugs early on, and these may be important.

M. Gent: It is nice to hear Dr. Crout's opinion, but it would be helpful if we could also hear some of the reasons.

It is my understanding that the FDA has some concern about the classification and cause of death, but we can respond to these only if we know its specific criticisms and see how it did its assessment. For example, in the Anturane Reinfarction Trial, all deaths were reviewed by three different groups. The Policy Committee made the final decision on these deaths, using all the information available, and we did this without knowledge of which treatment group the patient was in. Whatever the defects in the criteria for classification, they were applied in a blind and consistent way. I have no idea how the FDA did its classification, but it would be necessary for it to demonstrate that its review met the methodological standards of blindness and objectivity which we as investigators are required to follow.

Mustard: These trials are expensive, and a trial based on the "intent to treat" philosophy is the most expensive. If you apply the epidemiological criteria that were used in the AMIS trial, you involve yourself in a very expensive study.

You cannot examine the data to find the subgroup analysis. The PARIS study is being evaluated in the same way as the sulfinpyrazone reinfarction trial, in terms of "look-ins" at the data. The fundamental difference is between taking an extremely conservative epidemiological approach, which is enormously expensive, and not examining the data before the end of the study, or accepting the idea of trying to determine if treatment is effective during the course of the trial.

Gent: Again, I would like to make my position clear. For each trial, it is possible to define a sensible set of rules that impose the requisite restrictions and constraints—for example, which patients to count and which events to take into account. I am surprised that the PARIS group has been taking "look-ins," because our colleague co-ordinating that study is one of the strongest proponents of the "intent to treat" philosophy. But I agree with Professor Mustard that we cannot always afford the luxury of the "intent to treat" approach. One speaker expressed disappointment that none of the observed differences was statistically significant. However, we should remember that the average benefit (ignoring the AMIS study for the moment) of the other 5 studies was just over 20%—that is a clinically important difference. The only reason the observed differences were not statistically significant was because none of the studies were large enough to get around all the confounding factors of "noise."

Ian MacDonald: Could Professor Gent say a little more on the matter of clinical relevance and the *p*-value? He put clinical significance in seventh place. It has always seemed that there is something magical about a *p*-value of 0.05. Would it not be logical to develop some sort of theoretical way to derive a *p*-value for the clinical consequences of treating or not treating? In the treatment of bacterial endocarditis, one sometimes treats on suspician, because of the fatal consequences of not treating. Could you explain whether the *p*-value can be tailored to a particular clinical situation?

Gent: I agree with you entirely. The *p*-value is important because it gives an overall assessment of the likelihood that there is a real difference. But what is much more important is the actual value itself, and not whether it is greater or less than 0.05. For example, I can imagine situations in which all of us would be more impressed with a *p*-value of 0.1 and associated evidence than with a *p*-value of 0.01 without supporting evidence. I put clinical significance at the bottom, because I wanted to finish off by reminding everyone that it is *the* most important factor.

Mustard: Dr. Hirsh, I believe the male-versus-female difference in response to these drugs is real. John Kelton has convinced me that, as far as platelets are concerned, male and female cyclo-oxygenase is acetylated to about the same extent. We can postulate, then, that either a different process is at work in females, causing the clinical complications, or that whatever these drugs affect requires a higher dose in females. A higher dose of acetylsalicylic acid was used in the hip and knee study, and this might have produced the benefit in females.

Kelton: This is an important question. I do not have the answer, but will speculate. Initially, the sex difference in response to acetylsalicylic acid was thought to represent a biological difference between male and female thrombotic risk. The treatment of males with acetylsalicylic acid just lowered their risk to that of females. However, the fact that we observe this effect where the stimulus can be controlled suggests that this does not represent a difference in pathogenesis, but in reactivity.

We can demonstrate platelet accumulation differences in damaged microvessels and are now doing cross-perfusion experiments using male platelets in female animals. It is clear that there are some differences, at least in rabbits, between the reactivity of male and female platelets following cyclo-oxygenase suppression. With regard to cyclo-oxygenase, we can be certain we have total suppression.

I believe this represents a difference in reactivity rather than pathogenesis. As Dr. Mustard has demonstrated, there are a number of alternate pathways for aggregation and release. If the thromboxane or prostaglandin pathway is more important in the male than in the female, for whatever reason, this could explain the observed clinical differences.

Gent: It is not correct to say that sulfinpyrazone was shown not to be of benefit in the Canadian stroke study. The best estimate of potential benefit of treatment was made taking due account of any imbalance in patient characteristics on entry. The best overall estimate of risk reduction in stroke or death with acetylsalicylic acid was 35% and was statistically significant. The best estimate of risk reduction for sulfinpyrazone was 15%, a value that was not significantly different from zero. It is wrong to conclude that we demonstrated there was no benefit of sulfinpyrazone. The conclusion was that we were not able to demonstrate a significant benefit.

Mustard: In your analysis of the Canadian stroke study, you drew up four groups. You pooled all subjects taking acetylsalicylic acid versus subjects not taking acetylsalicylic acid and all subjects taking sulfinpyrazone versus all subjects not taking sulfinpyrazone. This means that the acetylsalicylic acid plus sulfinpyrazone group was lumped with the sulfinpyrazone group. I understand you chose this type of analysis because, in the initial evaluation, you could not demonstrate any interaction between acetylsalicylic acid and sulfinpyrazone. However, you have already pointed out to us that all these studies are full of "noise" and that this dilutes the ability to show differences. Therefore, you are now faced with the dilemma that failure to demonstrate interaction between the drugs could also be a problem of numbers and noise in the system. Indeed, if in setting up the study, you had taken the most susceptible group, namely males without a history of high blood pressure, you might have been able to show interaction between sulfinpyrazone and acetylsalicylic acid.

Gent: That is a fair question that has been asked before. John Kurtsky in the United States has persistently pointed out for the last 18 months that although we were not able to demonstrate any significant interaction between sulfinpyrazone and acetylsalicylic acid, that does not mean there is no interaction. However, we had to make that assumption in order to do the principal comparisons of acetylsalicylic acid versus non-acetylsalicylic acid- and sulfinpyrazone versus non-sulfinpyrazone-treated patients. We have described this in our publications, and Peter Armitage of Oxford has also done a careful appraisal of this problem. It comes down to an interpretation of what took place. If you look at the curves for stroke or death for each of the 4 treatment groups, it only makes sense to conclude that there was possibility for interaction if you accept the following premises: that sulfinpyrazone by itself is dangerous but when added to acetylsalicylic acid improves the efficacy, or that there is something wrong with the dosages, which singly are not of benefit but together are really very good. Unfortunately, neither of these makes sense. Given that there are a variety of possible interpretations, Armitage came to the same conclusion as we did about possible interaction.

Mustard: Although you may be skeptical, I am told that our industrial and clinical colleagues in Europe are very interested in the combined use of these drugs—that one company has patented the combined use of dipyridamole and sulfinpyrazone.

Acetylsalicylic Acid: New Uses for an Old Drug,
edited by H. J. M. Barnett, J. Hirsh, and
J. F. Mustard. Raven Press, New York © 1982.

Closing Remarks

J. F. Mustard

An overview for a meeting such as this is difficult, in that the field is broad and some of the data are patchy and inconsistent. This meeting has provided some documentation of what is known and, even more important, what is not known. The observation that acetylsalicylic acid inhibits the formation of prostaglandins from arachidonic acid has been a major development in our understanding of inflammation and the action of nonsteroidal anti-inflammatory drugs.

By now, everyone is familiar with the arachidonate pathway and the biochemical events that follow the freeing of arachidonate from membrane phospholipids. This appears to be the starting point of a fundamental biological reaction, and much work has been undertaken to determine how it is controlled and to identify the operative stimuli. Arachidonic acid is involved in at least three pathways and Dr. Weissmann has described a fourth, which certainly operates in leukocytes—namely, a non-enzymatic conversion of arachidonic acid to chemotatic lipids.

Acetylsalicylic acid blocks the arachidonate pathway by inhibiting the enzyme cyclo-oxygenase. Some workers have proposed that although high concentrations of sodium salicylate do not affect cyclo-oxygenase, they do affect the lipoxygenase pathway. Further investigation of this point is needed.

The arachidonate pathway is of interest because of the role of membrane phospholipids in the control of cell responses, the relationship of receptors to the various pathways, and the involvement of the phospholipids. Whether specific phospholipid classes are critically involved in some of these pathways is still questionable. I suspect that the platelet inositol–phospholipid pathway is critical in the process by which phospholipase C makes 1,2-diacylglycerol available and diglyceride lipase frees arachidonic acid.

In the near future, there should be substantial advances that will permit us to define the mechanisms by which arachidonic acid is made available. Do specific stimuli that cause cells to free arachidonic acid act through mechanisms that are different from those for the more generalized stimuli associated with ischemia or mechanical injury? Although PGI_2 is a key prostaglandin in many situations, other prostaglandins are critically important. Newly developed assays can now be applied for better identification of the prostaglandins and for reassessment of earlier results that were obtained with less sophisticated techniques. Such studies will give a better understanding of the specific prostaglandins that are involved in the different tissue reactions. For instance, the stable prostaglandins may have important long-term modulating effects which those in the thrombosis field have not recognized because of an overriding interest in "short-term" agents.

It is important to consider the effect of prostaglandins on cells in the vessel wall. In the field of thrombosis, we have been mesmerized by their effects on platelets. Surely, if PGI_2 is produced by endothelium and smooth muscle cells, a major effect must be on the tone of the vessel wall.

What happens to PGI_2 production by smooth muscle cells during the proliferative response of atherosclerosis? What effect do drugs such as acetylsalcylic acid have on this chain of events? What is the significance of Ruth Pick's findings that in monkeys given a lipid-rich diet, the administration of acetylsalicylic acid dramatically reduces the number of coronary lesions but does not affect the aorta? Is this because of an effect of acetylsalicylic acid on the arachidonate pathway or some other effect?

Another area requiring clarification is the relationship between inhibition of the cyclo-oxygenase pathway and increased conversion of arachidonate in the lipoxygenase pathway. As we learn more of the products of the lipoxygenase pathway, we shall probably find that they have important effects on different tissue reactions.

Consideration of attempts to control dysmenorrhea by inhibiting prostaglandin synthesis raises a fundamental question because acetylsalicylic acid is much less effective than some of the other drugs that inhibit cyclo-oxygenase. We know that acetylsalicylic acid is rapidly hydrolyzed when taken into the body. How well does it penetrate into the various tissues as acetylsalicylic acid? In some cases, tissues may not be readily perfused with acetylsalicylic acid, and the speed of its hydrolysis, along with competition for acetylation with other proteins, may diminish the amount of acetylsalicylic acid available to acetylate the cyclo-oxygenase in the cells. We require much better data on the tissue distribution of acetylsalicylic acid as acetylsalicylic acid, and its acetylation of the cyclo-oxygenase of different tissues.

With respect to gastric function, it is clear that in addition to any effect on prostaglandin synthesis, acetylsalicylic acid may have a direct action on the gastric mucosa. This has obvious implications for the design of agents that can pass through the stomach and still be absorbed without causing damage. However, it seems that if blood salicylate levels are high, the patient may experience mucosal irritation that does not result from the direct action of acetylsalicylic acid. We are just beginning to explore the question of tolerance to inhibition of prostaglandin production.

Although it has been stated that the nephrotoxicity of acetylsalicylic acid is not a problem in North America, there are many questions to be answered about the role of prostaglandins in the control of blood supply and renal tabular function. More information is needed on the effect of drugs, particularly acetylsalicylic acid, on the kidney.

It appears that the known prostaglandin pathways, although important, may not be essential. In certain conditions, inhibition of cyclo-oxygenase does not have a major effect. For example, although it has been shown experimentally that inhibition of prostaglandin synthesis leads to closure of the ductus arteriosus, this does not seem to have the impact one might expect if the prostaglandins represented a life or death factor. Furthermore, individuals with cyclo-oxygenase defects do not appear to have any major abnormalities. Nevertheless, available information indicates that we should be guarded in our approach to the use of prostaglandin inhibitors on the reproductive system.

The role of diet in the development of vascular disease and its complications will continue to receive attention in the next decade, partly because of the relationship between dietary unsaturated fatty acid type and the prostaglandin pathways. Eicosapentaenoic acid, a fatty acid found in some of the cold-water fish eaten by Eskimos, appears to prevent prostaglandin formation by inhibiting cyclo-oxygenase, although it was originally suggested that the conversion of eicosapentaenoic acid to thromboxane A_3 and PGI_3 was responsible for its effects. The possibility that this and other polyunsaturated fatty acids inhibit or modify cyclo-oxygenase activity raises the prospect that increasing the tissue levels of these fatty acids may allow us to influence the development of atherosclerosis and its thromboembolic events, as well as inflammatory reactions.

The effect of prostaglandins on smooth-muscle tone suggests a possible role in the control of blood pressure. In stressed rabbits, inhibition of cyclo-oxygenase results in a rise in blood pressure. Chronic treatment of rabbits with indomethacin causes a progressive increase in arterial pressure, but acetylsalicylic acid does not.

With respect to the prostaglandins' primary role in inflammation, it seems clear that they are involved in fever, although this may be facilitative rather than primary. In the production of pain, prostaglandins seem to augment other stimuli and this effect is on the peripheral nervous system. There is good reason why prostaglandins can contribute to erythema, but they are not essential for its development. It is interesting that inhibition of the cyclo-oxygenase pathway does not increase susceptibility to infection. Thus it appears that although prostaglandins contribute in some way to the inflammatory reaction and can augment some of its signs and symptoms, inhibition of prostaglandin formation does not worsen inflammation. Since no major effects are produced by this inhibition, one hesitates to conclude that the action of prostaglandins in inflammation is essential.

The role of prostaglandins in hemostasis and thrombosis is analogous to their role in inflammation. That is, prostaglandins may be facilitative but they are not essential. If thromboxane A_2 formation is shut off, the bleeding time is prolonged to some extent, but the disturbance is not as severe as that resulting from platelet deficiency. Given that the term "thrombosis" covers a multitude of events, how can the relative importance of thromboxane A_2 be compared with that of thrombin, for example? What are we to make of the observation that thrombi form when the neointima of the rabbit aorta is injured, but not when the endothelium is removed from a normal vessel? Certainly the circumstances for thrombus formation on the injured neointima are different from those dependent on exposure to collagen of the subendothelium. The former seems to be a more thrombin-dependent process, and the important point is that the thrombin stimulus is not easy to inhibit by blocking thromboxane A_2 formation with drugs such as acetylsalicylic acid.

All of this presents a very important challenge. How are we to determine the dominant thrombosis mechanism(s) in individual patients? Investigators have been comparing the rate of appearance in plasma of products formed from fibrinogen and materials released from platelets. However, many mechanisms may operate in patients suffering from advanced vascular disease. Those of us working in the field of thrombosis must increasingly concentrate on the process in diseased vessels rather than in the normal vessels of young animals, because there may be only a remote relationship between interaction of the blood constituents in these two types of vessels.

The matter of drug dose is very important in the field of thrombosis. It is probably wrong to assume that the only effect of acetylsalicylic acid and related drugs is on the thromboxane A_2 pathway. The Needleman–Majerus argument that low doses of acetylsalicylic acid are ideal for prevention of thrombosis is valid only if this pathway is the only one affected. Dr. Packham reviewed the effects that could not be attributed to the acetylation process. The salicylate effect on fibrinolysis may be important, but high doses of acetylsalicylic acid or salicylate may be needed to stimulate the fibrinolytic process. In order for a thrombus to stabilize and persist, fibrin has to form, and if this fibrin is lysed, the platelets will deaggregate and return to the circulation. For this reason, local stimulation of the fibrinolytic mechanism may be very important in limiting thrombosis, and differences in this may be one reason for sex differences. Although very high doses of acetylsalicylic acid may be thrombogenic in some animal experiments because they inhibit PGI_2 formation, there is no evidence that oral doses of 3 to 6 g/day are thrombogenic in man.

In our attempts to study in clinical trials the effects of drugs that inhibit cyclo-oxygenase, we are faced with some difficult questions. Professor Gent presented these as important challenges. They arise not so much because the clinical trials are begun with incomplete knowledge, but because the analysis of the trials is beset with all kinds of problems and, in some cases, considerable emotion. The methodology for measurement and evaluation must take into full account the knowledge base on which the trial was organized. He emphasized that we should establish trials that are efficient and present all the data in an open and objective manner. Because of limitations of knowledge when the trials are established, there should be clear guidelines for appropriate retrospective analysis of the data when the trials are completed. A criticism of the publications of the sulfinpyrazone and AMIS trials is their limited disclosure of data. The AMIS trial report, for example, does not indicate which patients dropped out of the study and why; the sulfinpyrazone study does not provide data for all the patients originally randomized to the trial. Surely the epidemiologists can agree on common approaches to the handling and evaluation of data that are acceptable to all and understood by everyone. This must be based on terminology that is understandable to those not working in the field of epidemiology. If this can be accomplished, not only will the efficiency of such trials be improved, but the amount of post-trial "noise" will be reduced and the understanding and support of non-experts increased.

Finally, let us ask some questions in the field of thrombosis. What are the principal mechanisms for thrombus formation in diseased arteries? Are there more sophisticated methods by which we can study the effects of drugs on this process? How do we determine whether a drug that affects a pathway in thrombosis has a significant effect on thrombosis? We discovered by accident that drugs such as sulfinpyrazone and acetylsalicylic acid block collagen-induced platelet aggregation. Therefore, because we thought that collagen was important to the initiation of thrombosis, we assumed that inhibition of its reaction with platelets might dramatically reduce thrombosis in man. We knew little about how an atherosclerotic plaque initiates the process and had not defined all the biochemical pathways in thrombosis when we started the clinical trials. Now we must question whether measurement of collagen-induced platelet aggregation is a relevant technique for screening for drugs. Should thrombus formation on the damaged lining of a normal vessel wall be used to study the antithrombotic effect of drugs or should we be testing whether the drugs inhibit thrombus formation on a reinjured surface? Can we study thrombosis and its modification by drugs using non-invasive techniques, such as radioisotope scanning? The development of non-invasive techniques may make it possible to study the thrombotic process in man and the effect of antithrombotic agents. Such developments would revolutionize the approach to determining whether a drug has antithrombotic activity. These approaches may even become useful for studying changes in the extent of atherosclerosis.

Most cells seem to produce prostaglandins under some circumstances. Drugs are going to affect other non-target-cell systems, with the results largely based on the response of cells in the tissue in which changes are taking place. Therefore, one must always keep in mind that the effect of drugs in modifying clinical symptoms may not be based on their action on thrombosis. For example, it is difficult to support the argument that the effect of sulfinpyrazone in preventing sudden death relates solely to its action on the thrombotic process. Its prevention of sudden death could be explained as well by its effect on other mechanisms, such as that causing ventricular fibrillation.

Resolution of the problems raised by observations concerning sudden death requires a much sharper definition of its nonthrombotic causes. In addition, there needs to be a better definition of sudden death that allows for something other than time of death to distinguish it from myocardial infarction.

The primary clinical question for the neurologist and cardiologist probably relates to the relative importance of different etiologic mechanisms. In the major drug studies to date, it is clear that patients with differing complicating mechanisms have been randomized to treatment and placebo groups. Retrospective analysis of the trials suggest that some subgroups benefit more than others. Is this because thrombosis is a more important clinical complication in some groups than in others?

Subgroup analysis of the trials yields very important data, and I hope the statisticians and epidemiologists can provide some means for deriving more information from these studies. This is why all the data have to be made available from all of the trials, making it possible to design improved studies, if nothing else.

In terms of thrombosis prophylaxis, some patient population groups benefit. Failure of the clinical trials to provide conclusive answers is not surprising. Indeed, one should be surprised by the degree of difference demonstrated in some trials, which were not designed to be efficient in demonstrating effects where subgroups of populations were not selected.

I would suggest that in 5 years' time we shall be meeting to discuss the testing of drugs that inhibit the prostaglandin pathway(s) for modification of thromboembolic processes, in designated susceptible subjects. We shall also be considering how to use these inhibitors to modulate important reproductive processes. We are entering a new era in the management of important biological processes, in which the relationship between drug effect and the biochemical definition of patient problems is much better understood.

Subject Index